Homoeopathy
and Science
Selected Writings

Elizabeth Wright Hubbard
MD

Edited for publication by
Maesimund B. Panos
MD
and
Della DesRosiers

BEACONSFIELD PUBLISHERS LTD
Beaconsfield, Bucks, England

British Library Cataloguing in Publication Data
Hubbard, Elizabeth Wright, d. *1967*
   Homoeopathy as art and science –
   (The Beaconsfield Homoeopathic Library; no.11)
   1. Medicine. Homeopathy
   I. Title II. Panos, Maesimund B. III. DesRosiers, Della
615.5'32

  ISBN 0–906584–26–4

The Beaconsfield Homoeopathic Library

Classical Homoeopathy, Dr Margery Blackie, 1986.   0906584140

Everyday Homoeopathy, Dr David Gemmell, 1987.   0906584183

Homoeopathic Prescribing, Dr Noel Pratt, revised 1985.   0906584035

Homoeopathy as Art and Science, Dr Elizabeth Wright Hubbard, 1990.   0906584264

Homoeopathy in Practice, Dr Douglas Borland, reprinted 1988 with Symptom Index.   090658406X

Insights into Homoeopathy, Dr Frank Bodman, 1990.   0906584280

Introduction to Homoeopathic Medicine (2nd Edition), Dr Hamish Boyd, 1989.   0906584213

Materia Medica of New Homoeopathic Remedies, Dr. O. A. Julian, paperback edition 1984.   0906584116

Studies of Homoeopathic Remedies, Dr Douglas Gibson, 1987.   0906584175

Tutorials on Homoeopathy, Dr Donald Foubister, 1989.   0906584256

Phototypeset by Gem Graphics, Trenance, Mawgan Porth, Cornwall in 10 on 12 point Times.
Printed in Great Britain at The Bath Press, Avon.

Acknowledgements

We would like to acknowledge our debt to Dr P. S. Krishnamurty of Hyderabad, India, for the encouragement he gave us while we were bringing together for publication the works of Dr Hubbard. His advice and practical assistance through the years have been invaluable. We thank the American Institute of Homeopathy for their permission to use copyright material.

We would also like to thank the following people for the help we have received from them: Mr Leonard Fox for his encyclopaedic knowledge of the author's work; Mrs Joy Richmond Martyniuk, research librarian at the National Library of Medicine in Bethesda, Maryland, for her valuable co-operation in our library searches; our publisher Mr John Churchill, whose command of our language and keen literary sense have greatly enhanced the work; and lastly, Anne Panos, whose constant support and encouragement have done so much to further this undertaking.

M.B.P., D.D.

Preface

Elizabeth Wright Hubbard has been called homoeopathy's strongest pillar and most brilliant flame of this century. Well-educated in the arts and sciences, and widely travelled, she had a rare clarity of thought as well as being unusually gifted as a teacher.

She studied homoeopathy in Geneva with Pierre Schmidt MD, and often referred to the inspiration of 'der alte Schlegel'. From these studies she brought an intense desire to share what she had learned with her colleagues and patients. For a number of years she taught at the Postgraduate School of the American Foundation for Homoeopathy, awakening in her students an understanding of the genius of homoeopathic remedies. As President of the American Institute of Homeopathy and as Editor of the Journal of the American Institute of Homeopathy, she waged a running battle against apathy. On her President's Pages and in her editorials she challenged her colleagues to contribute ever more of substance to homoeopathy. She dramatized, as no one else has done, 'the comfort of its order and the wonder of its law'.

She died on May 22, 1967. Her spirit lives on in her writings. To her, death was not a finality; it was a rite of passage in the partnership of the body and the soul, the one was always challenging the other to achieve perfection. Perhaps her contribution to homoeopathy was best expressed by a younger colleague, who, after many years of practice, realized: 'Had I studied Elizabeth Wright Hubbard early on, I should have been a much better homoeopath.'

Her entire life was meeting and overcoming challenges. She challenged Bryn Mawr when she was prevented from taking a course in free composition because she was a woman. In 1917 she challenged the established world of medicine by being in the first class that included women at Columbia University's College of Physicians and Surgeons. She was the first woman to intern at New York's Bellevue Hospital and the first to ride the night emergency ambulance. She challenged traditional Boston by making house calls in her Rolls Royce Roadster. As a woman she greatly challenged the society of her time by combining a career in medicine with marriage and parenthood.

She challenged homoeopathy to emerge from the past, be alive in the present and take hold of the future. She challenged her readers to understand that deep as her knowledge was, there was always much more to be discovered. She challenges us all with her sense of humour, her intelligence and her knowledge.

D.D.

Contents

Contents

Contents

PHILOSOPHY

What is Homoeopathy?

Homoeopathy is a science and an art of medicine. It differs from conventional medicine mainly in its concept of disease as a protective explosion – in acute instances as a protective attempt at exteriorization, and in many chronic diseases as an expression of symptoms (especially functional symptoms) asking for a remedy. It is based on the law of similars, first recorded by Hippocrates and developed into a system of medicine by Hahnemann, which states that 'likes cure likes'.

The fundamental proposition behind the homoeopathic materia medica is that remedies should be proved in potency on healthy human beings, and that the results, subjective and objective, of such provings form the drug pictures which are the primary 'likes'. Homoeopathy individualizes each case, realizing that an illness is not only a so-called disease but also the predisposition of the person attacked, as well as that person's individual reaction to the so-called disease. Homoeopathy therefore requires a case-taking which includes the totality of the symptoms – the patient's temperament, mental state, general reactions to heat, cold, storm, food and so on, any striking or peculiar symptoms, as well as his or her pathology. The picture of the sick individual must then be fitted with a proved remedy picture. This *simillimum* is then given in potentized form (the material quantity of the remedy being decreased, and the radiant energetic or vital properties of the remedy increased, by the potentization). Homoeopathy knows that cure proceeds from within outward, from above downward, and in reverse order of the appearance of the symptoms, and that when cases follow these rules of direction the remedy is truly curative.

1

What Does it Mean to be a Homoeopathic Physician?

It means double duty. First, one must undergo the rigorous training modernity requires to become an expert doctor; second, one must add to all this a study of homoeopathy, which includes therapeutics according to the natural Law of Similars:

- The unique concepts of individualization.
- The avoidance of suppression.
- The removal of obstructions to fundamental cure.
- Co-operation with the vitality of the patient.
- The perception of the totality of the patients' symptoms.
- The finding of the single most similar remedy.
- The administration of the minimum dose.
- The knowledge of the rhythms of repetition.
- Insight into chronic disease and its prevention by treatment at the *functional* stage.
- Coping with processes, not only end-products.

It involves a different study of substances which can become medicinal, controlled experimentation on human volunteers, and a novel method of preparing remedies which releases unsuspected beneficent powers without engrafting drug diseases atop natural ones.

It includes the means of improving the public health; and is the forerunner of psychosomatic medicine.

2

The Law of Similars

What, in connection with Hahnemann, most needs saying to a medical profession mostly not cognizant of him, and to the world of ailing humanity? Or, to those who are or might become medical students, and again to those who through bitter or monotonous results are alienated from usual medicine? Furthermore, to those who pursue every will-o'-the-wisp which someone claims as helpful, all the many 'paths' that lead up and down the garden, but surely not to the inevitable health, at least to the degree to which each ailing individual is susceptible?

One might think there should be a separate chapter for each of these categories. Not so – one simple, coherent statement of the laws of health should suffice. People know that Hippocrates said there are two methods of cure, by contraries and by similars, and the latter is the better. Unfortunately, from the days of Galen, the contrary method was espoused, and it had to wait for Paracelsus and later for Hahnemann to develop the similar aspect.

To the modern scientific mind let it be said, the law of contraries works in a chemical laboratory as acid neutralizes alkali, but it does not work in a biological or biochemical system in which there is a living factor (which Hahnemann was pleased to call the 'vital force').

According to the law of contraries, the substance chosen to oppose the disharmony works according to chemical laws, and then with material amounts of the chosen substance. However, in the matter of the law of similars, it is the substance worked out by Hahnemann's method that gives the impetus to Nature, or the vital force, or the ill human being. As soon as this nudge in the right direction is administered, the recipient, be it human or animal, carries on from there according to the specific pattern of the disease and of the host, until the vital force is exhausted. A new impetus must then be administered, and whether it be repetition or a collateral or complementary substance is for later comment.

Homoeopathy, in other words, is a symbiosis, a collaboration of whoever has a disease with whatever substance in the universe is capable of developing a similar pattern. During this constructive relationship there should be no suppression, no introduction of side effects, symptoms or conditions that are not germane to this healing symbiosis.

3

Nor must there be interference from masking medication, no failure to remove mechanical obstruction to cure, no further suppression of recurrent symptoms. True cure may then result, insofar as it is possible to the vitality of the individual case.

The Vital Force

Lord Chesterfield said that Christianity had never been tried and found wanting, because it was found so difficult that it was never tried. The same is true of homoeopathy. As usual, there are two methods of solution to this problem. Can we make real homoeopathy easier, simpler and faster for the homoeopath? Or must we change the patient, so that he takes a more distant view and appreciates the value of the bird in the bush over that in the hand?

In a similar way there are two methods of approaching illness. One is the popular warfare on germs, bacteria, viruses – the so-called 'attackers', and the other has to do with the strengthening of the beleaguered city – making human beings impregnable. The latter can actually be done despite years of wrong thinking, wrong living, wrong acting and wrong medication. Only homoeopathy profoundly understands how to raise the threshold of resistance, curing the allergy to sin and life which is a part of man's heritage on earth. Orthodox medicine cures in the Galenic tradition, by contraries, as in a chemical experiment. Here the substance administered is supposed to do the acting. In homoeopathy it is a biological laboratory – a human and not merely chemical set-up. The same chemical substances are in the corpse two minutes dead, and in the living body two minutes short of dying, and that invisible, unweighable difference, which we may call, as Hahnemann did, the 'vital force', or as moderns do, 'life', is a factor of basic and immense importance.

It is this vital force which, according to the homoeopaths, actually does the curing. The physician has only to give it an impulse in the exactly correct direction, according to the Law of Similars, and then it proceeds to cure until it has spent itself. The physician finds it most difficult to know when any given vital force is exhausted and needs another inspiration or push. This effort at the timing and repetition of a dose, and the matter of potency, is far more difficult, elusive, and important than the mere selection of the exactly similar remedy, even if that is possible. All fruitful research must take account of this vital force – otherwise it will degenerate either into gross materialism or else into superstition.

James Tyler Kent and others have provided astute observation

5

methods by which the person trained in homoeopathy can assess the quality of the vital force, and when it is flagging, spur it on again with a judicious repetition or change of potency, or else shift to a deeper remedy, or ultimately even to a nosode. Some patients ask if they must buoy up this vital force at intervals for the rest of their lives. Some must, if their health and inherited forces are poor. Others can be set straight with relative ease. It is extremely important to work on small children, expectant mothers, and indeed prospective parents in general. Such a clinic would make an invaluable contribution to public health.

Most acute illnesses recover of themselves. A few patients die. In people in poor health, serious and lasting sequelae may develop in the untreated. Chronic diseases do not tend to recover, although they fluctuate and relapse. Nothing of this kind should ensue with real deep homoeopathic therapy in the acute diseases. Immediately after every acute illness is a prime time to give the constitutional remedy. The Chinese are correct when they say, 'Go to your doctor when you are well, to be fortified.'

The Constitutional Remedy

It is a common saying that there is no absolute on this earth, and therefore no norm of complete health. Those who are familiar with Hahnemann's theory of the chronic miasms have some basis for understanding why this is so. A new-born baby carries the cumulative load of ill-health of all its ancestors, and the adult adds to this the weight of the drugging, bad hygiene, bad habits and sequelae of whatever diseases he has had, including the physical and emotional resultants of mental stress. Let anyone who is mathematically-minded calculate the sum total of these liabilities, compounded over many years, and he will be appalled at the apparently insoluble bankruptcy with regard to the health of every human being. Sensible living, sociological and emotional adjustment, abidance by the laws of spiritual life, and the correct cure of acute diseases by homoeopathic remedies will do something toward alleviating this condition. But these measures will only be palliative and preventive if they are not connected with chronic, constitutional medication in accordance with the law of similars.

What do we mean by the homoeopathic chronic constitutional remedy? We mean that substance which is similar to the totality of symptoms, spiritual, mental, emotional and physical, of our patient. We must take into consideration not only the present status, but also all shocks, illnesses, crises and tendencies in the life of our patient, and in so far as we can ascertain it, in that of the parents and ancestors. We must review the whole career of our patient from the time of conception.

With all this complicated history, can we reasonably expect to find one remedy which will be similar to such a galaxy of symptoms? In many patients, yes. We will clearly see how the appalling headaches from which our patient suffers today are the logical outcome of his condition in childhood, with his terror of thunderstorms, his fetid foot-sweat, his dislike of milk, his lack of stamina. In such a case, one dose of Silica in 200c or 1M potency may turn our patient into order, *from within outwards, from above downward and in the reverse order of the appearance of the symptoms.* The habitual headaches will give place to the return of perspiration, which in turn disappears, leaving our patient better balanced, more resistant and less likely to have future illness of any sort. In the majority of cases, however, it is not so simple. One must 'peel the onion', working back through layer after layer of engrafted and inherited disease by means of a series, not only of potencies of the same remedy but of several remedies, often related.

This is the age of prevention, of organized effort to get the children early and protect them. Let us make a special effort to prescribe fundamentally for all the children in our care. If we could treat the children of three or four generations by profound constitutional homoeopathy, our world would be a different place from the standpoint of health, prevalence of crime and human happiness.

I ask those who use mainly acute remedies to look into this matter of chronic treatment, to study Hahnemann's *Chronic Diseases*, Von Grauvogl's *Textbook of Homoeopathy*, Kent's *Lectures on Homoeopathic Philosophy*, and realise the tremendous value of giving every child and most adults their chronic constitutional remedy, one dose, repeated at long intervals when the self feels worse and symptom progress in accordance with Hering's three rules has ceased.

The scales are before us. In the one balance are the cumulative tendencies to disease, including excessive temperaments; in the other is one high potency homoeopathic dose of the true simillimum. Slowly sometimes, at other times swiftly, the balance will fall on the side of the weighty imponderable.

Health Checkups

With all the frightening information about cancer, polio, multiple sclerosis, leukemia, arthritis, and other diseases much before the public eye, a great many people undergo periodic health checks. Many of these are arranged by employers, others have to do with insurance policies, and still others are the periodic Papanicolaou tests for women or the general cancer detection programmes.

Most homoeopathic patients prefer to go to their homoeopaths, and their objective is quite different. They do not go to have a sad fact discovered early, but to receive constructive medication in regular periodic rhythm, so that they will be less likely to develop irreversible and often fatal conditions.

The homoeopath to whom one turns for such a check should be one versed in the philosophy as well as the treatment of day-to-day troubles. He or she must be capable of chronic constitutional prescribing, which is a specialty within a specialty. Many doctors now stress the threshold of resistance of the patient, and tend less and less to lay disease at the door of rampant bacteria. Susceptibility is perhaps the major and the most interesting factor in the health equation. Why will some members of a family come down with an epidemic, a current exanthem, or stray colds and viruses, whereas other members subjected to the same source of infection remain immune? The greatest single fact of homoeopathy is that it can improve individual health and prevent useless diseases. It does not *wish* to prevent diseases which have their places in the scheme of things, such as the exanthemata, which when properly homoeopathically treated, purify the individual and prevent the outbreak of some unexpected and fatal disease in later life.

A chronic case, properly homoeopathically taken and treated, is the best possible insurance towards long life and good health for any given individual. However, it is not enough for the homoeopath to give even this most specialized type of treatment. He must review the patient's habits and advise on hygiene. He must check into his blood chemistry and counsel accordingly about his diet. He must take into consideration structural or postural or positional defects and strains, and collaborate with an osteopath to correct these. A large majority of troubles in these apparently specialized fields can be corrected and prevented by proper constitutional homoeopathic prescribing, but the family doctor should not fail to have the patient checked by expert specialty opinion before and after the remedy. Do not forget that the dentist has a sphere which impinges on general health. The problem of bite and its adjustment is a serious one for overall wellbeing.

The allergist and the homoeopath are blood brothers if they but knew it. In the case of women, the doctor should enquire into their cosmetic habits and have a *Consumer's Guide* at hand to discover what is contained in various beauty products. Unfortunately, the regulation of cosmetics lags far behind that of food and drugs.

This whole approach to health is based on what should be done for people who do not consider themselves ill, but who wish to be sensible in the prevention of possible later trouble. The question arises as to what percentage of people need a constitutional remedy. The answer is: everyone, at least twice a year, whether he has a symptom or not. The further question arises: what percentage of illness, acute or chronic, is amenable to homoeopathic therapy? All are amenable in the functional stage, and much reversible pathology can be influenced. However, there are many cases of the type of broken-down constitution, where the gross pathology has reached the point of being a mechanical obstruction to cure. In those cases, mechanical means may be needed, and this may not be limited to surgery or splints, but may include diuretics, gross doses of heart medicines and other physiologic medicines.

Enlarging One's World

There are those who have a great love of strangers, the unknown, exploration, travel, curiosity, research. What a challenge in the meeting of the minds! Novelty, ingenuity, variety, the unexpected. How to make a fruitful and perhaps lasting, or at least unforgotten, connection to enlarge one's world. Psychiatrists explain the fascination of minorities for some natures. There is a snobbishness bound up with it . . . 'Caviar to the General'. Such a terrain is homoeopathy. One of the most learned physicians in that field says it is the medicine of the ten per cent. Yet children and the simplest people can understand and appreciate it. It fits in with the classical tradition, as well as with the most delicate of modern sciences.

'What', asked a young orthodox physician, 'is homoeopathy?' It is a method of healing in accordance with the law of similars rather than by contraries. What is its relation to the organization of ordinary medicine? It is a therapeutic specialty.

The same substances may be used by the homoeopathic method as are employed in ordinary medicine, but there is a homoeopathic way of administering and preparing them in microdilutions, succussions, triturations, or fluxion potencies. Any substance – vegetable, mineral, animal, natural or synthetic – can be prepared by the homoeopathic method. But even if so potentized or dynamized, it does not become a homoeopathic medicine until it has been 'proved', which means tested on relatively normal human beings on a voluntary research basis.

Medicines used homoeopathically do not have poisonous side effects nor, if properly given, harmful sequelae. They are biodynamic, not chemical; they belong not to the realm of physics but nearer to the realm of electronics. The body of the patient is an essential part of the circuit of homoeopathic cure. The patient, however, may be an animal, an infant, or an unconscious person.

Homoeopathic medicines are curative insofar as the case is curable – mechanical obstructions to cure being attended to or removed if possible – and they are not suppressive. The same natural substances are used in ordinary and in homoeopathic medicine (although the homoeopaths have an infinite range of possible remedies). But, according to

11

different laws and different dosage every natural substance – animal, vegetable and mineral, even inert ones – can and should be 'proved'; that is, subjected to research to learn its powers.

Usual medicine gives a drug for a *diagnosis*, whereas homoeopathic medicine is given for the *individual* who has the diagnosis, or disease. Homoeopathy individualizes – each case is unique, as in nature no two fingerprints are precisely the same.

Homoeopathy helps nature to cure, not just by naturopathic means such as diet, physiotherapy or manipulative adjustments, nor even by psychiatry. Usual medicine works against nature, or tries to make the patient feel no pain.

The nearest thing is the rousing of the allergens. In one case this is done with the substances at fault, whereas in the other case the resistance of the whole being is raised.

If drugs used homoeopathically do not work by the simple chemical formulae (acid neutralized by base, for instance), by what method can we discover their uses? By voluntary provings on relatively normal human beings, conducted with controls and using the double-blind technique.

Homoeopathy takes longer, requires far more, helps in all fields toward the limit of curability, and has a rationale and a philosophy. It offers huge assistance in functional cases where usual medicine knows only anodynes and hygiene, and in chronic diseases which do not tend to cure by themselves but only to remissions with downward cyclic course. It helps in every specialty.

Much in Little

Multum in parvo – 'much in little' – homoeopathy in a nutshell. In this quantitative age, where each man strives to raise his private Tower of Babel, and nations vie with one another to excel in dimensions of wrath and power, is it not refreshing that men of science turn their eyes to invisible vastnesses? Homoeopathy is such an inner world, lucid and unfailing.

One of its brotherhood sent me from a war-ravaged London a heavy ingot of metallic bismuth (used in munitions work), broken while molten hot and swiftly chilled till the slippery white sheen set in crystal patterns unique to that metal. They formed parallel steps and square patios, definite, architectural, at different angles to one another, like a miniature Acropolis at Athens, yet in colour, iridescent, purple, green, flame, gold. With the ingot, from that land of blackouts and bombing, came this message: 'To bring you the Comfort of Order and the Wonder of Law'.

This is what homoeopathy brings to medicine and to mankind, for all the ages – the comfort of order and the wonder of law. Yet to read the materia medicas, and especially to hear some of the learned papers on our remedies, who but an initiate with special powers and sight could perceive the pellucid simplicity of the healing agents given to our use?

Should we try for this hard beauty in our remedy pictures? There is much carbon, but few diamonds. Out of the milling herd of symptoms, what shall we rope and master? What is the essence to be distilled?

Mentals, Kent tells us. Modalities and concomitants, says Boenning-hausen. Objective symptoms, Stearns stresses. Generals, which pertain to the 'I', felt Boger. 'Strange, rare and peculiar', was Hahnemann's criterion. Pathology or endocrinological types, suggest some of the moderns. For the student all of these are necessary, until in his mind and very vitals a portrait grows, unique and sure for every substance. Until he sees remedial possibilities in each new substance of nature that he turns his thought upon, and learns to read earth's language in mineral, vegetable and animal.

To simplify this process one must ponder on the elements, of which all other substances and man are made. One must analyze plants into their component simple substances, at least the predominant ones, and feel

13

one's way into the relationship of remedies. Who is not helped by knowing that Lachesis contains much sulphur? or Lycopodium lots of aluminium? or Belladonna some magnesium phosphate, and Nux Vomica a share of copper? Over many years of materia medica teaching, varying methods of abridging have been tried. Dewey's *Quiz Compendium*, Boger's *Cards*; ditties like Stacy Jones' *Similliads* or MacAdams' verses; *Keynotes* such as Lippe's, Allen's or Guernsey's, or Nash's *Leaders*, save our time. Pierre Schmidt of Geneva lists ten generals, ten mentals (if available) and five rare, strange and peculiar, with an epithet or key word and portrait. Boger gives locations and sensations.

Without doubt an artistic, pictorial representation of a remedy will stick in the learner like arrows in Sebastian. Who can forget the ragged philosopher, the unsuccessful inventor, the great unwashed which is Sulphur? Or the washerwoman, the unwifely wife who is Sepia? Or the harrassed accountant, in Renaissance days a tyrant, a Malatesta, typified by Nux Vomica? Or the pretubercular Irish fey, Phosphorus? Or Paul Dombey, dour, precocious, spindley, as Kent calls Lycopodium? Or pampered Miss Ignatia, falling for the cab driver? Or the Arsenicum dandy, with his goldheaded cane? Or the whimsical April Pulsatilla? Or Aurum's beefy, desperate taciturnity? Or the ovoid, proliferative, discharging Thuja? Or the creaky hinge – Rhus Tox. – and the barometric brutal Mercurius?

There is no royal road to homoeopathy save honest toil; but there is a primrose path of dalliance with the remedies both beguiling and rewarding. May this brief glimpse along it lead you, in profitable leisure, to contemplation of the comfort of its order and the wonder of its law.

Children in Difficulty

We are all children in the sense that few adults achieve maturity. We are all in difficulty of some sort, the laws of Karma being what they are. The man in the street would say that many children 'in difficulty' are abnormal, subnormal, idiots, morons, retarded, backward or stunted personalities. Anthroposophists who work with them prefer the phrase 'children in need of special care'. You do not have to be among them for long to realise that most of them are people to whom one becomes very partial.

What kind of difficulty do we discuss? These are people who cannot get along without protection, temporary or permanent. We are not discussing poverty, acute illness, passivity, violence, juvenile delinquency, the status of orphans, the condition of being maimed, the plight of the unwanted child, or of those smothered with false love or psychologically warped from parental mishandling. The diagnoses on these young folks that are made in schools for backward children or mental institutions vary from presumed birth injury, cerebral palsy, epilepsy, post-encephalitic syndromes, Mongolism, inability to learn in school, stuttering or unintelligible speech, deaf and dumb mutism, even schizophrenia. And finally, arrested development following diseases such as typhoid, measles, rubella, mumps and meningitis.

Are such children remediable? If so, what special means does homoeopathy offer for their understanding and handling, and towards their cure?

There is the tender tradition of the village idiot, protected by all, molested by none. It is a known fact that the difficulties of many of these children are in the sphere of the intellect or the will, and that in a compensatory way they are often unusually rich in heart forces. They have often been kept in the background, considered a nuisance and a disgrace, sent to various custodial institutions and deprived of the co-operative love of a normal family unit. The spontaneity, the warm response, the courtesy, the tolerance, the intuition and the humour of these children, when in an understanding and warm environment, is notable.

Rudolf Steiner, the founder of the anthroposophical movement, had a special feeling for these children. He even said that in the last previous or the next incarnation they were, or will be, great people. His attitude toward them reminds one of Bergson, the philosopher of Creative Evolution fame, who revolutionised the cruel and ugly treatment of the insane in France by showing that the normal approach to experience and the beauty of living is not open to those whose brain is injured. Hence they need to be in a more sensitive and more artistic environment than the normal human being, where they can take in experience and sound nourishment at a subconscious level.

What are some of the factors behind these difficulties in children? First, and obviously, heredity. The second factor, to ordinary thought, would be environment. Our present civilisation entirely omits training for love, marriage or parenthood.

The third great element in these children's difficulties is their Karma, upon which Steiner has many lectures. This subject is not within the scope of this book.

Let all mothers remember that the womb is the cosmic workshop. The time of the first breath of a baby marks its actual entrance from the womb world to the outer world. Some babies have been separated from the mother's body sometime before they breathe. In others there is a time lag between the first breath and the first cry. An infant that is overdue shows a strong Karmic connection with its mother. Cosmic forces are thereby able to stay with the child longer. No one should induce or hold back labour for anyone's convenience; if however the labour is dangerous, it can be helped with remedies from the vegetable kingdom, such as Caulophyllum, Chamomilla, Gelsemium, Nux Vomica, and Pulsatilla.

One element to be considered in the development of children is that which Alfred Adler calls the family constellation. What would you say is the first great division in life? Rich and poor? By no means. Cultivated and ignorant? Indeed no. Believers and non-believers? Far from it. Workers or parasites? Still not, though closer. The two main divisions are male and female and position of birth in the family. Dr Koenig has written a book called *Brothers and Sisters*, combining Adler's thesis with Rudolf Steiner's spiritual insight. He gives a picture of the first child, the second child and the third child in any family, and if there are more than three children the cycle recapitulates – the fourth child having the pattern of the first, the fifth of the second, the sixth of the third, the seventh again of the first, and so on. He also gives an initial chapter to the only child. So, to the things you need to know about any child or person, add their position in the family constellation.

In brief his thesis is: the only child is an observer. No quarrels, no fondness, no friction. Ambivalent, rigid, often unmarried. Eccentrics like John the Baptist share the nature of the first child, in that it is a ruler, traditional, oriented to the past. Cain was a first child. The first child in a way represents the Father in the Trinity.

The firstborn child is often neurotic. He is full of guilt. Wishes to reform the world. He is the gate between the parents and the children. Janus with the two faces of Saturn and Jupiter is related to door, stick and key. Christ was a first child. They are often sacrificed. They become judges, lawyers, doctors.

The second child is born modern. He is neither a conquerer nor a defender. He shatters conventions. Abel is the symbol of the second brother. Divine acceptance. A girl with an older brother is of the Artemis type. Second sisters are companions rather than wives or mothers and are often tough and rebellious. The second child is unconcerned, the child of the present, the artist.

The third child is the outsider. The stranger with a complex nature. Great saints are third children. Death is nearer to third children. Third children are men of the future, like Seth. They are too high in the air, and irrational. In the Trinity they correspond to the Holy Spirit.

There is a movement started under Rudolf Steiner's direction called the Camphill Movement, with schools and homes for young people in difficulty. They are graded by age: one for children between the change of teeth and puberty (approximately 7–14); another for teenagers, 12–18; and a village for those in need of special care from then until 30. The medical work on these young people has followed some of Dr Steiner's indications and their chronic constitutional cases have been studied in the profound homoeopathic sense. Certain strikingly good results have been apparent. It is interesting to see the proposition of remedies from the different kingdoms which apply to this type of case. In usual illness the vegetable kingdom predominates. Here there were nine different remedies (Ignatia, Gelsemium, Lycopodium, Nux Moschata, Nux Vomica, Pulsatilla, Staphysagria, Stramonium, Thuja). In this work the mineral kingdom leads in frequency, probably because it corresponds to the ego. Eighteen different mineral substances were employed, ten of them elements: Aurum, Cuprum, Graphites, Iodum, Mercurius, Phosphorus, Palladium, Silica, Sulphur, Zinc. Seven salts or acids: Antimonium Carb., Argentum Nit., Baryta Carb., Calcarea Carb., Magnesia Carb., Natrum Mur., Nitric. Ac. One mushroom: Agaricus. One chemical substance: Methyl Alc. Nine nosodes: Medorrhinum, Morbillinum, Mumps, Syphilinum, Pyrogen, Tuberculinum Bov., Typhoidinum,

Variolinum, Scarlatinum.

Meanwhile what can you do to help in this one of the important problems of today? You can hold respect and affection for these folk in need of special care. The so-called retarded child perceives intuitively whether we are equipped to cope with him. Be on the lookout for this type of condition early, and tell your friends that such places exist. We have many children improving there who have previously been institutionalised. Realise that this is the age to be conscious. We must cultivate inner vitality and feel nothing but joyous compassion. Enthusiasm is the experience of truth. Have patience. Remember that the cosmos gives itself time to work. Promote beautiful speech, splendid posture and gait, like a guiltless animal. Remember that the voice is the expression of the ego. We need wonder, reverence, gentleness and humour. Whisper to children. Let them point out what torments them. Cure by imagination, tales, irony, rhythm and laughter. Show them in a story that thieving and war end in absurdity. Fantasy and ingenuity create union. Allow them to learn the inevitable consequences of natural laws. Realise the uses of absurdity, not only of adversity. Remember the Negro proverb, 'Sing at the door, so that the child passing by may learn wisdom'.

VISIONS

Mass Medication

Whatever one's profession – lawyer, prelate, teacher, engineer or physician – one is first a human being. What does it mean to be a *human* being? It means having restrictions imposed by the physical instrument which we call our body. It also means the unique privilege and obligation of at least a budding self-consciousness, and a partial ability to control our instincts by rational thought. Furthermore, it implies the dubious privilege of the knowledge of right and wrong, the freedom of choice, and hence the ability to help mould not only ourselves but also the environment in which we find ourselves. In this we are privileged above the animals, and even above such higher beings as have not received the dire boon of freedom.

The political ideology of democracy in its original form may or may not be the wisest vehicle for human freedom, but the cause of the protection of the individual and the rights of minorities is the fundamental, precious heritage. More and more we are permitting ourselves to be bereft of this hard, sweet core of the spirit. Technical progress, efficiency and legislative efforts to raise standards by outward pressure – all in themselves good and necessary things – are blinding us to the encroachment of selfish forces. We are being led by fear, conformity, and advertising. There are earnest struggles for some aspects of human freedom, and real efforts against prejudice and segregation in fields political and economic, just as there were a century ago in religious realms. The medical profession is feeling the brunt of coercion, and partly by a portion of itself, but even more by an aspect of big business which has to do with the universal commodity – health. Only a section of our population goes to school, or votes, or earns a living; but everyone from the cradle to the grave needs health help.

We, the people, as patients, must protest at the exploitation for financial reasons of our individual health. We protest at the use of hormones to caponize poultry and 'wonder drugs' to fatten cattle. Enlightened groups are battling mass fluoridation. Because of our special approach to science and to medicine, we homoeopaths know what serious illness can be engrafted onto people through the administration of minute doses, unconsciously and repeatedly, to the susceptible. The public is deeply alarmed at the possible results from radiation fall-out. They are not, however, sufficiently alarmed by the constant poisoning from supposedly beneficial sprays, fertilizers, preservatives and purifiers, nor by the long-range effects of sedatives, synthetic drugs and tranquillizers. If the spirit is to survive, its vehicle, the body, must be unclogged. If we cannot survive the pace of modern living without being drugged, we must, for our self-preservation, revise our life pattern. Homoeopaths, an enlightened minority, must join strongly in this battle for the preservation of human beings in their full state of awareness.

The Osmosis of Homoeopathy

What is osmosis? In science, it is the process by which one substance diffuses into another through a semipermeable membrane. Figuratively, the term describes any gradual process of assimilation or absorption that resembles this diffusion. How is this applicable to homoeopathy? The two substances concerned in the osmosis, let us call homoeopathy and for lack of a better term, organized medicine.

Let us first consider the nature of the symbolic membrane which separates the two camps and yet permits of interchange between them. The constituents of this membrane are four:

Laziness – due, not only to overpressure of work, but to the habitual lack of concise thinking on the part of the human being.

Prejudice – on both sides. Inherited from the early days of homoeopathy when there was persecution, and indeed some protection, from being a sect (persisting in some quarters today as back-biting and a 'holier-than-thou' attitude). The persistence of this sect mentality has been partly due to the intense specialization in materia medica needed to do good work in our art – the specialist, as the saying goes, 'knowing more and more about less and less'.

Worship of 'science' versus contempt for 'science'. The difficulty here is not in the facts of science. The difficulty and the danger is in the *interpretation*. One of the most moot points, for instance, is the attitude toward bacteria. Are they a cause, a product, or merely a concomitant of disease? Can they be separated from what *we* call the intangible 'miasm', whether acute or chronic, which goes with them; and what is the relation, if any, of this 'miasm' to a filterable virus? We tend, furthermore, to depend solely on the action of our remedies as we have inherited them, overlooking the necessity of testing them by all known laboratory means and of keeping ourselves up to the mark by the checks of modern science.

Questions of *worldly advantage*.

So much for the membrane, over which we must all co-operate to keep passable. The question is, which way will the osmosis take place? This depends on the relative richness of the substance on the two sides, in

21

other words, on the comparative powers of homoeopathy and organized medicine of today.

What can we do, not only to show to others that this is so, but to prove it to the sceptics in our own ranks, as well as to that most honest and often subterranean part of ourselves? We can prove it empirically by our cures. But these, at best, are subject to that most tantalizing of facts, the impossibility of one person being both an experiment and its control. We should, however, take special care to support our cures, not only by laboratory data but also, when possible, by consultation for diagnosis and corroboration with a non-homoeopath. Also, by giving diet and hygiene and a mental boost to patients whose condition permits, at first, *without* the indicated remedy. Then follow with placebo given in one's best manner, carefully noting the effect of each of these two procedures; then give the carefully-studied simillimum, and note whether the result is not a startling improvement. If it is not, let us be sure that it is *our* fault and not the fault of homoeopathy.

As a further sign that the remedy is acting and the improvement not fortuitous, we have Hering's three laws of cure: (i) the action of the remedy from within outward, (ii) from above downward, and (iii) in the reverse order of the appearance of the symptoms. A further control check can be made after our single dose has worked itself out, (or rather, when the reaction of the body to the dose has run its course). If the symptoms agree, we can then repeat and see a new improvement and the continued action of Hering's laws. Last but not least, we may regard any remedy aggravation, especially if the symptoms aggravated appear strongly under the remedy in the materia medica, as a further control.

Furthermore, we can record these data and publish them.

But this is not enough. No amount of painstaking work, or re-presentation, or collation of classical material from homoeopathic authors, will suffice to put us on the map. We must do original research, consistent with the accepted vehicles of the modern scientific mind. We must bridge the gap between the laboratory person and our clinical therapeutist. We must strive to establish a Foundation with laboratory, hospital and clinic, which can check records and conduct experiments on a basis of pure homoeopathy over a series of thousands of patients and many years.

This Foundation must correlate endocrinology and morphology with homoeopathy. It must work out the relation between remedy types and disease diagnosis. Its work should include measurable psychological tests of different remedy types (such as a group of typical Sulphur patients, or Phosphorus, or Lycopodium patients). Its laboratory work should include provings on animals with remedies in both low and high potencies, as has already been done in the case of fruit flies and guinea pigs by the New York Foundation, and especially experiments on the physiological effects of high potencies on sensitive human provers. Our best thoughts could turn to some of the puzzling questions. What would be the effect of remedies given in *high* potencies according to the law of *contraries*? In what way does the homoeopath who prescribes for diseases or for organs differ from the usual physician, except in his effort at individualizing; unless, of course, he prescribes for organs and diseases on the basis of the totality of similar symptoms? If these things were accomplished, the unique sphere of homoeopathy would be demonstrated and *we* would permeate, tranquilly and irresistibly, the entire realm of medicine.

Let me remind you of the five uniquenesses of homoeopathy:
1) Cutting short acute diseases.
2) Curing chronic diseases.
3) Removing hereditary taints (prophylaxis against chronic disease).
4) Individualizing each case, and
5) Utilizing energies on a plane not otherwise used in drug medicine.

'The future of higher homoeopathy', said Compton Burnett, '*lies in behind the symptoms.*' The degree of our osmosis into organized medicine will, in the last analysis, depend on what each of us homoeopaths perceives 'behind the symptoms'.

Potencies High and Low

You may have heard the fable about two plumed knights who approached an inn from opposite directions. In front of this inn there hung a beautiful shield. The first knight said, 'What a beautiful *silver* shield!' and the second knight exclaimed 'What a beautiful *golden* shield!' They fell to disputing as to whether it was made of gold or silver, and were about to enter into mortal combat when a peasant nearby suggested that each should first look on the other side of the shield. This they did, and behold! one side was of gold and the other of silver.

It is of real benefit to hear the varying opinions of representative and successful prescribers on the moot point of potency. Surely the selection of a remedy by the law of similars is the fundamental tenet of homoeopathy. Even if one were to practice wholly with tinctures selected homoeopathically, one would get better results than are obtainable with tinctures prescribed according to any other method. Many allopathic successes with quinine, iron, arsenic or potassium iodide, for example, are due to their being homoeopathic to the case.

We feel, however, that the power in potentization is the next greatest asset to homoeopathy. This is the second great tenet. We are sure that if prescribers would learn to use the high potencies they would, themselves, be amazed at the far-reaching curative results, and the number of their successes would be increasingly great. Undoubtedly there are instances in which the medium or lower potencies act better, or even succeed where the high potencies fail. This especially appears to be the case where there is much pathology, sometimes in recent injuries, or where there is hypersensitivity to the remedy to be used. In cases of poor reaction some prescribers find that very high potencies stimulate recovery, while others hold that lower potencies are more successful repeated at short intervals until reaction sets in. The more chronic work any prescriber does, the more he needs and uses the high potencies, although in very dyscrasic chronic conditions potencies as low as 30c or 12c may be needed in single dosage, handled as though they were high potencies.

It is recorded that Digitalis in tincture is indicated in certain decompensated heart conditions. Does that mean that it is prescribed homoeopathically, i.e. for a slow pulse with the other homoeopathic indications of Digitalis, or that it is given for its so-called 'physiological' effects on the allopathic indications of rapid pulse and so on? Homoeopaths have had some very pretty results in decompensated hearts, previously digitalized by allopaths, with such remedies as Apocynum, Crataegus, Naja and Natrum Mur.

Would that all homoeopaths could use the silver of the lower potencies and the gold of the higher potencies, seeing both sides of the shield and keeping the intuitive open-mindedness of the peasant in the fable. Tolerance, however admirable, is not enough. One must master the technique of those with whom one disagrees, welcoming successes by their method.

A Programme of Research for Modern Homoeopathy

Developing the science pertaining to homoeopathy is necessary, not only that it may give a deeper backing to our work than the empirical one, but also that it may clarify our own conceptions, discipline our minds, and lead to the evolution as well as the continuance of homoeopathy. Nothing in this world is static, and surely Hahnemann, with a vision far ahead of the age in which he lived, and with his colossal fecundity of mind, would have been the first to have led medicine into further development. Nothing of what is true, precious and marvellous in homoeopathy should be overlooked or unemployed, but should be further worked out by the aid of present-day science, which homoeopathy can and must guide and inspire.

What opportunities for experimentation and investigation into homoeopathic problems are there today which were not possible to the scientists of Hahnemann's time?

1) The law of similars can be statistically proven, not only through clinical results with strict controls, but also through experiment in laboratories of physiology, pharmacology, pathology, bacteriology, botany and zoology.

2) The subject of dosage offers an enormous field for experiment. In accordance with the Arndt-Schulz phenomenon, the stimulative threshold of every remedy used homoeopathically on healthy subjects must be determined. This in itself is a lifelong task. The various factors influencing the amount of any one remedy needed to stimulate any one healthy human subject have so far not even been enumerated. If animals are used for experiment, the threshold will vary for each kind of animal and for each individual of a given kind. If this were worked out, it may be that we could determine scientifically that certain remedies act best, on the average, in certain strengths or potencies. Allied to this is the determination of the degree of hypersensitivity caused by diseased conditions of different sorts, as well as the hypersensitivity induced by previous drugging of various kinds. The individuals so tested, both healthy and diseased, for stimulative threshold, would have to be

classified and standardized according to the criteria of modern laboratory methods, and also according to the criteria of symptoms such as we use as a basis for a homoeopathic prescription. At first the relatively low potencies would probably have to be employed. Experimentation on the value of high potencies would at first have to be carried out in physics laboratories and would have to include the detection of power in high potencies. This would lead towards hypotheses as to what actually produces the empirical effects, quite possibly involving the transmutation of material substance into energy which is still specific, and by which the effect is produced. Might this not be analogous to Hahnemann's spirit-like force which acts on the same plane as that unknown entity, the vital force of the living human being?

The relation of dosage to aggravation must also be determined. Experiments must also determine the actual power content of our potencies, especially the high ones, and some method of standardizing these, both during and after their manufacture. The main problem would be the detection and prevention of impurities (the so-called oligodynamic effect of Kotschau). Some of the material being potentized is absorbed by the container, whether it be porcelain, glass or whatever, even if an absolutely clean container is used for each manipulation. In any dilution a certain very small amount of substance from the container must necessarily get into the solution. Furthermore, any impurities in the potentizing media (Sac. Lac. or alcohol or distilled water), add complications. Other impurities in the remedy substance itself may be present. For instance, many metals and elements are almost inseparable from traces of other substances; and plants may be contaminated with dirt or with salts in the water used to wash them, and so on.

3) Botanical laboratories are needed for the identification and classification of plant remedies; and field botanists should be sent all over the world collecting accurate specimens for drug manufacture. A herbarium and complete homoeopathic garden, including greenhouses for such of the remedial plants as need different climates, are essential to complete homoeopathic study.

4) The same is true in the field of zoology.

5) Chemical laboratories are essential, in which every remedial plant should be analysed into its constituents. At present we have fair analyses of a very small number of our plant remedies, such as *Phytolacca* and *Pulsatilla*. The animal remedies must be similarly analysed, as must the nosodes and sarcodes.

Extensive experiments in synergy and catalysis offer another field, and might elucidate some problems of remedy relationship. Laboratory studies should be made in an effort to demonstrate and explain inimical, antidotal and complementary remedy relationships. The allotropic forms of elements should be studied and compared with the varying or contradictory actions of those same elements in homoeopathy. The problem of isomers and that of reaction to polarized light, and many other similar problems, should be attacked for the same purpose. The field of colloidal and physical chemistry should be explored by an expert with thorough homoeopathic training, or collaboration, to devise methods from this approach of learning about our remedies.

6) A geologist should give data on the composition of the soil of the natural habitat of our different remedies, and also of the composition of so-called geological remedies. The effect of the composition of fertilizers on plants and foods grown by their use should be tabulated.

7) A meteorologist should collaborate in the study of why certain remedies, like certain people, are sensitive to seasonal, climatic and meteorological conditions. This includes the phases of the moon.

8) Endocrinological studies should be made to determine the action of the various homoeopathic remedies which are used to correct such conditions.

9) Thorough studies of the actions of our remedies from lethal doses up to the highest known potencies shoud be carried out on organs, tissues, animals and humans. A comparative tabulation of the action of each remedy as used in ordinary medicine and as used homoeopathically in different potencies is especially necessary, with a view to working out the laws that govern the apparent paradoxes of such actions.

10) The pathological laboratory should fully develop Hinsdale's scheme of proving the pathological effects of our remedies on animals and humans, insofar as it is safe to induce pathology. In connection with this come the studies of the toxicologist and the changes in clinical pathology brought about by our remedies.

11) The bacteriological laboratory should demonstrate the effects of our remedies in varying potencies on the different bacteria, being guided in their experiments by the symptom similarity between the remedies used and the bacterial diseases. This must probably mean testing the bacteria from humans and animals before and after suitable homoeopathic dosage, since presumably it is the vital force stimulated by the similar

remedy which acts on the bacteria. Experiments must, however, be made with remedies on bacteria in vitro. Immunological experiments must also be done.

This leads us to some of the most moot points, such as the use of homoeopathic remedies for prophylaxis and treatment in place of many of the vaccines and antitoxins. Long and careful studies in hospitals for contagious diseases must be carried through to determine the relative efficacy of the two methods.

12) A study of the influence of food substances and their adulterations, including preservatives and condiments, and different kinds of metal cooking utensils, should be undertaken, as well as research into the influence of fumes and water impurities – all regarded from the homoeopathic standpoint.

THE RELATIONSHIP OF HOMOEOPATHY
TO ORTHODOX MEDICINE
Towards a Sound Medical Peace

Homoeopathy has had a checkered career, doing its miraculous good in quiet ways. At the onset, and for many years after, it was marked by belligerency and even persecution. Later, when medicine in general had absorbed some of its obvious good points and ceased to battle it, homoeopathy went into a period of unmolested, quiet work. But rarely did people properly understand or believe in its fundamental tenets. Slowly through the decades science has discovered things about nature and its laws which were a part of homoeopathy, or allied to it, such as vaccines and sera, colloids, the use of radioactive substances and the powers of atomic energy. Each of these many discoveries was acclaimed and yet not connected with homoeopathic philosophy. Today there is a great upheaval in thought, and the time is ripe for the assertion of the invaluable and fundamental principles behind homoeopathy.

We who have been lax, prejudiced and absorbed in our private results, too busy to give even a modicum of thought and effort to the presentation of our wonderful tools of healing, must now unite and put some of the devotion of which we have shown ourselves capable into the making of a sound medical peace, and contribute our forces toward the founding of a healthier and better world.

Individualization is the essence of homoeopathy. It is ironic and troublesome, but perhaps also a vital fact that homoeopaths have great difficulty in agreeing on anything except the remedy. Let us now define the issues on which we must agree if we are to make a forceful presentation of homoeopathy. We must make a living portrait of homoeopathy just as we would make one of a remedy, searching out the totality throughout all the realms of science and humanity. We must evaluate, as we evaluate our symptoms in case-taking, and be precise and profound, both objective and subjective. I would like to offer a series of propositions, Hahnemannian instead of Pythagorean, but clear as any from mathematics.

Homoeopathy is scientific. That we cannot escape. It copes with the same facts as the rest of the scientific world, but interprets them in so different a manner as to be startling. We need to have succinct statements of the homoeopathic viewpoint on each of the departments of medical knowledge, so that anyone ordinarily trained would be electrified and their minds galvanized into deeper thinking. We should endeavour to control our results in the scientific sense of experimental controls. We should use every known harmless scientific method of diagnosis and laboratory research to make our findings judgeable by other scientists.

We should work indefatigably to increase the knowledge of our intricate art among its professed practitioners, supporting and devising methods to promote its better practice. We should be constructive, full of enthusiasm based on well-grounded data, filled with such a vivid spirit of power in the art of healing that our contagion spreads like wildfire among the groping and disappointed honest servers, both of the sick and of the cause of science.

The Dragon's Teeth

Dr Hubbard wrote these lines in 1930. It is salutary to consider them now. — Ed.

This year homoeopathy has lost by death a large number of its élite, including Drs Close, Thatcher, Perez, Loos, DeFriez, and many more, and there are a number of others, well known to our readers, who are so seriously ill that they will not be able to serve longer for homoeopathy. On the other hand, the office of the Hahnemann Institution of Chicago tells us that they have requests from 672 communities for competent homoeopathic physicians. The State Insane Hospital at Westboro, Massachusetts, is in urgent need of a homoeopathic resident psychiatrist. Some of our greatest masters have no one to train as their assistants and successors. How are we to fill these needs? How can we recruit the ranks? Whence will the new blood come?

The Summer School of the American Foundation for Homoeopathy is training a few each year. This summer the Hahnemann Institutions in Chicago are opening a postgraduate school for this same purpose. These movements are wonderful but they are only a drop in the bucket. How can we make young men and women see that whereas ordinary medicine is overcrowded, and the first years of such practices are hard sledding, the homoeopathic field has nearly seven hundred known openings, with practices of devoted patients large in numbers? This is merely the practical side. How can we impress upon the young that a faithful study of homoeopathy will so enhance their powers of curing as to make such cures seem miraculous? This, to our mind, is the greatest problem in homoeopathy today.

Mythology tells us of Cadmus, Prince of Phoenicia, whose army was destroyed by the dragon. This monster was difficult to overcome because of his many invulnerable scales, but Cadmus slew him and sowed his teeth, from which sprang, fully armed, a new host of vigorous warriors. Homoeopathy is a Cadmus of today. Consider some of the scales of the dragon against which it must contend – inertia; the inaccessibility of homoeopathic knowledge; the lack of training in the appreciation of scientific medicine by many masters of the homoeopathic art; their

32

hindering and ignorant animosities; the impurities of homoeopathic practice among many of its self-acclaimed vassals; the dissensions in its ranks; the lack of willingness, ability and financial backing to carry out the research on its scientific background (for, with any new discovery, the burden of proof is with the discoverers); and the ignorance and prejudice of the uninitiated.

Let us systematically demolish these scales, slay the dragon and sow his teeth far and wide, for then, and then only, will a new army be raised up for homoeopathy.

On Enlightened Minorities

Enlightened minorities must contribute insights on the problems of daily life. Only so does the spirit level rise. It is not enough to function splendidly in our own back yard. Consider what we, with our specialized knowledge and training, can offer to our colleagues, our politicians and the general public. For there is a service of ideas as well as of hearts and hands, and the expressed thoughts of today become the deeds of tomorrow.

The world is engaged in a perilous struggle for human freedom, for fuller consciousness, for the privilege not just of liberty and the pursuit of happiness, in any outer sense, nor even for the development of the individual, precious as that may be. It is fighting also for the privilege of seeing the ideal latent in the real, the connection of mankind and the microcosm of this earth upon which we incarnated, and its ensuing responsibilities.

Homoeopaths should understand, perhaps more keenly than anyone, the *total* view and its relation to the *individual*. The naturopath clears the way by detoxifying and using the forces of ingestion of water and air. It is the realm of hygiene. The osteopath regulates the muscular system and the chiropractor aligns the spine to free nerves and blood supply.

The biodynamic agriculturist presents us with proper, natural and full foods.

Conventional medicine gives us refinements of diagnosis and nomen-clature and enables us, through laboratory techniques, to gauge progress and prognoses; and through surgery to correct and remove mechanical obstructions. Thus we know the *physical* aspect of our health problem.

Herbalists use nature's healing vegetable kingdom substances for our aid. Psychiatry tries to give us self-diagnosis and teach us control. Faith-healing groups attempt self-cure and aid from spiritual sources.

Homoeopaths should be aware of the necessity of healing on all these levels, and of the synchronization of our three-fold being. They must perceive the tendency to over-intellectualization, its virtues and its dangers, to over-emotionalization and to over-metabolization – the Will run riot. They must take this runaway and enable it to stabilize and, consequently, to free itself.

Giving the most similar remedy promotes this by inner impetus, through co-operation with the vital force inherent in each human being. We must take great care not to give similar remedies in any but a profoundly homoeopathic way . . . *otherwise we are prescribing nominally homoeopathic remedies according to the usual law of contraries.*

Among all the paths to healing, the homoeopath is heir to the deepest and most fruitful answer to the dilemma of our time – the undue accent on the physical fragment of the whole human being.

EDITORIAL

As Editor of *The Homoeopathic Recorder* and as President to the American Institute of Homeopathy, Dr Hubbard found a forum to express her strong feelings about the needs of the homoeopathic movement and to urge again and again remedial action. Her voice repeatedly called out for an end to animosity, defensiveness and inattention. She tried to promote international co-operation among homoeopaths as well as striving to develop communication among homoeopathic physicians throughout her own country. She constantly battled against apathy. — Ed.

Educating the Patient

To cure your patient with a few sugary powders and an arresting certitude of manner, conveying a faith in his improvement, is not enough. After such cures your patient will believe implicitly in you and send his friends to you, but the credit he will give you belongs largely to homoeopathy.

The first duty of the homoeopath is to cure, but surely the second duty is to inculcate a concept of homoeopathy. Why should this be so? First, because we can create an intelligent demand for homoeopathy. Second, because we can safeguard our patients. They must learn to understand, for their own sakes, certain of the principles underlying our art. If only the public knew the results of suppression, how much suffering would be saved. If only they could be made to realize what a bar to recovery surgery may be, when it intervenes before the condition behind the pathology is cleared up. If only people could realize why the indiscriminate taking of drugs on a so-called physiological basis hinders real cure.

Every homoeopath should undertake an educative campaign with each patient. This does not mean that you should teach him to dabble in self-medication, but that you should initiate him into some of the fundamental tenets of health. If your patient already has experience of homoeopathy this may be so from tradition or from experience, rather than from an intelligent understanding of the laws of cure. In this instance he will be with you from the beginning and will be pleased to be taken into your confidence, to be allowed to understand what is being done to help him. If he is one who has never heard of homoeopathy, you must first convince him that you are 'scientific', by thorough physical examination, attention to hygiene and diet, and the use of the appropriate laboratory tests. Next, you must perceptibly help him with your remedy. Nothing is so convincing to the patient as a definite improvement in his sense of well-being.

These two things being accomplished, you can then safely begin to explain some of the principles of cure, without at first using the term homoeopathy. Our fundamentals are very appealing. The fact that you can help a patient, even though no organic change is detectable and no diagnosis possible, is reassuring and important to him, for he has probably had many experiences with modern therapeutic nihilism. He will be intrigued with your interest in what he has tried to tell his previous doctors, and of which they have taken no account. You can present the process of individualizing the case so strikingly that he will say, 'That is what I always said – people cannot and should not be treated alike.'

You can go on from individualization to an explanation of what modalities are, and teach him the sort of things he must tell you when he writes to ask you for medicine. Every homoeopathic patient should be trained to give a sufficient picture of his symptoms that a homoeopath new to the case could make a prescription without asking a single question. Explain thoroughly those factors which interfere with the action of the homoeopathic remedy and warn him against them. Explain the direction of cure, the possibility of aggravation, and the difference between the temporary intensification of symptoms and the general increased sense of well-being. He must understand the importance of mental symptoms, as well as the spiritual inferences consequent to the fact that the inner and the higher are always the most important. He must also understand the necessity of telling you the mental causes of many of his disturbances, not in detail, but so that you can classify them. For instance, your patient need not tell you why she had the argument with her husband that gave her a headache, or what mortification preceded her bilious attack, but she must let you know the general nature of the mental factor in the case.

Furthermore, you can easily interest your patients in chronic constitutional remedies, indicating their variances from the normal from childhood up. Annoying symptoms which they have accepted and disregarded can be shown to be curable. Let them see that emotional and mental traits, as well as physical distresses, are subject to our remedies. What a relief to the mother of a chronic bed-wetter, or of a child with offensive excoriating foot sweat, or of one with jealous tantrums, to know that these things can be modified and often cured.

To explain these matters to patients takes time and clear thinking, but even from a selfish point of view it is a good investment, and is surely one of the greatest aids to the cause of homoeopathy and the common good.

The Value of Provings

In this age of scientific research homoeopathy makes a unique contribution, both as to method and to findings. It believes, not only in the Law of Similars, but in the fact that all natural substances from the three kingdoms – mineral, vegetable and animal – are potential instruments of healing. To be available for use in homoeopathy, each of these substances must be tested in experiments upon relatively healthy human beings. This we call proving. The human being is the most delicate instrument, and thanks to its self-consciousness can report all shades of symptoms, subjective and psychological. There is a much wider range of individual difference between man and man than between mouse and mouse. Moreover, proper proving is not only wholesome but positively improves the health, putting the system into order and raising resistance.

Substances to be proven produce only fleeting symptoms. These may be objective only, such as perspiration or diarrhoea. A good proving subject must be honest and painstaking, and able to follow instructions accurately. One does not have to be in perfect health but must be able to agree, over the month or two of proving, to take no medicinal substances. One can work during the proving and continue one's usual habits, if moderate. Not all people are sensitive to all substances, nor equally sensitive to all strengths or potencies of the same substances. The symptoms of a remedy do not appear all at once, nor necessarily in the same series, nor all in each experimenter. The later a symptom appears in the course of a proving, the more characteristic it is likely to be. The more individual a symptom is, the longer it lasts. Individual symptoms, especially if peculiar, must never be discarded, even though appearing in very few provers. They cannot be accepted as a part of the materia medica of the substance unless shown by three or more provers, but are kept for confirmation. We have the duty to mistrust any symptom, but never to reject it until repeated experiment has shown it to be untenable.

The proving experiments are conducted on a double blind basis. This means that not even the people in charge of the proving know the nature of the substance being administered to the group of provers under their supervision. Controls are given in the same form as the remedy – this not only establishes the scientific value of the proving but helps to eliminate those provers who are too imaginative. A medical research statistician should be enlisted to approve the technique.

Second or third trials of the same medicine may produce different effects on the same prover. Only by comparison and standardization does the picture of the remedy emerge. Symptoms do not arise spontaneously while health is under the influence of a medicine being proved. Hence, symptoms that a prover may have had a considerable time prior to the experiment should not be discarded, but noted as being recurrences. No single prover is likely to produce the whole gamut or symptoms in a remedy. Re-proving should be done on the same prover at suitable intervals until no new symptoms arise, and only the original symptoms recur. There must be a relationship of trust and co-operation between the provers and those who are in charge of the proving.

The Importance of the Individual

People are animals plus. The difficulties that veterinarians encounter are different from those met by physicians working only with human beings. The animal cannot speak in words, although to the trained ear its cries, like those of a baby, are significant of feelings. Fortunately, neither can it intentionally mislead you, nor malinger. Astute observation is a prime necessity for the homoeopath, as it is for the veterinarian. There is a saying that if the patient says one thing and the gesture is contrary, believe the gesture. Those who claim that the apparent success of homoeopathy is due to faith or autosuggestion should watch the results with animals, infants, and unconscious humans.

There is a wider background for a homoeopathic interest in animals, in that some of our most important healing medicines are made from animals. What would our armamentarium be without Sepia, the cuttlefish, Apis, the honey-bee, Crotalus Horridus, the rattlesnake, Lachesis, the bushmaster snake, and Cantharis, the beetle?

There is a similarity, often of type, between human beings and animals, and mythology is full of allusions and parables involving animals and humans. In teaching materia medica we point out the resemblance between certain animals and certain remedies. For instance, Antimonium Crudum is a true picture of the human pig, from its sour odours and sensibility to the full moon, enormous appetite and sour, swill-like indigestion; Pulsatilla resembles the sheep – followers, not leaders, able to stay huddled together in the snow, timid and bleating, yet at times whimsical and playful; Arsenicum Album is the remedy for the horse, making its coat glossy and improving its wind – both remedy and beast being nervous, restless, sensitive and fearful.

From a public relations point of view, the veterinary aspect of homoeopathy is of great interest. Cure a beloved pet and you may win four generations of a family of patients. Recently I was on a cattle ranch where they also bred quarter horses. One of the prize foals had curious symptoms. It would try to run away and was unusually susceptible to any acute trouble, particularly respiratory. It seemed so frail and tired, although beautiful in conformation. The breeder feared he would lose it. One dose of Tuberculinum 30c changed the animal's actions, looks and susceptibility. A boxer dog was beset with huge black warts which recurred many-fold if any were removed. Thuja 10M was followed by a dropping-off of the warts and a healing of a chronic catarrh which had bothered the animal for months.

'Little Sunday'

The next best motto to *Similia similibus* is *Festina lente*. Homoeopathic physicians are relatively few in any community and their practices are large. Moreover, they must do double work; all the diagnosis and scientific investigation of the up-to-date physician, and the careful research and study into modalities and the depths of chronic disease in addition. For them life is even busier than for the average practitioner, and as they believe in the primary importance of the mind and spirit they must be integrated, replete with power, centres of radiation of health, emotional and physical. How to fill this role in the pressure of modern civilization is a vital question.

On the Continent of Europe, in some parts, they have the charming habit of 'little Sunday', usually Thursday afternoon. Where week-ends are so popular as they are with us in America, it would seem better to hold 'little Sunday' on Wednesday.

Do this, fellow-practitioners, as a spiritual investment. Make it an ironclad rule not to do your usual hectic routine on 'little Sunday' afternoon, but to save that time for constructive thought, original writing, meditation, solitary contact with nature, or play along these lines with your proverbially neglected families. *Festina lente* on all days, but especially at the mid-week. Let 'little Sunday' be a refreshing oasis amid the strenuousness of our doctorial desert.

WHIMSY

The pages of *The Homoeopathic Recorder* and the *Journal of the American Institute of Homeopathy* were enlivened from time to time by articles best described as whimsical. Here are three samples. — Ed.

A Homoeopathic Bouquet

Rarely does one have the opportunity of being as expansive as the heart and the imagination wish. Not often can one play with deep and serious knowledge and enjoy its colourful facets. Only infrequently is ingenuity challenged to the limit. All these fortunate releases were invoked, in fact required, by a simple situation in which British Royalty, knowledgeable in homoeopathy, permitted tribute.

In other words, Princess Margaret came to America! and your Editor, who had been trying for weeks to obtain the necessary permission to send her a gift on behalf of the American Institute members, was suddenly called to the telephone; where an ebullient British gentleman, a member of the British Information Service, gave permission for the Institute to send its floral tribute next morning.

What an orgy to look at the profusion of blooms in one of the great florists preparing for Thanksgiving, and to choose only such specimens as had homoeopathic uses. They were usually redolent, often shy and quiet. And the emphasis at that season was for greens rather than showy blooms. The flowers themselves included: violets, *Viola odorata*, useful for sinus and ear trouble; acacia, *Robinia*, for acid stomach; *Cyclamen* for the thirsty Pulsatilla patient; anemone, *Pulsatilla*, for puberty troubles, femininity, and indigestion from fat; *Calendula*, the homoeopathic iodine; daisy, *Bellis perennis*, for bruises, the gardener's remedy; rose, *Rosa damascena*, for hay fever; lily of the valley, *Convallaria*, in skipping heart; *Iris versicolor*, with burning migraine; bittersweet, *Dulcamara*, for autumnal diarrhoea; Star of Bethlehem, *Ornithogallum*, for gastric cancer; broom, *Cytisus scoparius*, relative of our *Baptisia*, for grippe; eucalyptus for some coughs; geranium, the tonic; mistletoe, *Viscum*, of tumour fame; barberry, the *Berberis* of kidney stone virtue; ivy, *Hedera helix*, for convulsions; lemon, *Citrus limonum*, for haemorrhage and neuralgia; and the sovereign cedar, *Thuja occidentalis*, for tumours, catarrhs, hair and nails; huckleberry foliage, *Vaccinum myrtillus*, so useful in diabetes; yew, *Taxus baccata*, for gout; *Magnolia glauca*, and laurel leaves, *Kalmia latifolia*, both notable in heart trouble; the speckled, brilliant leaves of the *Croton tiglium*, famous for bowel and skin complaints; and oleander, *Nerium*, of paralytic fame.

Whimsy

It seemed incredible that delphinium, *Staphysagria*, was not to be found, nor hydrangea, rhododendron or peony. No delicate primrose, no homely pansy, no clematis, lilac, crocus, ecchinacia, gentian, foxglove, candy tuft, squill jasmine, monkshood, yarrow, lobelia, dandelion, morning-glory, forget-me-not, honeysuckle, dogwood, hawthorn, bella-donna, rue, capsicum, mint, poppy, plantain, goldenrod, buttercup, *Ranunculus bulbosus*, for shingles, not even juniper, *Sabina*, of gin and haemorrhage import.

Just one or two of each of these available in a great sheaf, and so that something might go with the princess on the plane, a corsage of *Cypripedium*, lady-slipper orchids which bring tranquillity and rest.

Appended is the letter thanking you all for that delicate attention. How comforting, as in its incipience, so now, after nearly a hundred years, that the Royal Family of the great English Commonwealth is still being cherished by nature's helpers, the homoeopathic remedies.

Kensington Palace
W.8
8th December, 1965

Dear Dr Wright Hubbard,

Princess Margaret has bidden me write to thank you most sincerely for the lovely bouquet of flowers used in homoeopathic medicine, which you so kindly sent when Her Royal Highness was staying in Manhasset.

This delightful and fascinating gift gave The Princess great pleasure during her last day in the United States, and she would be most grateful if you could pass on a message of her warm appreciation to all who joined with you in sending it.

Yours sincerely,
Francis Legh
Private Secretary to
The Princess Margaret,
Countess of Snowdon

Thuja

The cedar is a formal tree
It peoples the gardens of Tivoli.
The tree of the dead it's supposed to be
And stands guard in a cemetery.
It protects both from moth and rust,
To its chest or closet treasures you entrust,
In ancient Egypt they used it to embalm
To keep majestic Pharaohs from time's harm.
The cedar is a healing tree,
Its battles against redundancy.
All things oval and all things dark –
Waxy buds and striate bark.
Only the wax-wing sits silently
Atop the tree of life, the Arbor Vitae.

With Apologies to
Gilbert and Sullivan

I've got a little list, I've got a little list,
Of homoeopathic doctors whom we won't admit exist –
They never will be missed, they never will be missed.

The one who ruins everything by too quick repetition,
Whom all single dose enthusiasts condemn unto perdition –
       He never will be missed . . .
And he who gives the second best and oft likewise the third
In one shotgun prescription – if he is never heard
       He never will be missed . . .
And he who, short of patience, changes horses at the stile,
In your august opinion will never be worthwhile.
The alternating fellow; he who gives an intercurrent;
Or the drainage drugs the French use – all are equally abhorrent.
They never will be missed, they never will be missed.

The user of a Kent is to Gehenna bent:
The Boenninghausen djinn is in original sin:
The users of the Field no man of us will shield:
The devotees of Boger try hard to put him over.
       This motley repertorial
       Of wisdom senatorial
       Deprived of yearly bickerings
       And philosophic dickerings
       Oh! how they would be missed!

The resigners and decliners, the correctors and objectors,
The procrastinating people who to letters don't reply,
Those with chips upon the shoulder visible to each beholder,
And those who give fine papers audible to those near by –
They are on my little list, they are on my little list.
The awaited opportunity to cavil with impunity,
By force of intuition to bring cases to fruition –
Through giving the Simillimum to hasten the millenium,

48

With Apologies to Gilbert and Sullivan

The I. H. A. Convention seems to thrive upon contention!
But HOW it would be missed!

From Hippocrates and Hahnemann and Boenninghausen too,
   You may learn what you should do . . .
From Paracelsus to Swedenborg and Boger, Kent and Close,
   You may learn to give a dose . . .
From Hering and the Nestor of us all, good Dr Knerr,
To whose monumental learning as a family we defer;
From Roberts' lore of serpent balm and Underhill on diet,
You learn to do no harm and yet to keep the patient quiet.

The user of a Kent must be a knowing gent:
The Boenninghausen crew needs a secretary or two:
The wielders of a Boger need no repertory to put it over.
   This motley repertorial, of wisdom senatorial,
   With symptoms in totality both general and modality,
   With potency adjusted to avoid an aggravation,
   With camphor and the coal-tars banished from the nation,
   Are giving the Simillimum to hasten the millenium!

REPERTORY

Editorial Comment

In the early years of homoeopathy, Hahnemann and other scientists tested and studied each remedy they developed, thus coming to know them intimately. As they began to use them clinically, they saw how human bodies responded to each of the substances they prepared and potentized, and carefully recorded this information. Often, we are told, they experimented upon themselves with these remedies, gaining a special insight into the nature and symptomatology of each one.

The work continued over the years, the materia medica growing with each addition until the accumulated mass of information about the homoeopathic armamentarium obviously required some sort of codification. Thus was the concept of the repertory born – an index to the growing materia medica. The ability to use a repertory effectively greatly enlarged the practitioner's scope, as in time there were too many with all their remedies, symptoms and indications, for anyone to carry in his head.

The creation of a repertory is an interesting story in itself. We are told that Adolph Lippe made the first one, but as the materia medica continued to grow and new proving symptoms were added, students of homoeopathy realized that more organization of the information was sorely needed. Dr James Tyler Kent, of Chicago, Illinois, put his medical students to work to help him produce an expanded repertory, interleaving the Lippe book. When a sizeable manuscript had been produced, it became clear that using symptoms from various sources was not going to result in a satisfactory repertory, due to the varying ways in which the several authors had organized their work; so the whole thing was abandoned and they started again from scratch. The result was the world-famous *Repertory of the Homoeopathic Materia Medica*, by J. T. Kent, A.M., M.D., which stood nearly alone for many years as the indispensable aid to the practitioner trying to find his way to the elusive simillimum. This monumental work went through several editions, carefully revised from time to time by Kent, and subsequently by others: Pierre Schmidt of Geneva, Diwan Harish

Chand of New Delhi and, most recently, by Barthel and Klunker and by Jost Künzli.

Ever since computers first came on the scene as practical equipment for the small office, computer-wise patients have exclaimed, as they watched the tedious process of fingering through the Repertory for the pertinent symptoms, 'You need a computer for such work!' Who could deny that? But who could find the time to work out a program? The *British Homoeopathic Journal* published an article by Dr E. E. E. A. de Ruyter of Australia on the computer in homoeopathy. Someone had found the time and possessed the necessary skills and presented the profession with HOMREPAN . . .

Since that time ever more sophisticated programs for finding the remedy indicated by the symptom picture of the patient at hand have been developing. There now exist a plethora of choices for mechanical aid in this difficult task, but one serious reservation remains: it is more than ever vital to take the case well and thoroughly, and to select the right symptoms for repertorizing. As we used to admonish the students in the American Foundation Postgraduate Course: prepare your case properly for presentation to Dr Kent. Elizabeth Wright Hubbard was one of the all-time experts at doing just that, and taught it most effectively. — Ed.

Proposal for an
Abridged Kent's Repertory

As a true classical homoeopath, Elizabeth Wright Hubbard considered Kent's *Repertory* to be essential to her prescribing. One of her projects was the design of a 'portable' version of it. As a writer, she painted wonderful remedy pictures with her words. She would say, as did Margery Blackie, the renowned British physician, that it was 'the patient who mattered, not the disease.' — Ed.

From a teaching standpoint, and for those learning to use homoeopathy, one of the greatest obstacles is connected (as is so often the case) with a most precious aid. We mean the Kent *Repertory*. Invaluable, magnificent and fascinating as it is, there is no denying that there are a great many rubrics in it that are rarely used, others which are repetitious, and still others which are confusingly placed. Its size makes it unwieldy for carrying on the daily round. Many people have expressed the desirability of a small Kent *Repertory*, available at a modest price, containing the main rubrics and following the general present arrangement.

Such an abridged edition should, we strongly feel, contain the three classes of remedies as at present. There should be neither change nor curtailing in the remedies given under any rubric. Under the rubrics to be omitted should be not only those which repeat, and those which are rarely used – such as many under 'Delusions, etc.' – but also those containing so many remedies and in their nature so general as to be practically useless to the user, i.e., rubrics such as 'Sadness', 'Restless-ness', or 'Vertigo'. This edition should have a brief index and some scheme of collating rubrics having to do with diagnosis, such as suppressed gonorrhoea, scarlet fever, haemorrhoids, etc., and rubrics relating to mental causes which are at present sprinkled all through the book.

The first step, however, would be to ask a number of veteran users of the *Repertory* to specify those rubric titles under one section, say 'Mentals', which they most often use and consider to be most important. This book would not supplant the present *Repertory*, but would be a handbook to it for beginners and for ready reference in a hurry. One cannot carry to the bedside one's entire cabinet of homoeopathic remedies, but one can certainly carry a compact little case of chosen ones. This is no discredit to those of our remedies which are left in the office. In the same way, the portable edition would be of great use on a large number of occasions, and one would always have to refer to the fuller original book when necessary.

Thoughts on
Revamping The Repertory

The greatest single book in homoeopathy is perhaps Kent's *Repertory*. To the ever-increasing number of physicians who use the Kent method of repertorizing, it is absolutely indispensable. Every prescriber needs this mammoth index, this concordance of our craft, not only to work out chronic cases in his rare hours of leisure, if any, but also for immediate reference at the bedside in acute, desperate or obscure cases. The student and the novice need it constantly, although no master mind is retentive enough to dispense with it entirely. Yet, how unwieldy a book it is! – five pounds in weight, large and very expensive. These disadvantages in format, harassing as they are, are as nothing compared to the obstacles to swift and precise prescribing in the text itself.

For the sake of those who are not thoroughly familiar with the Kent *Repertory* I explain its present plan:
1) MIND, being the innermost and most important, stands first.
2) VERTIGO, unreasonably enough, comes next.
3) HEAD, which includes scalp, follows.
4) EYE and VISION.
5) EAR and HEARING.
6) NOSE.
7) FACE, including lips, salivary glands and sinuses.
8) MOUTH, including tongue, taste and speech.
9) TEETH.
10) THROAT, including uvula and oesophagus, but not larynx.
11) EXTERNAL THROAT, including thyroid, glands, torticollis.
12) STOMACH, including desires and aversions.
13) ABDOMEN, including groins, hernia, liver, dysmenorrhoea (also found under GENITALIA, FEMALE).
14) RECTUM, including constipation and diarrhoea.
15) STOOL.
16) URINARY ORGANS: Bladder, including urination; kidneys; prostate gland; urethra; urine.
17) GENITALIA, MALE and FEMALE (menses are also found under Generals).

18) LARYNX and TRACHEA, including throat-pit and voice.
19) RESPIRATION.
20) COUGH.
21) EXPECTORATION.
22) CHEST, including heart, lungs, breast and axillae.
23) BACK, including cervical region and spine.
24) EXTREMITIES.
25) SLEEP, including dreams.
26) CHILL.
27) FEVER.
28) PERSPIRATION.
29) SKIN.
30) GENERALITIES, including physical generals; pathology; convulsions; fainting; aggravations or ameliorations from food; certain sensations; types of pain, direction of pain, pain in certain tissues, such as bones, cartilages, glands, muscles, periosteum; pulse; aggravations before, during or after sleep, menses, coition, etc.

Let me enumerate a few of the obstacles:

1) Many rubrics are out of place from the point of view of common sense. For instance, things pertaining to the neck are found both under External Throat and under Back; pulse is under Generals instead of being with heart under Chest; sinuses are divided between Head, Face and Nose; salivary glands are found under Face; lips are also under Face, instead of under Mouth. These are matters of anatomical classification which should be simplified and corrected. There is no section for the circulatory system, the glandular or lymphatic system, nor for the nervous system.

2) Even under the existing arrangement certain headings are misplaced: Awkwardness under Generals when it is a Mental; desires and aversions to food under Stomach when they should be under Generals, for they indicate the whole patient; and the type of menses, so characteristic of the whole person, should be under Generals instead of under Female Genitalia as at present. These, of course, are only a few examples.

3) Pathological and diagnostic headings and many objective symptoms are now sprinkled through the book. These should be collected, classified and placed in a special section by themselves.

4) Many common symptoms, such as vomiting, restlessness, sadness, etc., have such large rubrics as to be practically useless. Moreover they consume much space. These should either be deleted or put in at the head of the particulars related to them, with only the third or highest degree remedies given. (*Editorial Note:* I would challenge her on this. Some feel that the presence of a remedy in such a list is significant, regardless of degree.)

5) Repetitions abound. These are often due to the use of synonyms in different places with somewhat different remedies. These could either be cross-referenced or else combined under the most usual synonym, or grouped under the most usual heading, with the other synonyms as sub-headings and the varying remedy rubrics distinct under each. By this last method one does not blur the shades of meaning and would thereby promote discrimination on the physician's part. Examples are: haughty, insolent, contemptuous, defiant, scornful, arrogant, dictatorial, presumptuous, domineering, dogmatic.

6) The *Repertory* is based on only about 540 remedies. This should, of course, be brought up to date, but that is a herculean task, not really within the scope of an abridgement and rearrangement of the present *Repertory*. There are some important remedies, however, which should be added.

7) Confusion arises in the mind of the novice until it is realized that where nothing is mentioned after the heading of the rubric it often means 'aggravated from'. For instance, 'GENERALITIES, FASTING' means 'aggravated while fasting'. The ameliorations are always mentioned, whereas the aggravations are only sometimes mentioned, which makes it a bit confusing.

8) Many rubrics could be omitted with profit from an abridged version of the *Repertory* to be carried in one's bag – consider a rubric such as 'Cheerfulness'. It is the abnormalities of cheerfulness that are noteworthy, for example over-exuberance, which might be classed as hilarity, or too little cheerfulness, which should come under depression.

9) Last, but by no means least, comes the lack of an index and cross-references. These are essential for the proper use of the *Repertory*. At present the prescriber has to write in the page number of the cross-references for himself.

These are some of the main criticisms, although there are many others. Every systematic physician would have his own preference as to arrangement, his own evaluation of the meaning of words, especially in the section on Mind, and his own ideas of what would constitute a workable repertory.

In proposing the following schema for an abridged working *Repertory*, we proceed from the premise that it should be arranged in a logical and common-sense order which, while true to the best of homoeopathy, should also be consonant with current medical knowledge. The basic arrangement of our new *Repertory* would be according to the value of symptoms, emphasizing those which pertain to the patient as an individual personality. This implies that the Mental Generals come first, the Physical Generals next, and the Pathological Generals third, as indicative of the tendency of the constitution. Immediately after these, and before the details of any systems or organs, should come the other general sections such as Vertigo, Sleep, Chill, Fever and Perspiration. Ideally the 'Strange, Rare and Peculiar' characteristic particulars should come next, in a separate section. It may seem insuperably difficult to winnow these out from the chaff of common symptoms, but at least a very helpful and suggestive 'keynote' section of them could be compiled. There should then be an index, with certain essential cross-references.

All of the above, we feel, should constitute Volume 1. Volume 2 would be devoted to the symptoms of the separate systems, anatomical regions and organs, with the modalities, sensations and so on separated. This second volume would be of special use in acute work, whereas the first volume would almost be sufficient for the working of a chronic case, at least in the first stage, based on the generals.

At the back of the first volume would be a list of synonyms, not only in English but also in French, German and Spanish. This would make the work internationally useful. A list of correct remedy names with pronunciation marks and standardized abbreviations, plus a brief section on remedy relationships should be appended.

It is not possible in this context to give complete details, even as far as already worked out, but this tentative schema is offered.

1) MIND, or MENTAL GENERALS.
   a) The Will, which includes: the loves, hates, emotions, suicidal thoughts, loathing of life, lasciviousness, revulsion to sex, sexual perversions, fears, homicidal tendencies, jealousy, suspicion, greed, obstinacy, depression, loquacity, impatience, conscien-

tiousness, dreams, (which, though highly indicative of the patient's mental state, are now listed under sleep), desire or aversion to company, family, friends, etc. Under this heading should come ailments from emotions, now scattered throughout the book, and aversions, similarly dispersed.

b) The Understanding, which includes delusions, delirium, hallucinations, loss of time sense, mental confusion, etc., and some pathological mental conditions such as idiocy, imbecility, insanity, hysteria, mania.

c) The Intellect, which includes concentration, memory, mistakes in writing and speaking, precocity.

d) Certain Objective Symptoms such as biting, desire to hide, grimacing, and others.

2) PHYSICAL GENERALS.

a) Constitutional Types, which include such rubrics as dwarfishness, emaciation, lack of excess of vital heat (cold- or hot-blooded), obesity, blonde or brunette (rubrics from earlier edition of Kent), sensitiveness, and lack of reaction.

b) Suppressions – emotions, discharges, eruptions, diseases, pathology.

c) Menses, habitual type and recent changes in type, aggravation or amelioration before, during or after menses.

d) Other Discharges, type, better or worse from, and other modalities.

e) Modalities of the patient as a whole, including time, periodicity, seasons, moon phases, temperature and weather (scattered in numerous places), bathing (dread of bathing should be put under Mentals), rest, motion, position, external stimuli (touch, pressure, clothing, light, noise, etc.), eating and drinking, coition.

3) PATHOLOGY, including disease diagnoses.

4) OBJECTIVE SYMPTOMS.

5) VERTIGO, FAINTING.

6) SLEEP. Dreams, see Mentals.

7) CHILL and FEVER.

8) PERSPIRATION.

9) STRANGE, RARE AND PECULIAR SYMPTOMS. This should be placed here because, when present, they are of great value in pointing to the remedy.

All the rubrics should be classified, combined and arranged alphabetically, and scattered rubrics should be brought under one heading. The second volume would contain the PARTICULARS, arranged under anatomical locations, systems and organs. The missing systems, such as circulatory, nervous and locomotor, should be added and the rubrics belonging under them reclassified in their proper places. Certain regions such as neck or breast should be separated for readier reference. Certain rubrics such as sinuses, pulse and glands should be rationally placed. All the pain section rubrics, and rubrics on sensations, should be carefully reviewed and standardized.

Although it is manifestly impossible to fit a repertory to the needs of every individual mind, the proposed revision would at least make a workable and lucid reference book for a larger number of homoeopaths.

James Tyler Kent Prize Case

From time to time *The Homoeopathic Recorder* published a case presentation, inviting readers to submit their working out of the case. On this occasion, a prize was offered for the best solution to the *James Tyler Kent Prize Case*, here reprinted, followed by E.W.H.'s *A Method of Working out the Kent Prize Case*.

CASE

Mr B., age 28, slight, blonde, 10 pounds underweight, singer.

Chief Complaint
Hay fever annually since 4 years of age, August and September only.
Sneezing paroxysms until exhausted.
Worse strong light, motion and heat (can't stand sun). Better at night.
Watery nasal discharge, bilateral, excoriating.
Itching eyes.
Asthma, from 10 to 14 years of age, at night, wakening him at 2–3 a.m.
Skin test showed sensitivity to ragweed. Courses of ragweed injections and corticosteroid sprays under previous allopathic physicians did not aid.

Family History
Father, mother, 1 brother and 2 sisters, living and well.
No tuberculosis, no cancer, no epilepsy, no hay fever in family.
One uncle had asthma.

Past History
Typhoid at 18 (four doses of 'Serum').
Influenza at 19.
Operations: Deviated septum at 21. Tonsillectomy at 21.
Vaccinated once, which took.
No history of eruptions, acute rheumatic fever, diphtheria, scarlet fever, malaria, pneumonia or pleurisy.
Frequent styes.
Train and car sick.

Takes cold every month or two.
History of gonorrhoea (treated by protargol).
Hair falls out (sulphur and resorcin used on scalp).

Present Illness
Depression.
Lascivious thoughts bother him.
Childhood scenes recur, broods over them.
Patient wants to be hypnotized or magnetized.
Homosexual experiences.
Exceedingly conscientious; neat.
Says sleep is his only salvation; sleeps on the left side with head low.
Weepy recently.
Shortness of breath, on stairs and in singing.
Sensation of clenched jaw often.
Abdominal cramps from cold milk; not from hot milk.
Never suicidal; fears nothing but himself; very social.
Warm-blooded, but loves hot weather.
Worse in sea air and fog.
Worse on damp days.
Eats anything, but lately has an aversion to milk; however, craves ice
    cream; always loves fats and dislikes starches.
Afraid of undertaking things.
Always blaming himself.
Dry feeling behind sternum causes cough.

Examination
(Only positive findings stated.)
Skin of the face greasy-looking.
Nasal polyps, bilateral.
Silver fillings in teeth.
Fissured tongue.
Thin skin with prominent arm veins.
Split first heart sound.
Left lung apex posterially somewhat dull; no definite râles.
Palms of the hands very hot and sweaty.
Slight eczematous condition between toes.
Blood pressure 160/90.
Urine negative except for smoky odour.
Blood count normal except for 3% eosinophiles.
Chest X-ray negative.
Sputum not obtainable.

A Method of Working out
The Kent Prize Case

This case is judged on the following points:

1) Homoeopathicity.
2) Evaluation of symptoms.
3) Repertory rubrics, corresponding to the symptoms.
4) Reason for the final choice of remedy or remedies.

It is obviously a deep chronic case, because all hay fevers in childhood are. It shows underlying psoric and sycotic miasms. The psora is shown by the hay fever and the eczema; the sycosis, by the suppressed gonorrhoea, the over-conscientiousness, the worse on damp days, and the frequency of taking cold. We should ultimately expect Psorinum and Thuja to aid us.

We would first disregard the acute attacks of hay fever and do the chronic case on the basis of the generals, first evaluating the symptoms – mentals stand highest. The most fundamental mentals are those having to do with the love of life, suicidal tendencies and disgust, and which are not present in our patient. You could never give him Aurum. Second among the mentals come the fears and phobias, the sycotic mentality. Our particular patient has had a rather recent sycosis and his fears are not many nor profound, but that trend of mind shows in his lack of confidence and compensatory conscientiousness. Next in importance after the fears come the reactions to the love life and sex matters. Ailments from emotions, such as mortification or anger, are lacking in this patient; after that are the marked traits of the ego such as jealousy and obstinacy, which in this case are also lacking. Last under the mentals would come certain desires and aversions, such as to company. The food aversions come under generals.

1) Lasciviousness, which I place first because it was his absorbing mental difficulty.
2) Conscientiousness.
3) Homosexuality.
4) Lack of confidence.
5) Desire to be magnetized.

Next come the generals. One must never forget the importance of suppression of diseases, discharges and eruptions, so let us put:

6) Suppressed gonorrhoea.

The fundamental general, and to our thinking, perhaps the only one to be used as an eliminating symptom, is the warm-bloodedness or chilliness of a patient. I do not include this in the list of rubrics for repertorizing because the number of remedies in it are so large, but you would never give a warm-blooded patient like this one Kali Carb. or Arsenicum Album. You might, however, give him borderline remedies on either side, such as Phosphorus or Sepia, which are chilly but only mildly so, and not always.

One of the most important generals when well marked is time – time of day, entirely absent in this case. Next after time come the general reactions to weather, heat and cold, dampness, open air, season and periodicity. Of these, his only marked one is:

7) Worse in damp weather, again a sycotic symptom.
8) Better from sleep, a very marked symptom in this case.
9) Frequent colds.

Next under generals come the aversions:

10) To milk, recently. (Recent changes in cravings and aversions are valuable remedy pointers.)
11) Craved fats always.
12) Averse to starches.

Let us take the hay fever, which is so chronic as to become an important general:

13) Hay fever.
14) Tendency to polypi. (These are not used here as a pathological entity but rather as showing the constitutional tendency.)
15) Train and car sick.

Numbering the remedies by degrees under these rubrics, 1, 2, 3, (3 being the large black type), we then total the numerical values of the fifteen symptoms for any given remedy, making that total a numerator of a fraction, the denominator of which is the number of symptoms under which that remedy appears in any degree, i.e., Calc. Carb. 19/9. We then choose the four or five highest remedies. In this instance there are seven which come fairly close together, as follows:

Calc. Carb. 19/9
Silica 19/8
Phosphorus 17/9
Pulsatilla 16/9
Sulphur 14/9
Nux Vomica 14/8
Sepia 14/6

Calc. Carb. is first, Silica second, and Phosphorus third in the generals, numerically. Actually Phosphorus is much more similar to our patient.

In a case with generals as full as this, we really do not need the particulars, but for completeness will put them in as follows:

1) Abdominal cramps from cold milk.
2) Styes.
3) Greasy face.
4) Falling hair.
5) Fissured tongue.

The particulars repertorize as follows:

Sulphur 8/3
Phosphorus 7/3
Sepia 6/2
Pulsatilla 6/3
Calc. Carb. 5/3
Nux Vomica 3/2

In the particulars Sulphur leads, Phosphorus is second, and Calc. Carb. only fifth. We then add the generals and particulars as follows:

Calc. Carb. 24/12
Phosphorus 24/12
Silica 24/10
Pulsatilla 22/12
Sulphur 22/12
Sepia 22/12
Nux Vomica 17/20

Calc. Carb. and Phosphorus are tied for first place. It will be noted that some of the leading symptoms are not present in this case, for example the craving for salt and aggravation from thunderstorm of Phosphorus, the scalp perspiration, glandular involvement and obstinacy of Calc. Carb. So much for the chronic constitutional remedy.

An acute remedy should be selected for the attacks of hay fever, since in a singer they cannot be permitted to run their course.

We have the advantage over the competitors in that we have the clinical results of the treatment of this case. Being a novice at the time, I gave this patient Phosphorus 10M, after which he promptly went into acute tuberculosis with fine apical râles, cloudy left apex on chest X-ray, night sweats, loss of weight and lassitude. Needless to say, the doctor was worried. Of course the remedy could have been antidoted, but with a sharp reaction even that may be dangerous. But if the patient's vitality would 'stand the gaff', and the environment were made favourable, the very fact of an aggravation will ensure a marked improvement. I arranged for my patient to go to the mountains for six weeks complete rest, with no medication of any kind. The symptoms subsided in two or three weeks, and on his return the chest X-ray was practically normal. X-rays, chest and sputum examinations every six months since then have been entirely negative.

About five months after the initial aggravation I ventured Phosphorus 30x; one month later Phosphorus 200c; two months later another Phosphorus 200c; and four months after that, Phosphorus 1M. The improvement during this time was steady without aggravation in each instance, until a week or ten days before the administration of the new dose. He has since had Silica and now Sulphur at long intervals.

The acute remedy chosen for the hay fever was Natrum Mur. 200c, three doses one hour apart, which cut the attacks short in two days. After two of these attacks, thus aborted, he has had no further hay fever during the two subsequent summers, for the first time in twenty-four years.

Two of our veteran homoeopaths were discussing this case. One said offhand, 'Give Calc. Carb.', and the other advised Phosphorus as the chronic and Allium Cepa as the acute. This is quite reasonable, since Phosphorus often follows Allium Cepa.

Case 1 – Kent's Method of Repertorizing

A good example of the working of an orderly mind is this discussion of Case 1, in which Dr Hubbard demonstrates her approach to a difficult case, displaying her passion for thoroughness. This case has been used as an example of the potential danger of improper prescribing of high potency homoeopathic medicines. Her handling of the severe aggravation is of special interest.—Ed.

Mr E. W., aged 60, complains of burning heat in the right thigh, which seems to be located in the skin, and which, during the past fifteen years, has spread to the right arm and hand and foot. It is present during sleep as well as in the daytime. There is an almost complete paralysis of his entire right side. He is slow and deliberate in his speech, of good intellect and in good spirits, although not a little suspicious, especially so of all doctors.

Some fifteen years ago he developed a series of ulcers on the groin, from one of which a sequestrum of bone discharged. He treated himself by a home remedy of chewed lead, which he prepared himself. Eighteen years ago he had typhoid but remembers no other disease. He denies venereal infection. He has no children and has been separated from his wife for more than ten years. He has a lack of facial expression but no Argyll pupil or Romberg, although the reflexes in the right extremities are lacking. He cannot repeat the words 'Methodist', 'Episcopal', etc. There is very little atrophy of the muscles, although his strength on this side is gone. He has to eat with his left hand, and has a shuffling gait.

DISCUSSION

It is said that more than half the battle in any cure is a case well taken. We all know that the cases with few outstanding or characteristic symptoms (except pathological changes) are difficult to treat and of bad prognosis, and usually show a profound miasmatic disturbance. This case is so incomplete as to be impossible of a satisfactory solution. It may be that the individual actually shows no other symptoms and could give no more, but we should like to have a check-up, especially on the following:

Other mentals, such as suicidal tendencies in the past, fears, whether the cheerfulness was euphoric or grandiose or merely normal, whether the suspicion was paranoid in trend or only the result of unfortunate experiences with physicians, and so on.

The general type of the patient, which is not mentioned, and many other little objective points such as tongue, ears, warts, moles, condition of nails, colour and character of discharges, if any; condition of the external glandular system, type of build, skin quality, warm-blooded or cold-blooded type, sweat in general, and sweat of affected parts in particular; sleep, conditions of aggravation and amelioration, time of aggravation, such as after sleep, morning, night, etc. The case as given presents no individual picture that might make the patient either a living entity or a drug entity to the physician. There is a conspicuous absence of Generals, no mention being made of reactions to wet weather or dry, heat or cold, position or motion, or to any of the desires or aversions in food.

Even from a general medical point of view the case is incomplete. One would like to know whether the groin ulcers followed buboes, whether at any time there was a urethral discharge whose venereal character was either unknown or unadmitted. This might be revealed by discovering what kind of treatment he had ever received. No mention is made of Wassermann tests or Neisserian smears. One would like to know the cause of the paralysis. From the brief description given little hint can be gained, but it makes an enormous difference in the choice of the remedy whether the paralysis is from a blood clot in the brain due to cerebral haemorrhage, or to a possible lead poisoning with resulting degeneration of nerve tissue, or to a luetic lesion in the cerebrospinal mechanism. Under the paralysis, is it progressive, as it would be if of syphilitic or lead origin, or is it stationary or retrogressive, as would be more likely in apoplexy?

The only really characteristic symptom in the whole case is the sensation of heat in the paralyzed part, although, being a particular, this should not be placed first. A careful inquiry is needed as to whether other symptoms throughout the life have been right-sided. We would call attention to the fact that the lesion in the brain, if any, is left-sided. Right-sided paralysis alone is not sufficient to give great weight to right-sidedness as a general symptom, although in so barren a case one clutches at straws.

The question of suppression of the ulcers, which may well have led to the paralysis, should be stressed. A check up of symptoms for lead poisoning, both in the gums, good and paralyzed side, should be gone into. No mention is made of trembling, formication or numbness.

In any case where there is a paucity of available symptoms it is important to get as clear a picture as possible of the childhood, whether fat or thin, rickety, amiable, with a tendency to glandular troubles, suppression of eruptions, foot sweat or discharges, susceptibility to frequent colds. In other words, the type of the child prior to any possible venereal, pharmacological or suppressive complications.

CHOICE OF RUBRICS

(Page numbers refer to the 4th Edition. — Ed.)

1) My first would be *Generalities, syphilis*, p. 1406. 'Generalities, gonorrhoea suppressed' is tempting in view of the history of ulcers in the groin but is not justified without further data.

2) *Generalities, ulcers, glands*, p. 1410, combined with

3) *Skin, ulcers*, p. 1333. We must get a clear description of the ulcers to make this a valuable symptom. It is vital to the case. Bleeding, itching, burning, lardaceous, bad odour, colour of discharge from, punched-out edges. Without these particulars we must use the two rubrics above, combined.

4) *Suspicious*, p. 85.

5) The only other mental given is *Speech, slow*, p. 82, which we use, lacking others.

6) *Paralysis, one-sided*, p. 1390.

7) *Paralysis, one-sided, right*, p. 1390.

8) *Extremities, pain, burning, right thigh*, p. 1095.

9) *Skin burning*, in general to cover other parts showing this symptom, p. 1303.

10) *Paralysis, heat in part*, p. 1390.

11) *Bone necrosis*, p. 1375, *Caries, bone*, p. 1346.

The following remedies come through, the numerator of the fraction indicating the numerical value of the remedy and the denominator the number of rubrics in which it appears.

Case 1 – Kent's Method of Repertorizing

Phosphorus...... 23/10	Belladonna........18/8	Mezereum.........12/7
Merc. Sol. 19/9	Phosphoric Ac....14/8	Natrum Carb. 10/7
Rhus Tox. 16/9	Thuja 12/8	Plumbum 9/7
Ars. Alb. 22/8	Silica 18/7	Causticum 14/6
Lachesis.......... 19/8	Sulphur.............18/7	Opium 11/6

Remedies such as Belladonna and Rhus Tox. should be thrown out as they are not deep enough for this case. Lachesis can be thrown out because of the absence of the marked Lachesis personality, characterized by loquacity, aggravation after sleep, sense of constriction, extreme sensitiveness, marked suspicion. Phosphoric Ac., Thuja, Mezereum and Natrum Carb. do not present a similar picture. Plumbum appears in low degree in a large number of rubrics. As this remedy rarely comes through in repertory work, and as the patient chewed lead to cure his groin ulcers, it should be kept in the back of the mind. Plumbum has marked trembling and is subject to gastrointestinal disturbances. Sight unseen, we should say it does not fit the case. Causticum and Opium should also be kept in the back of the mind. This reduces our list of remedies to five:

Phosphorus 23/10	Ars. Alb. 22/8
Merc. Sol.......... 19/9	Silica 18/7
Sulphur............ 18/7	

The patient should be gone over again with these remedies in the foreground and Plumbum, Causticum and Opium in the background. Each of the five is a searching miasmatic remedy, and careful observation should enable a fairly certain choice among the five. Without further data it is impossible to prescribe accurately.

I had a case very similar to this one. Owing to the paucity of symptoms I gave one dose of Sulphur 30c as the opening remedy, with the result of a return of a previous suppurating discharge and the slow but steady amelioration of the paralytic symptoms. It must never be forgotten that when in doubt, and when Sulphur stands among the first five, it is a good opening remedy to develop symptoms and bring the case into order.

Case 2 – Kent's Method of Repertorizing

Mrs L. P., aged 50, married. No children, never pregnant. Complains of a soreness over the region of the liver, a burning, referred to the right scapular region and thence downward. Frequent headaches, preceded by blindness of the right eye, with nausea but no vomiting. Has no modalities. Is an aspirin fiend. Generally she feels better lying down. Most of her attacks begin in the morning. She has a sweetish taste in her mouth. She is fair and stout, has many gold teeth and a chronic naso-pharyngeal catarrh. She may be said to be of the lymphatic constitution. Her bowels are regular but there is a frequency of urination. Some years ago she was subject to eczema. She is sore to touch in the region of the gallbladder and clothes annoy her there. She is better in the open air. Has periodic nosebleeds. Ten years ago she was operated upon for polypi of the nose. On several occasions she has had a cessation of menses which returned after some months with a severe uterine haemorrhage. Examination of the uterus shows it to be large and boggy, adnexae normal. There is a small red teat in the cervical orifice. She was advised against operation and a remedy was given. This produced a haemorrhage of dark, watery fluid from the uterus, and old stagnant blood. The teat from the cervix proved to be a polypus. She remains well to date.

DISCUSSION

From a diagnostic point of view this case is prettily given. From the description of the patient I should judge that marked mental symptoms are lacking, but I should like to hear about timidity, absorption in details, and so on. Only a couple of vague generals are mentioned. Surely more must be obtainable, particularly in the realm of cravings and aversions in foods, menses, sleep, etc. Modalities as to pressure, motion, sides easiest to lie on, relief from hot or cold drink or food or applications, and similar modalities as to the headache are really needed, as well as amplification of the morning aggravation symptom. However, despite these omissions in the case history one can prescribe with fair certainty on the few symptoms given.

As to 'Generals', to my understanding, worse in the morning applies only to the attacks. Better in the open air is vague, and better lying down I take to apply to the attacks rather than to the woman at all times; but if it did apply to her it could be easily explained by the abnormal pelvic condition. In this case as given I prefer to start with some of the things of which we are *sure*. So we have taken the following symptom rubrics:

1) A combination of the four following:
   a) Abdomen, pain, hypochondria, right, p. 563.
   b) Abdomen, pain, burning, the general rubric, p. 572.
   c) Abdomen, pain, sore hypochondria, right, p. 590.
   d) Abdomen, pain, sore, liver in, p. 591.
2) As modalities of the above I have taken:
   a) Abdomen, pain, sore, morning in, p. 589.
   b) Abdomen, pain, sore, clothing aggravates, p. 589.
   c) Abdomen, pain, hypochondria extending to back, p. 563.
   d) Back, pain, sore, dorsal region, scapulae, extending downward, p. 933.
3) Polypus in nose, p. 349. Combined with polypus in womb, p. 743.
4) Sweet taste in the mouth, p. 426.
5) Eczema, p. 1312.
6) Chronic nasal catarrh, p. 324.
7) Epistaxis, p. 335.

Polypi is a general of the patient. The tendency to produce any kind of pathology in different organs is an important general, whether it be warts, wens, polypi, fibroids or whatnot.

As I interpret the case, the frequent headaches are not concomitants of the abdominal pain. The headache, which is so characteristic, should be treated acutely in and for itself. As described, it is typical of Kali Bich., the only other remedy given in the repertory in headache preceded by blindness being Sarsaparilla, although Iris is to be compared. The temperament of the patient as given and the 'chronic catarrhal' would incline me to the use of Kali Bich. for the acute headache attacks, although further study of the location, modalities and quality of this head pain itself would be imperative.

The sweet taste in the mouth may be only a symptom characteristic of the abdominal attacks, or it may be a symptom of the patient herself. If it is the latter, it should be included as a particular of the patient.

The frequency of urination I take to be a result of the pelvic pathology, and so do not use it.

Then the remedy finally chosen should have power over eczema, but details are essential to a proper decision. The most revealing symptoms of this particular case are pathological, as follows: tendency to polypi, periodic nosebleeds, chronic catarrh, old eczema. It is a good illustration of how pathological findings do influence our choice of a chronic remedy. As given, this case is a good object lesson that it is easier to repertorize a case which is mainly pathological in common symptoms by the Boenninghausen method than by the Kent method. It also particularly illustrates the necessity of combining rubrics in the Kent, and shows that the Kent method, when properly handled, can find the remedy in a case poorly taken and full of pathology.

On repertorizing, the acute attack is clearly Chelidonium, and this remedy ranks fifth for the whole patient. In chronics the chief remedies rank as follows:

Lycopodium
Calcarea Carbonica (a very close second)
Sepia
Phosphorus
Chelidonium

The description of the type of the patient is clearly Calc. Carb. Lycopodium is not blonde, stout and lymphatic, but is dark, thin, irritable and haughty. Sepia is also the swarthy personality and not lymphatic, and would probably have much more marked mentals. Phosphorus is a different personality.

We should give this patient Calc. Carb. as a chronic remedy with confidence. Remember that Calc. Carb. also has marked power over acute gallbladder attacks in Calc. Carb. personalities.

Further Case Studies

A five-year-old boy is upsetting his parents by screaming, crying tantrums. Nothing is right. He is usually an amiable and gentle child. He is not teething. No fever, not apparently ill. Not thirsty, though he will drink sour fruit juice. He twitches in his sleep. His face is red in blotches. He has apparently no other symptom until he finally and shyly says that he sees a 'funny man' in his room at night. He does not ask for a nightlight, nor appear afraid of the man as you would expect him to be. Prescription: Belladonna 10M, one dose. The mother telephoned the next day to report that peace had descended and the boy is his usual serene self.

Arthritic woman of over 70, healthy, with an absurd and overpowering fear of apoplexy. Is usually a poised and sensible person. Has a stiff leg following an old injury. No other symptoms except that she feels her head will burst at night. Kent 'Mind, Fear, Apoplexy of' page 43 gives Argentum Met., Asterias Rub., Coffea, Ferrum Met. Under 'Apoplexy, night, at, with feeling as if head would burst', Asterias Rub., the only remedy.

The patient was given Asterias Rubens 200c, the red starfish, which has the collateral interesting symptom 'Muscles refuse to obey the will' (Boericke, page 95). Her undue fears were completely banished by the starfish. This is a dangerous as well as an unusual example, in that the prescription was based mainly on the *one* symptom.

Woman of 52 has had, as she called it, a 'life history' of earaches and headaches since age 10. She had been seen only once before by me, at which time she complained of a foul rotten-egg odour to her stools and declared that she smelt badly to herself, although no one else could detect her body odour. She was chilly and worried. Prescription: Psorinum 15c, one dose. Her right ear discharged the next day and she felt marvellous in herself. But in a couple of days she returned complaining of her old headache pattern, giving the following symptoms: pain like a knife in the vertex on coughing (Kent, page 172 'Head, pain, vertex, coughing on' – Alumina, Anacardium, Apis, Causticum,

Conium, Cuprum, Kali Carb., Sabadilla, Squilla, Sulphur.). She had severe pain in the left temple on coughing (Kent, page 170 'Head, pain, temple, on coughing' – Alumina, Causticum, Kali Carb., Sulphur.).

She also asked me if there was any objection to her eating a great deal of starch, as she was (most unusually) longing for it (Kent, page 486 'Stomach, desires, starch' – Alumina.).

Who would ever think of a dose of Alumina for such a violent headache, which she claimed had been untouched in the past by the usual pain-killers as well as by low potencies of Spigelia? After the Alumina she was completely free from pain for ten hours. In two days it began faintly to return. Three more doses, and no headaches since.

Man of 49 years has a violent pain in right shoulder. He is astonished because although he has no particular cough, sputum suddenly flies forcibly out of his mouth. When told that no stool will stand without at least three legs, he finally said that when he coughed there was a sore spot under the sternum. Kent to the rescue: page 1052 – under 'Extremities – pain, shoulder, right', and Kent – page 862, 'Chest, pain, sore, sternum under, coughing on' – only one remedy appears in both these rubrics; Kent, page 815 – 'Expectoration flies forcibly from mouth' has only three remedies: Badiaga, Kali Carb. and Chelidonium, of which Chelidonium is the only one which appears in both the other symptoms. Chelidonium 10M, one dose was given. Two weeks later the patient says the bursitis pain had completely gone in twenty-four hours, and that he has been continuing his heavy work with no recurrence of symptoms. The sternum pain and forcible expectoration are gone.

Boy of 5 with a violent cough.
Angry when consoled, Kent p. 2: Arsenicum Alb., Chamomilla, Natrum Mur.
Cough, better standing, Kent p. 806: Mag. Sulph.
Cough, better erect, Kent p. 806: Natrum Mur., Stannum.
Cough, worse lying on the back, Kent p. 797: Ammonium Mur. Arsenicum Alb., Natrum Mur., Nux Vomica, Phosphorus, Sepia
Expectoration green in the morning, Kent p. 816: Ferrum, Lycopodium, Natrum Mur., Nitric Ac., Psorinum, Silica, Stannum.

Natrum Mur. – an unexpected remedy for cough – came through clearly, and cured in short order.

Rubrics in Boenninghausen
Not to be Found in Kent

Elizabeth Wright Hubbard seemed to possess a remarkable capacity for detailed work. In addition to several published studies, in which she collaborated with other homoeopathic physicians in compiling and analyzing consecutive cases, she prepared lists such as the following material from Boenninghausen, and the valuable 'Index to Remedies in Kent's *Materia Medica*', also reproduced here. — Ed.

To the Kentian Clan and Boenninghausen Band, Greetings and News! The Mouse may help the Lion. In Boenninghausen's 482 small pages are 335 rubrics which are not to be found in Kent's 1423 large pages.

The homoeopathic student is taught both methods of repertorization – by Kent and by Boenninghausen – and is warned not to mix the methods, not only because the remedy grading is different, but because the ideology is so disparate. These repertories, like most of life, are full of paradoxes. The Kent repertory claims to be based on generals and yet is a maze of particulars; Boenninghausen's is very factual and classified: every symptom that refers to a part may be predicated of the whole. The interrelationship of symptoms and of remedies and the sequence of remedies are brought out. It opens a way into the wide fields of combinations. For Boenninghausen, the totality is made up of the general characteristics of the particular symptoms plus the condition, under the four general categories of locality, sensation, modality (aggravations or ameliorations) and concomitants. Roberts in his brilliant *Principles and Practicability of Boenninghausen's Therapeutic Pocket Book* says it is based on the doctrine of concomitants, a concomitant being an attendant circumstance existing or occurring with other symptoms, having always a relation in *time*. The concomitant is the differentiating factor. Hahnemann says that 'the *characteristic* symptoms represent that which is *curable* in each case of disease'; in other words, the common symptoms of the diagnosis do not point the way to cure. Boeninghausen called chronic symptoms *concomitants in acute ailments* and often prescribed exclusively on them, although it should be possible to find a remedy covering both acute and chronic.

The Boenninghausen method shines in cases without many mental symptoms; without rare, strange and peculiar symptoms; with few particulars; in cases where modalities predominate and concomitants are marked; cases showing pathological symptoms and objective symptoms. Roberts used to say that it was as good as *Sensations As If*, though in *larger* terms.

Some of the features of Boenninghausen are unique, such as the use of sides of the body throughout; rubrics of *troubles associated with* stool, urination, etc.; *accompanying symptoms of* nose, leucorrhoea, respiration, cough, menses, stool, fever, etc.; sleep and waking; and *aggravations and ameliorations before, during and after* cough; vertigo, fever, menses, stool, urine, sleep, sweat, and so forth.

The last section on Relationships of Remedies, pages 322 to 482, is the most difficult for the novice and the most unusual part of the book, but discussion of it is outside the scope of this book.

The whole repertory is built on generals, yet there is no section for Generals, as there is in Kent, and certain *general* rubrics are interspersed, with quite hilarious, unintentional humour. For instance: under Aggravations is the rubric for Children, and that for Women (What is worse for Women? or Women are worse for what? or are the remedies worse for the Women?).

There are a few 'Ameliorated by' rubrics in Kent, but there are 58 in Boenninghausen which are not in Kent.

Certain symptoms crop up frequently in case-taking which are baffling or impossible to find in Kent, except by combining rubrics or taking the nearest, but not the exact, symptom. Boenninghausen uses common sense rubrics, such as 'Falling asleep late', 'Can't get to sleep again after waking', 'Becomes chilled easily'. Rubrics of anatomical parts – often obscure ones – such as Loins, Groins, Perineum, Inner Gum, Tendo Achilles, Nape and the elusive Antrum are to be easily found alphabetically.

Among the gems are the rubrics on the *moon* phases which are not in the 5th Edition of Kent; the *wind* rubrics, the 'blondes and brunettes', the pregnancy rubric and the puerperal state, and such a frequent complaint as sebaceous cysts.

Although Boenninghausen only has 342 remedies against Kent's 591, it often has a much larger rubric than the Kent. On the other hand, it has none of the enormous and useless rubrics such as unmodified 'Vomiting'.

Even if you never repertorize by the full Boenninghausen method, you can save yourself much time and trouble with specific rubrics for short-cutting in office or bedside work by the use of these unusual sections.

Rubrics in Boenninghausen Not to be Found in Kent

When a remedy does not appear in certain definite rubrics in Kent, check the equivalent one in Boenninghausen; you may find it there. Let us use the best of *both* methods in arriving at the simillimum.

Repertorizing An Imperfectly Taken Case

Girl, aged 3 years. Parents claim that ever since vaccination at the third month of life she has had this trouble: eruptions which began on the head and behind the ears, spreading over the entire body with local treatment. The eruption was first discrete, then confluent, oozing, scaly, watery fluid, yellow; very itchy, and after scratching becomes pussy and crusts over with raw flesh beneath. The child is fair, chubby and has blue eyes. She develops asthma each time local treatment is tried. Her nose runs constantly and the head is always stuffed; she breathes through the nose. The cervical glands are enlarged.

This is an example of imperfect case-taking. There must be any number of possible symptoms to be found in this child. Even those that are mentioned are not given fully; for instance, the odour of the oozing, and whether or not sticky or gluey as well as watery. No description is given of the modalities of the asthma, although since it is secondary to suppression it is not as important as though it were a primary symptom. Further description of the coryza is lacking. The symptom of cervical glands may be merely a resultant of the scalp infection, or it may be characteristic of the child.

This case exemplifies the fact that a case poorly taken from the homoeopathic standpoint is difficult to repertorize by the Kent method and easier by the Boenninghausen. It further demonstrates the fact that one must combine rubrics.

For lack of Mentals and Generals the case must be repertorized on the eruption itself and the concomitant nose symptoms. For rubrics we have taken:
1) Bad effects from vaccination
2) Head eczema in general, the large rubric
   (a) Head, eruptions, crusty
   (b) Head, eruptions, moist
   (c) Head, eruptions, yellow

The four head rubrics are combined into one:
3) Ears, eczema behind

4) Eczema in general, under skin
  (a) Skin, eruptions, crusty
  (b) Skin, eruptions, moist
  (c) Skin, eruptions, yellow
5) Skin, eruptions suppressed
6) Nose, sense of obstruction combined with
7) Nose, discharge copious with stuffiness
8) Nose, discharge fluent and watery

Numerically the remedies repertorize out in the following order:

1. Sulphur	7. Petroleum	13. Calc. Sulph.
2. Graphites	8. Mezereum	14. Causticum
3. Silica	9. Lycopodium	15. Hepar Sulph.
4. Arsenicum Alb.	10. Natrum Mur.	16. Mercurius
5. Calc. Carb.	11. Kali Sulph.	17. Viola Tricolor
6. Psorinum	12. Staphysagria	

Out of these seventeen the first twelve were considered, and Viola Tricolor was studied because it is an unusual remedy to come out so high. Whatever remedy we choose for this case must be one that can cope with bad effects of vaccination, and it must be both psoric and sycotic.

It is criminal to give a case of this kind leaving out any symptoms of perspiration, and not telling us whether the child is chilly or warm-blooded, its disposition, its fears, etc. For instance, sight unseen, we incline to give this child Silica, which would be the remedy if there had been offensive sweat of the feet, brow perspiration, mildness, timidity, fear of thunderstorms, etc. If on the other hand the child is hungry an hour before lunch, averse to milk, craving sweets, always warm with burning feet, averse to washing, not the angel child type, it may be that Sulphur would be a better choice. If Arsenicum is the remedy the child will be restless, frightened, chilly, liable to aggravations at one or two o'clock, day or night, an orderly, fastidious type with no messy sweat. The Calcarea child has sour sweat, is rickety and obstinate. Natrum Mur. is late walking, although not rickety, and craves salt. The description of the child as given does not sound like the Natrum Mur. type.

As far as type is concerned, Kali Sulph. is typical of this child. Psorinum stands unusually high for it and the child is obviously very psoric, but Psorinum does not have bad effects from vaccination and is odorous, messy and very chilly. If the child contains its anger, suffers from keeping things in and tends to eye troubles, we would think of Staphysagria.

Kali Sulph. and Viola Tricolor rank high, and are unusual remedies to come so high. They should be considered because of this fact, for Viola, especially, rarely ranks so high.

In judging remedies after repertorizing, one may be justified in choosing any remedy among the first five, even the fifth, if it seems to best fit the case in question.

We repeat, sight unseen, that we incline to Silica.

Index to Remedies in Kent's Materia Medica (Third Edition)

Elizabeth Wright Hubbard seemed to find time for endless detailed sorting and classifying of homoeopathic information. Many of her articles were co-authored by other physicians, and much useful material was made available to the profession in this way. One of her works, undertaken apparently alone, is offered here not only as an example of her painstaking labour, but for the use of the prescriber as well. — Ed.

The Numbers in Parentheses Give the Main Reference.

ABIES NIGRA 762.
ABROTANUM (17-18) 34, 570, 624, 824, 906.
ACETICUM ACIDUM (18-19) 850.
ACONITUM NAPELLUS (19-32) 55, 60, 62, 103, 131, 144, 161, 162, 218, 250, 256, 257, 260, 273, 282, 341, 345, 403, 508, 509, 533, 538, 576, 624, 700, 733, 850, 852, 904, 925, 928, 940, 941, 943, 961.
ACTÆA RACEMOSA (BLACK COHOSH, see CIMICIFUGA).
ÆSCULUS HIPPOCOSTANUM (37-42) 60, 72, 240, 374, 413, 826, 903.
ÆTHIOPS ANTIMONIALIS (BLACK ANTIMONY) 107.
ÆTHUSA CYNAPIUM (42-44) 808, 896.
AGARICUS MUSCARIUS (44-51) 41, 125, 755, 774, 898.
AGNUS CASTUS (51-52).
AILANTHUS GLANDULOSA (52-56).
ALLIUM CEPA (CEPA) (56-60) 479, 760, 822, 856.
ALOE SOCOTRINA (60-64) 47, 379, 583, 762, 806, 809, 814.
ALUMEN (64-69) 69, 75, 77, 128, 133, 152, 318, 875, 897.
ALUMINA (69-82) 64, 69, 128, 135, 223, 333, 438, 630, 687, 735, 752, 757, 804, 813, 814, 875, 897, 907.
ALUMINUM METALLICUM 69, 72.
AMBRA GRISEA (82-88) 178.
AMMONIACUM GUMMI 104, 202.
AMMONIUM CARBONICUM (88-93) 94, 331, 650, 826.
AMMONIUM MURIATICUM (93-95).
ANACARDIUM ORIENTALE (95-97) 415, 454, 855, 963.
ANAGALLIS ARVENSIS 454, 455.
ANCISTRODON CONTORTRIX (COPPERHEAD, see CENCHRIS CONTORTRIX).
ANTHRACINUM 450, 832.
ANTIMONIUM CRUDUM (97-102) 104, 105, 106, 107, 237, 331, 413, 661, 672, 791, 900.
ANTIMONIUM TARTARICUM (102-108) 68, 92, 122 (Tartar emetic). 130, 288, 331, 575 (Tartar emetic), 666, 814, 878, 879, 900, 907 (Tartar emetic).
APIS MELLIFICA (108-116) 45, 116, 117, 118, 119, 120, 232, 260, 440, 445, 532, 582, 651, 657, 696, 697, 752, 767, 807, 809, 914, 935, 940, 980.

81

Repertory

APOCYNUM CANNABINUM (116-122).
ARGENTUM METALLICUM (122-130) 79, 80, 96, 682, 685, 755, 875.
ARGENTUM NITRICUM (131-138) 48, 124, 125, 248, 511, 541, 542, 703, 735, 752, 753, 758, 851, 852, 971.
ARNICA MONTANA (138-144) 32, 152, 171, 257, 280, 373, 450, 474, 555, 556, 557, 558, 651, 652, 681, 763, 773, 814, 831, 845, 850, 853, 880, 905.
ARSENICUM ALBUM (144-163) 40, 46, 74, 75, 92, 98, 100, 105, 119, 135, 140, 141, 163, 164, 171, 190, 199, 222, 259, 267, 287, 288, 289, 301, 313, 314, 330, 331, 336, 340, 406, 413, 440, 450, 475, 477, 480, 481, 487, 488, 529, 567, 568, 574, 587, 596, 671, 675, 677, 681, 688, 700, 701, 713, 714, 726, 753, 755, 782, 785, 822, 823, 826, 828, 832, 850, 856, 864, 865, 867, 871, 872, 879, 880, 886, 890, 894, 902, 904, 905, 929, 930, 935, 943, 947, 954, 958, 959, 961, 976.
ARSENICUM IODATUM (163-169) 823.
ARUM TRIPHYLLUM (169-173) 56, 221, 232, 265.
ASAFŒTIDA (174-178) 540, 711, 915.
ASARUM EUROPÆUM 630.
ATROPINUM 602.
AURUM METALLICUM (178-186) 17, 96, 174, 176, 188, 301, 464, 487, 532, 533, 564, 624.
AURUM MURIATICUM (186-190) 176.
AURUM MURIATICUM NATRONATUM 344, 753.
BACILLINUM 970, 971.
BADIAGA 133.
BAPTISIA TINCTORIA (190-195) 52, 55, 221, 232, 265, 450, 681, 814, 831, 832.
BARYTA CARBONICA (195-205) 65, 75, 274, 315, 316, 318, 893, 896, 897, 979.
BARYTA IODATA 200, 305.
BARYTA MURIATICA (205-209) 201, 202.
BELLADONNA (209-234) 32, 55, 56, 62, 96, 103, 143, 144, 194, 203, 251, 255, 256, 257, 258, 259, 262, 282, 283, 284, 290, 291, 307, 308, 310, 342, 345, 354, 391, 393, 401, 403, 419, 428, 437, 440, 466, 472, 480, 508, 509, 519, 531, 549, 550, 551, 578, 593, 624, 647, 679, 685, 703, 733, 795, 809, 813, 815, 830, 852, 859, 896, 908, 909, 915, 916, 917, 935, 939, 940, 941, 980.
BELLIS PERENNIS 776.
BENZOICUM ACIDUM (235-239) 239, 240, 624.
BERBERIS VULGARIS (239-244) 898.
BORAX (245-250) 75, 196, 316, 413, 612, 661, 726, 727.
BROMIUM (250-256) 677, 828.
BRYONIA ALBA (256-273) 17, 30, 32, 62, 103, 113, 130, 143, 148, 171, 190, 213, 229, 230, 250, 287, 290, 291, 341, 391, 393, 431, 461, 471, 480, 482, 486, 489, 509, 510, 624, 701, 733, 759, 760, 761, 762, 795, 823, 828, 834, 849, 850, 864, 877, 878, 879, 880, 883, 908, 910, 941, 942, 943 980.
BUFO (BUFONES) (273-280).
CACTUS GRANDIFLORUS (280-286) 66, 510, 624, 664, 717, 908.
CADMIUM SULPHURATUM (287-289) 701.
CALADIUM SEGUINUM (289-293) 654.
CALCAREAS IN GENERAL 968.
CALCAREA ARSENICOSA (313-314).
CALCAREA CARBONICA (293-312) 45, 65, 82, 85, 119, 142, 156, 183, 196, 197, 202, 231, 234, 268, 313, 314, 316, 327, 338. 395, 412, 413, 477, 504, 506, 541, 543, 555, 556, 559, 614, 624, 632, 671, 675, 684, 710, 753, 762, 808, 809, 815, 849, 853, 888, 890, 893, 897, 898, 900, 913, 924, 925, 927, 930, 942, 967, 969, 971, 977, 979.
CALCAREA FLUORATA (CALCAREA FLUORICA) (315-316).

DULCAMARA (BITTER SWEET) (474-482) 32, 224, 308, 674, 683, 685, 697, 700, 828, 834, 930, 942.
ELAPS CORALLINUS 91, 449.
EUPATORIUM PERFOLIATUM (BONESET) (482-488) 171, 831.
EUPHRASIA OFFICINALIS (488-489) 57, 685, 822, 852, 856, 928, 981.
FERRUM METALLICUM (490-495) 40, 136, 161, 495, 496, 501, 545, 683, 828, 864, 865, 942.
FERRUM PHOSPHORICUM (495-501) 480.
FLUORICUM ACIDUM (502-508) 42, 48, 49, 699, 828, 831.
GAMBOGIA 583.
GELSEMIUM SEMPERVIRENS (508-513) 260, 486, 520, 563, 597, 892, 906, 907, 980.
GLONOINUM (513-519) 813.
GNAPHALIUM POLYCEPHALUM 852.
GRAPHITES (521-528) 64, 76, 77, 197, 203, 362, 458, 477, 671, 682, 684, 733, 755, 772, 773, 774, 775, 795, 863, 887, 898, 900, 962.
GRATIOLA OFFICINALIS (519-521) 319, 791.
GRINDELIA ROBUSTA 906.
GUAIACUM OFFICINALIS (528-530).
HAMAMELIS VIRGINICA 354, 868, 877.
HELLEBORUS NIGER (531-535) 564, 980.
HEPAR SULPHURIS CALCAREUM (535-544) 23, 28, 64, 135, 178, 184, 203, 216, 229, 324, 326, 341, 342, 567, 600, 601, 603, 622, 624, 673, 708, 710, 735, 737, 752, 795, 811, 813, 814, 820, 894, 902, 904, 906, 917, 945, 946.
HYDRASTIS CANADENSIS (544-546).
HYDROPHOBINUM (LYSSIN) 550, 917.
HYOSCYAMUS NIGER (546-555) 96, 335, 440, 564, 685, 916, 917.
HYPERICUM PERFOLIATUM (555-560) 142, 401, 651, 652.
IGNATIA AMARA (560-565) 36, 37, 86, 256, 258, 261, 403, 510, 711, 728, 730, 763, 886, 906, 907, 963, 975.
INULA HELENIUM 762.
IODINES IN GENERAL 823.
IODUM (IODIUM) (566-573) 163, 164, 507, 603, 657, 822, 823, 855, 904.
IPECACUANHA (573-579) 32, 103, 122, 144, 288, 345, 354, 411, 454, 471, 596, 700, 734, 860, 890.
JACARANDA CAROBA 701.
KALIS IN GENERAL 579, 580.
KALI ARSENICOSUM 128, 314, 521.
KALI BICHROMICUM (579-586) 61, 62, 339, 347, 423, 541, 631, 646, 666, 823, 878, 879, 887, 965.
KALI CARBONICUM (586-599) 39, 150, 203, 378, 579, 580, 683, 710, 759. 826. 886, 905, 948.
KALI IODATUM (KALI HYDRIODICUM) (600-604) 347, 566, 569, 582, 599. 657, 698, 710, 823, 962.
KALI NITRICUM 133.
KALI PHOSPHORICUM (604-613) 128, 314, 521, 540.
KALI SULPHURICUM (613-620) 104, 188, 905.
KALMIA LATIFOLIA (620-624) 17, 133, 904, 906, 908.
KREOSOTUM (625-628) 259, 638, 762, 913.
LAC CANINUM (629-632) 528.
LAC DEFLORATUM (632-637) 629.
LAC FELINUM 903.
LACHESIS (637-649) 47, 55, 56, 75, 90, 91, 139, 156, 175, 184, 223, 234, 254, 301, 359, 378, 425, 445, 447, 448, 449, 450, 470, 479, 518, 527, 541, 552, 582, 591, 629, 630, 632, 651, 654, 668, 684, 691, 699, 716, 717, 718, 772, 807, 817, 823, 848, 854, 867, 868, 878, 883, 885, 900, 903, 905, 906, 908, 924, 940, 963, 981.

Repertory

OLEANDER 814, 886.
ONOSMODIUM VIRGINIANUM 305, 797, 852.
OPHIDIANS IN GENERAL 450.
OPIUM (764-767) 21, 109, 138, 215, 347, 381, 403, 427, 429, 516, 667, 756, 761, 804, 815, 941.
ORIGANUM MARJORANA 319, 520.
OXALICUM ACIDUM (768-770) 661, 975.
PÆONIA 753, 827.
PARIS QUADRIFOLIA 452, 453.
PETROLEUM (771-775) 41, 49, 271, 299, 411, 455, 477, 753, 914, 979.
PETROSELINUM SATIVUM 965.
PHOSPHORICUM ACIDUM (788-793) 159, 291, 316, 420, 496, 498, 713, 714, 756, 856, 875, 907.
PHOSPHORUS (775-788) 40, 55, 56, 80, 114, 122, 133, 136, 151, 173, 188, 190, 200, 220, 229, 232, 255, 273, 288, 310, 311, 335, 341, 356, 423, 424, 450, 460, 470, 486, 493, 496, 498, 520, 526, 545, 560, 569, 576, 582, 589, 595, 624, 638, 664, 666, 669, 674, 675, 680, 682, 685, 687, 701, 703, 710, 759, 775, 792, 804, 837, 848, 852, 854, 861, 863, 866, 877, 879, 883, 884, 886, 900, 902, 903, 906, 907, 909, 924, 943, 979, 981.
PHYTOLACCA DECANDRA (793-796) 227, 854.
PICRICUM ACIDUM (796-798) 291, 505, 683.
PLATINUM METALLICUM (798-801) 133, 319, 403, 429, 520, 659, 684, 914.
PLUMBUM ACETICUM 804.
PLUMBUM METALLICUM (801-806) 68, 76, 77, 368, 454, 684, 712, 736, 800.
PODOPHYLLUM PELTATUM (806-809) 63, 152, 159, 406, 460, 791, 796, 976.
POTASSIUMS (see KALIS).
PSORINUM (809-815) 17, 32, 321, 481, 521, 650, 664, 684, 728, 757, 823, 861, 866, 892, 931, 940, 966.
PTELEA TRIFOLIATA 373, 677, 745.
PULSATILLA NIGRICANS (815-831) 17, 32, 35, 36, 37, 39, 40, 46, 49, 56, 58, 79, 115, 132, 174, 182, 188, 216, 218, 221, 260, 267, 310, 389, 417, 429, 466, 474, 489, 491, 502, 503, 504, 506, 519, 528, 564, 571, 597, 614, 615, 618, 624, 631, 632, 654, 655, 657, 659, 685, 761, 767, 850, 855, 858, 863, 866, 891, 892, 893, 895, 900, 907, 909, 910, 928, 942, 946, 963.
PYROGEN (831-834) 320, 450, 850, 879, 942.
RANUNCULUS BULBOSUS (834-837) 415.
RHODODENDRON CHRYSANTHUM (837-839) 685, 775, 899.
RHUS TOXICODENDRON (839-846) 17, 30, 80, 97, 140, 141, 142, 143, 171, 173, 190, 218, 233, 260, 267, 268, 316, 336, 379, 415, 416, 454, 455, 553, 555, 556, 558, 559, 574, 602, 603, 624, 674, 681, 685, 686, 700, 714, 733, 752, 774, 802, 803, 828, 831, 834, 849, 850, 851, 853, 854, 878, 892, 935, 962, 970, 972, 973, 979.
ROBINIA PSEUD-ACACIA 947.
RUMEX CRISPUS (846-850) 255, 879, 908.
RUTA GRAVEOLENS (851-854) 405, 557, 900, 902.
SABADILLA OFFICINARUM (854-858) 823.
SABINA (JUNIPERS SABINA) (858-862) 225, 466, 940.
SACCHARUM LACTIS 495.
SAMBUCUS NIGRA 903.
SANGUINARIA CANADENSIS (862-867) 237, 373, 884, 892, 908.
SANICULA AQUA 52.
SARSAPARILLA (867-870) 379, 504, 632.
SECALE CORNUTUM (870-873) 40, 122, 147, 158, 328, 335, 345, 354, 401, 407, 408, 450, 576, 650, 703, 830, 861, 867, 868, 976.

Index to Remedies in Kent's Materia Medica

SELENIUM (873-875) 291, 736, 792.
SENECIO AUREUS (Var. GRACILIS) (875-877) 863.
SENEGA (877-880) 202, 850.
SEPIA (880-890) 37, 49, 62, 334, 344, 347, 453, 454, 477, 484, 504, 505, 506, 510, 542, 596, 726, 728, 734, 762, 809, 813, 814, 827, 830, 854, 892, 900, 904, 905, 906, 907, 940, 962, 979.
SILICATES IN GENERAL 969.
SILICEA (SILICA) (890-900) 32, 52, 76, 218, 296, 299, 316, 339, 396, 503, 504, 506, 507, 537, 540, 541, 542, 543, 558, 614, 636, 662, 676, 678, 683, 685, 696, 699, 773, 775, 795, 811, 813, 823, 854, 863, 864, 880, 910, 915, 917, 926, 927, 966, 967, 969.
SINAPIS NIGRA 857.
SODIUMS (see NATRUMS).
SPIGELIA ANTHELMINTICA (900-903) 624.
SPONGIA TOSTA (903-906) 29, 133, 538, 878.
SQUILLA MARITIMA (SCILLA MARITIMA) (907-908).
STANNUM METALLICUM (908-911) 92, 130, 311, 875.
STAPHISAGRIA (DELPHINIUM STAPHISAGRIA) (911-915) 142, 178, 181, 261, 378, 504, 540, 555, 559, 601, 698, 753, 814, 905, 962.
STICTA PULMONARIA 823.
STRAMONIUM (DATURA STRAMONIUM) (915-918) 96, 210, 258, 440, 531, 549, 550, 667, 703, 907.
STRONTIUM CARBONICUM 560.
STRYCHNINUM 402.
SULPHUR (918-945) 23, 31, 32, 41, 46, 48, 55, 61, 62, 63, 64, 65, 67, 75, 76, 128, 156, 197, 205, 221, 240, 296, 304, 321, 325, 327, 341, 342, 390, 458, 470, 477, 504, 522, 529, 543, 583, 589, 596, 598, 599, 614, 658, 666, 667, 671, 672, 675, 682, 684, 685, 700, 728, 733, 737, 763, 764, 775, 781, 785, 809, 813, 814, 815, 817, 819, 849, 854, 861, 863, 864, 875, 880, 890, 892, 893, 897, 898, 900, 913, 917, 950, 951, 959, 966, 969, 970, 972, 979.
SULPHURICUM ACIDUM (945-949) 62, 247, 582, 920.
SYMPHORICARPUS RACEMOSA (596).
SYPHILINUM (949-954) 686, 966.
TABACUM 462, 582, 773.
TARENTULA CUBENSIS (TARANTULA CUBENSIS) 832, 850.
TARENTULA HISPANICA (TARANTULA HISPANICA) (954-959) 914.
TARTAR EMETIC cf. ANTOINON TARTARICUM.
TELLURIUM 287.
TEREBINTHINA 771.
THERIDION (959-961).
THUJA OCCIDENTALIS (961-965) 52, 79, 292, 396, 541, 558, 661, 706, 708, 736, 814, 855, 860, 898, 900, 907, 913, 914, 927, 928.
TUBERCULINUM BOVINUM (966-973) 50, 119, 201, 321, 529, 614, 675.
VALERIANA OFFICINALIS (973-975) 711.
VERATRUM ALBUM (975-978) 90, 144, 330, 459, 460, 554, 856, 906, 916.
VERATRUM VIRIDE 54.
VESPA VULGARIS 807.
WYETHIA HELENOIDES 835, 856.
ZINCUM METALLICUM (978-982) 18, 47, 76, 113, 216, 287, 461, 520, 534, 632, 732, 963.
ZINCUM PICRICUM 798.

REMEDIES

One of the most telling comments on Elizabeth Wright Hubbard came from Dr Arthur H. Grimmer in his discussion of one of her presentations: 'Dr Hubbard has a way of making homoeopathy seem so easy. You can see the remedy right there, and that is why we should picture our remedies as living entities of sick people.'

On another such occasion, Dr Grimmer, referring to the part on Intellectual Remedies said, 'I don't know how we can discuss this paper. It is perfect. It is a wonderful, brief, concise, clear-cut picture of the mental phase of our remedies, which we see almost every day in our practice. Yet, Dr Hubbard has brought that mental phase out so clearly and beautifully that there is nothing to discuss. All we can do is just admire and thank her for it.'

Sometimes the discussions were as interesting as the papers presented, and it is a temptation to share some of them with the reader. — Ed.

Garden Remedies

Once upon a time, in the peaceful town of Tübingen, there dwelt a seer, the Nestor of homoeopathy, a famous student of Paracelsus, and to him came a devoted novice from across the seas who begged to become apprenticed to him. Crowds who got off at the little railroad station divided into two streams, one for the University, and one for Dr Schlegel, to be healed. His home was half way up a hillside, with a porch overlooking a valley to far hills; and he fetched a great magnifying glass and led his novice out on to the sunny porch. Concentrating the sun's rays by the glass onto her hand until they burned, he said: 'If you will let what I teach you burn into your heart, I will take you for my student.' Then the old man led her up the hillside behind the house, and it was all a garden of herbs and plants that are used in homoeopathy.

Daphne mezereum was there, and *Berberis vulgaris*, blue *Squilla* and *Convallaria*. With each he made her acquainted as with a friend; *Daphne* for crusty eruptions and neuralgia, *Berberis* for urinary distresses and skin, *Squilla* for coughs and bladder weakness. Lily of the Valley for hearts. Through the weeks of work which followed, until he succumbed to the fibrillation which he termed his 'Heldenhexameter', his 'hero's rhythm', he fostered this deep intimate feeling for the plants of healing.

Recently I rejoiced anew in an American garden at seeing so many growing friends and tools, pointing out to my patient the stormy monkshood, purple *Aconite*; the stately delphinium, *Staphysagria*; delicate columbine, *Aquilegia*, tremulous, overwrought, sleepless; yellow broom or genester, *Baptisia*; the tiny English daisy, *Bellis perennis*, so trod upon, hence of use in the tumours from bruises; dainty *Clematis*, not yet blossoming, which the ancients used on beggars' ulcers; the gracious dogwood, *Cornus florida*, drowsy and frail, of help in malaria; the purple foxglove, *Digitalis*, just coming up; the lusty sun-flower, *Helianthus*, vulnerary like *Calendula*; the blazing star, *Helonias*, famed for its pruritis and backache; sturdy *Hydrangea*, of aid in gravel and kidney colic; *Iberis*, the bitter candytuft, a notable heart tonic; *Iris*, the blue flag, with its sour burning and eye migraines; mountain laurel, *Kalmia* of heart and rheumatic fame; even a stray burdock, *Lappa major*, for skin, styes and womb; tiger lily, vivid as its symptoms; *Lobelia*

89

with its vomiting and asthma; *Sabadilla* and *Salvia* with their night sweats; and in the rock garden *Sempervivum*, the modest house leek, of tongue ulcer and cancer fame.

Returning, we passed the fragrant *Valerian*, and *Vinca* the periwinkle, by *Viola odorata* and *Viola tricolor* in the shade of the house; and the evergreens, *Taxus* for gout and skin, *Thuja* and *Sabina*.

May this brief garden fantasy prompt each of you into remembrance and add zest to your zeal, that you may be mindful of healing in your summer hours.

The Intellectual Remedies

In the course of our friendship with our remedies, as with our acquaintances, we learn their qualities and who can be depended on for charm, for fun, and to do the work of the world. I would like to introduce to you the coterie of the intellectual remedies.

It would be difficult to select from any one thousand people the dozen or so noted for their qualities of mind, so I beg your clemency for the fragmentary group that I present here. They are selected, not with an eye to numbers, but from two viewpoints: first, the practical clinical one, on the basis of patients with unusual mental ability whose symptomatology had called for these remedies; and secondly, from a theoretical standpoint, by running through the mental pathogeneses of our frequently-used remedies. By mere chance I found twenty-five remedies which I should put pre-eminently in this class, and I want to offer just a highlight on their mental processes.

We seem fated always to begin with Aconite. Like *Genesis*, it is the beginning, and like the nature of the remedy what can be said of its intellect is strong and swift: brainy people, full of power and vigour, with a plethora of ideas, sudden in decision, swift and accurate in carrying out. Hypersensitive, yes, but in a robust way, capable of ecstasy and even of clairvoyance, but not in an effete form. Subject to fears and anguish, strong as their natures, and, strangely enough, with a dash of malice which in them is a spice rather than a habit.

Argentum Nitricum is next. This may surprise you, because we associate silver with failure of the intellect, but in this remedy there is an intellect to fail. This is the prototype of public performers, lecturers, flatulent mentally as well as physically, folk full of drive, hurried by the pressure of work and public contacts. They become apprehensive, fidgety, full of fear and anxiety. Strange conduct crops out as they urge themselves to more and more effort to compensate for their failing confidence, and they are nimble at devising queer reasons and excuses for their erratic mental processes; to use modern parlance, they rationalize par excellence.

Belladonna, has been intellectual from its childhood, these vigorous, plump, large-headed boys with a high I.Q. Here again the force shows itself in sudden violent complaints; the mind is so active and fertile that the irritation of illness drives it quickly into the realm of delirium and violence. Unexpected acts crop up, which in normal circumstances are piquant and refreshing, and which in mania may appear as biting, physical violence, boisterousness and destructiveness.

Next we come to one of the very few remedies of the people who carry on the world's work. We are speaking, of course, of our businessman, Bryonia. Rich and competent though he is, he fears poverty. He may be slow on the uptake, but how persistent he is; he can follow through with large projects – his obstinacy is an aid, his choleric disposition an added strength. The Bryonians are not negative, they are a bursting people, which their pains symbolize. They are better under pressure, in mind as in body. They are a mighty folk and can produce real end results in the world.

You may disagree with me about my next type, Calc. Phos. To be sure he is a slow starter, but he makes up for it. He begins with the trifling weakness of Calc. Carb., but he develops some of the brilliance of Phosphorus and in the end he approaches the mental range of Tuberculinum.

Intellectuality and insanity are relatives. Consider the beatific state of Cannabis Indica – its grandiose ideas, its wonderful theories, its thrilling and prolific mind, its enthusiasm to the point of exaltation and clairvoyance.

Coffea is a great worker. Its power to think and to debate are heightened; it has a super-sanity, its memory is phenomenal; it will quote you appositely from the poetry of any period. It labours incessantly for some great cause and then breaks down with insomnia, thinking of a thousand things in bed. Hypersensitive to noise, to joy, to the pain of its neuralgias.

You may not think of Fluoric Acid as intellectual, for in a way it is the gigolo of remedies, the male Sepia. But consider it in the trilogy of Silica, Pulsatilla and Fluoric Acid. It is the businessman, hungry for thought as well as for emotion, with a curious mildness like Pulsatilla, and a reticence commendable in one so emotional.

On Ignatia we need barely touch. We all know its over-educated refinement, too much cherished in mind and body, fed on Chopin instead of porridge, but capable in its changeable way of great things in the arts.

Consider the mental veracity of Iodine, the typical thyroid, zealous, restless, often literary, feeling that if it stopped its active brain it would go mad; at the same time over-careful, exigent, impulsive; a great driver of itself even more than of others.

Kali Carb. has a more complicated and intriguing mentality, witty, whimsical, sensitive to changes of mental atmosphere; also a ticklish proposition in spirit as in body, impossible on committees because of its touchiness, trying in the family, quarrelling with its bread and butter but ingenious and vastly capable.

Its relative Kali Phos., whom we usually meet in nervous prostration before prolonged sorrow drives it into indifference and sadness, is an interesting type, its competence shot with unexpected cruelty, contrariness and passions.

You have all suffered from the uplifters, the compensatory social workers who need Lachesis. Like Josephus in the Good Book, they never finish anything, but Oh, what they do begin! Brilliant in comprehension, always a lap ahead, their loquaciousness a form of alleviating discharge, self-conscious, conceited, jealous of prominence – what promoters they are. A brilliant group, they must fight to the end succumbing to their own temperaments.

What would the profession of the law or indeed the teaching ranks do without Lycopodium? Here from the outset the mind has been developed at the expense of the body; incompetence, dread of new or even of familiar roles, infinite procrastination coming from this sphere; indecision, misanthropy, the imperiousness of weakness, the personification of the inferiority complex, or as one of my patients once put it, of mental impotence.

Nitric Acid, with its deep lines of suffering, its sensitiveness, its vindictiveness and taciturnity, shows you its mental calibre less than the others, but it is there beneath the obstinacy, beneath the physical sufferings, a vivid brain.

Natrum Phos. has the solidity of Natrum Mur. with some of the scope of Phosphorus, abundant ideas but easily distractible, hurried, angry at trifles, discouraged, fretful.

Phosphorus, at its best, has perhaps more brains than any remedy. It is over-active, vehement and suffers from its own vehemence; excessive throughout, with a disorderly strength, it has the element of immodesty, a sort of mental exhibitionism which makes all its traits, both good and bad, show up to their full value. It also has ecstasies and clairvoyance, although these are of a more tenuous and Celtic type than those of Aconite. Train and restrain Phosphorus and it will go to any heights.

Another of the builders of our modern civilization is Nux Vomica – the certified public accountant, charged with detail of which he is a perfect master but which irritates him into fault-finding, vehemence and even spite. He must have an outlet from his sedentary and exacting occupation, he cannot bear reading or conversation; he takes to dissipation or lets out in spells of touchiness. He will kick the chair and rip off the button from irritable weakness; he has too many irons in the fire and they are always hot; he is harried by a thousand details until he is tortured and takes it out on the family. His mental peristalsis is reversed; he is full of perversity; he strains not only to vomit, to stool and to urination, but to forcing things his own way. He suffers and makes all about him suffer from mental tenesmus.

Staphysagria we think of in other spheres, but he is one of the cultivated gentlemen of the earth, controlling himself at any price, brooding over his chagrin, soured by his pent-up wrath, to the point where he has to let the bank handle his business because repression has fatigued him until he can no longer cope with it.

Of the exasperating prowess of Sulphur we need hardly speak; the scholar, the bookworm, the inventor, the great unwashed – ill-shaven, threadbare, with soiled collar, his room full of papers and books, his closet full of boxes, his mind full of metaphysics. The first time you meet him he is a genius, the next time a nuisance, and subsequently a pest.

Silica, with its neat, clean, orderly mind, with its firm yet delicate perceptions, has a mental fibre of which we need more – if only he had the confidence and the personality to impose his thought on the community.

Tuberculinum, the traveller, the great cosmopolite, ever in search of new people, new excitement, new ideas – the faddist, the consumer of cults.

Veratrum Album, the dowager, unkindly witty, loquacious, malicious, working destruction with rapier ability in the Women's Club, of which she is the president.

One less well known to you, perhaps, is Viola Odorata – thin, fair, mild, impressive-looking, with a marked increase of mental activity, over-intellectual and suppressed in emotions with her aversion to music, especially the violin.

And lastly, another of the brains of the outfit, Zincum, who vies with Nux Vomica for hard work, docile yet irascible, the keynotes to whose nature are oversensitivity and the inability to throw things off, either mentally or physically. The eruptions in the spirit of Zincum as well as in the skin cannot be thrown off, and its natural fidgetiness and activity are turned into a slow and desperate prostration.

Here you have them – some of them – the group whom it pays to cure; who, when they have received their remedies, are capable of doing great work in any field, as well as in the support of homoeopathy.

DISCUSSION

Dr G. B. Stearns: It is very interesting to try to classify these remedies. Iodotanin, Phosphoric Acid, Phosphorus, Silica, Lycopodium and Belladonna are all in one group. They all go together, and they apply to the same kind of people. Coffea, Iodine, the Kalis, Sulphur and Zinc are in another group. The others are scattered around.

Dr G. Royal: I want to add a little bit to her Kali Phos., for two reasons. First, because I proved it upon myself thoroughly in different potencies; secondly, because I have used it a great deal and I know it is one of the best of our mental friends in the materia medica.

There is an expression that rules all through the remedy covered by the word 'tired'. You will also find it under the expression 'brain fag'. It applies to the brain especially. It does not make much difference what the cause is – the makeup, as far as the neurotic individual is concerned, is excellent. But how or what produces the tired feeling or the brain fag is of a great deal of importance. For instance, it may have been a busy day and a large number of patients have come in, old patients, perhaps one or two new ones, with a lot of peculiar symptoms. You have had to think and think hard. There is not much irritation in this, but there is hard thinking. Then again, you attend a meeting. You get into a discussion. Parliamentary rulings, by-laws and constitutions have to be set aside. The mind becomes just as tired from this kind of activity as it does from the other. And in addition to that tired feeling we become irritated and almost disgusted. Kali Phos. comes in well in such a condition.

Even though I may be off the question a little bit, I want to compare the word 'tired' under Kali Phos. and also Echinacea. 'Tired' is the word in both remedies which should be emphasized, tired in the different organs of the body. Echinacea does not make your head or your brain tired. (I have proved and used them both.) Echinacea makes you tired physically – muscular tiredness; Kali Phos. makes you mentally tired. There is a difference between the two.

Dr G. Royal: The important three Zincums are the metal, the phosphide and the valerianate. Dr Hubbard spoke about the fidgety condition under Zinc. She is correct, if she will include it in all three of them, because it is very marked under Zinc Val.

Take Zinc Phos. There is where you go down, way down in deep. I had a case that was led into my clinic and put down in the chair, a farmer about forty-six years old. His wife had to sit him down. He had as blank an expression as you ever saw. The family history was good. The personal history was good until he had an encounter with a mad animal that gored him fearfully and he lost an immense amount of blood. A short time after that he began to have what his wife called spasms. The family doctor made a diagnosis, a very incorrect one, of epilepsy. He did not take into consideration all the four symptoms. Then, having made his diagnosis he put him on heavy doses of potassium bromide.

When I saw him at the clinic he did not know what his name was and could hardly walk. The examination proved that he was impotent – gone, as you might say.

That was the case. We gave him 3x of Zinc Phos., four times a day. For auxiliary treatment we put him on a meat-free liquid diet. It took a good deal of time to build him up so that his blood was what it should be, and to overcome the effect of the prescription of bromides. Gradually he got better, but it took a year before he could get out and do the business of a large farm.

Again and again I have had conditions where there is deterioration of the nerve, especially the optic nerve. That is where Zinc Phos. comes in.

Dr G. Stevens: Dr Hubbard's description of Lycopodium made me think of a case that I had, a boy about twelve or thirteen, large and overgrown – a boy with an exceedingly good mind but difficult to manage in school because he was so absent-minded. It was difficult for him to concentrate. He had a very decided inferiority complex. He was apt to be cross and fussy in the morning, teasing his younger brother and sisters abominably at times, and teasing the grownups of the family too, when he could. But the inferiority complex, the lack of confidence, I think, was what especially led me to think of the remedy, and his mother said that Lycopodium made him over, for awhile anyway.

Results With Unusual Remedies

Case 1. Insomnia. Elderly woman with nervous prostration, unable to get to sleep until seven o'clock in the morning, week in, week out; restless, sensitive to noise, mentally over-excited, lively and gay during the night with occasional twitchings, has tried all sorts of sedatives without success. I compared Scutellaria, Valerian and Cypripedium and gave one dose of the latter in 1M, and placebo each night. The patient slept ten hours the first night, only a very occasional night until 2 a.m. for six weeks, then return of insomnia. Repeated Cypripedium 1M, one dose; sleeping well since.

Case 2. Headache. Violent headaches, as if the patient would go crazy, with loquacity, sensation as if the temples were in a vice, and as if the skull opened and shut, or as if waves in the head, changing to penetrating pain on motion, numbness of the vertex. Carboneum Sulphuratum 200c., one dose, with almost immediate relief. This patient's chronic remedy was Sulphur. Return of similar headache again yielded to Carbo Sulph. and has not returned since.

Case 3. Heart trouble. Frail, delicate, exquisite lady of sixty with a weak heart. Electrocardiograph showed bundle branch block. Apprehensive, drowsy; sensation as if the heart stopped with faintness; relief in the cold air and from lying. Sore feeling in the abdomen with heart distress. Convallaria 10M, one dose. Relief of symptoms and gradual increase of strength. This prescription was almost an intuitive one, Crataegus and China Sulph. having been given before without marked improvement. She resembled Lily of the Valley (*Convallaria*).

Case 4. Facial neuralgia. Acute swelling and redness of one side of the face with swollen gland under the chin, pain and tightness of the occiput and neck, worse putting the head back, extreme sensitiveness of the bones of the nose to touch, dryness of the mouth and throat, no sweat. Cinnabaris 1M, one dose. Face normal in a couple of hours and relief by nightfall of all symptoms, which had been severe for several days.

Case 5. Varicose ulcer. Stout German woman with a varicose ulcer over the lower right shin, shallow, black, offensive, her one complaint 'terrible burning'. Anthracinum 50M, one dose. Burning relieved within the hour and ulcer healed in a few days and did not return, although she had had it months and had even had a small haemorrhage from it. Her chronic case came out to Graphites, which has since been given her. She has lost twenty pounds and walks miles, and stands all day at her work without recurrence.

Case 6. Acute sinus trouble. Young woman with a history of pneumonia and pleurisy came for sudden obstructive coryza, constant blowing of her nose but nothing comes, pain at the nose root with stuffed feeling, dry, harassing night cough, sensation as if floating in the air. Sticta Pulm. 10M, one dose. Next morning patient reported first good night's sleep in a week and nose almost cleared.

Case 7. Mammary tumour. Middle-aged woman with almond-sized tumour in her right breast near the nipple, stitching pains shooting inward, chill after stool, burning vesicles on the right side of the tongue. Phellandrium Aquaticum 10M, one dose. Symptoms swiftly cleared and lump gone in three weeks. No return in two years.

Case 8. Heart trouble. Middle-aged man, hypochondriac, palpitation on first lying down, choking sensation in morning, heart troubles him whenever he thinks about it, excessive weakness, must lie down, feeling as if the heart were temporarily paralyzed, burning sensation in the lower throat. Oxalic Acid 10M, one dose. Relief of heart symptoms and extreme prostration, more cheerful outlook.

The range of remedies a prescriber uses is sometimes singularly hackneyed. However, especially in acute prescribing, repertorization of three or four symptoms of a more-or-less peculiar or keynote character may bring you to a relatively unusual remedy which will fit the case. Go over your prescriptions for the last year or for any month and see what the gamut is, and what remedies are frequently repeated. Meteorological conditions also influence the remedies indicated. I have often noticed that a certain remedy or group of remedies will be called for on the same day. Constant study of the less familiar remedies will widen the scope of our usefulness.

DISCUSSION

Dr Grace Stevens: I am very much interested in the point about finding indications for the same remedy several times in succession. I have noticed that a number of times and I have heard other people speak of it. I am sure it is not necessarily because you have the remedy in mind.

Dr Grimmer: There are three more of us who have confirmed the same observation, that many days we prescribe the same remedy, on cases which occur close together.

Dr Hubbard: Do you three wise men give any reason for that?

Dr Grimmer: Well, I have a theory – you may accept it for what it is worth. I believe the astrological conditions that prevail at any given time bring people with similar complaints to the doctor at that time.

Dr Hayes: There is one point which I think should not be forgotten or overlooked: that a little repertorization of peculiar and unusual symptoms, rare symptoms, many of them, will turn up the unusual remedy.

Dr Hubbard: I am glad you brought that out, because when one uses the expression 'keynote remedies', I felt a little worried lest I gave it because of the keynote, which I practically never do; but it is perhaps fair to use some of the keynotes as a basis for repertorization with a few symptoms.

Dr Harry B. Baker: Speaking of that case treated with Sticta Pulmonaria, about ten years ago we had a run of influenza cases, with that heavy feeling at the root of the nose. I have not seen it since then at all. One thing I have noticed is that cases in epidemics seem to call for different remedies in different parts of the country, even parts more or less in the same latitude.

In the epidemic of 1918 I remember seeing some of the men use Arsenicum. In the fall of 1918 I believe we gave but one remedy and that was Gelsemium. We did not have to give anything else.

Dr Underhill, Jr.: There is such a thing as intuition, which we all possess latently and which is developed in some people. Many consider intuition to be something we should rise above, but it is really a higher attribute of mind, perhaps, than ordinary reasoning. Some of the most brilliant prescriptions I have ever made have come about this way – chronic cases which have been extremely puzzling and in which I failed to achieve success for a considerable time. I have gotten right down and plugged on them and still did not see daylight. Then, after having almost given up in despair, I have seen the patient and perhaps just touched him, or listened to the heart, or touched the pulse, and the remedy would pop into my mind right out of the blue. It is nearly always correct if I go through that particular sequence, but if I have not worked on it, it does not amount to anything.

Dr Hubbard: I had a case this past winter I was particularly anxious to cure. Those are always the ones I have trouble with. I repertorized her with the utmost faithful care, and never in the repertory study (and I re-studied her three times) did she come anywhere near the remedy I was itching to give her. I have never given her the remedy I was itching to give her, which is Aurum, and why I wanted to give her Aurum I can hardly even tell you except to me she has been Aurum.

She has not done well on the many I felt justified in giving her, but I could not give her Aurum on just a hunch, do you think?

Dr Underhill: I would think so.

Dr Hubbard: But it does not come out, even eighth or ninth.

Dr Grimmer: Are any of the mentals present at all?

Dr Hubbard: She will not admit to them at all, and I think now they are not present. But she is a Russian, and I feel that somewhere in her background they were definitely there.

Dr Grimmer: I would not hesitate to give it to her with those antecedents.

Dr Moore: I think some of us practice by intuition without knowing it. I had done a cataract extraction on a trance medium. I was doing a dressing and she said, 'Someone comes in with you every day'. I asked for a description and she gave an excellent description of an uncle of mine who was a surgeon, dead a while before, and I said, 'What does that man do?' She said, 'He tells you what to do'.

So, in the practice of medicine, all I have to do is be there. Somebody tells me what to do. It is easy.

The North Pole to the Rescue

A merry, pretty, mid-fifties schoolteacher, who had been under appalling strain for years without complaint, developed a constellation of vesicles on the left side of the brow and scalp, which burned and itched quite unendurably, and spread to the left eye. She had very little fever and few constitutional symptoms. She described the pain as 'frightening' and had sat bolt upright in a hard chair all night. She panted with the pain. She wanted to be let alone and not talked to, and was sensitive to people moving about in the house, both from the jar and the noise. Difficulty in keeping the legs still. Numb sensation in the left temple. Some relief from cold. Diagnosis: Herpes zoster. Initial prescription based on numbness of the left face, Kent p. 379 and the flippancy of the lady even in her anguish: Graphites 1M.

No relief. Quite desperate with pain. I asked her if she could not describe better how she felt. She said there was a sensation of coldness in the painful eye. Kent p. 236. The only remedy Thuja. The larger heading – Coldness in the Eye – includes Graphites and also Calc. Phos. The pain, by the next day, had concentrated in the left temple, where it throbbed. Spigelia 200c gave slight relief. On further questioning she said she felt as if the eye were separating from the head. Robert's *Sensations As If*, p. 131, suggests Lachnanthes, but on reading it in the materia medica it does not fit at all. Finally the patient said, 'It feels as though there were lumps of ice behind my eyeballs'. Roberts, p. 119, 'as if a lump of ice lay in the orbit of the eye', one remedy only: Mag. P. Arct. (Magnetic Polus Arcticus) 1M, 3 doses. Next morning, she phoned and said: 'You have hit it'. The pain had lessened almost immediately. I have never used Mag. P. Arct. before, although I once used the southern magnetic pole, Mag. P. Aust. for an ingrowing toenail.

Why do I quote this case? Partly to show how indispensable are the sensations 'as if'. Next to my Kent, I would rather have the Roberts *As If* for frequency of use and accuracy of prescribing. One could discuss this case for a long time from many viewpoints. For instance, to be pathological for a moment, Kent, p. 1314, has a rubric on zona which includes Graphites, Ranunculus Bulbosus and Thuja. Oddly enough, it does not contain Spigelia, which is primarily a nerve rather than a vesicular remedy, and it does not mention our North Pole, which alleviated the condition because of its exact and unique symptom similarity.

A Tissue Remedy – Calcarea Sulphurica and its Relation to the Nosode Pyrogen

I wonder how many people, if asked to give the names of the nine Muses, would remember them, or the Seven Wonders of the World, or even the Seven Labours of Hercules – but I am sure that every homoeopath would be able immediately to give the twelve Tissue Remedies, so I will not repeat their names here.

The very caption 'Tissue Remedies' is a moot point, because it is not an exact statement. Of course, a tissue remedy means a remedy which appears 'as is' in the tissues of the body. Other remedies than these twelve appear in the tissues of the body, and, moreover, the term 'double salts', which some people apply to them, is not correct either. One of the tissue remedies is Silica, which is silicon dioxide, not a double salt but an oxide, and therefore the term 'tissue salt' is incorrect. I do not know what would be the purist's term for these substances.

Of these twelve, Calcarea Sulphurica is the most questionable. It appears in only one of the tissues of the body, namely the bile, and it does not always appear there, according to Bunge, the physiologist. In the second revision of his book, Dr Schuessler leaves out Calc. Sulph. entirely and divides its symptoms between Silica and Natrum Phos. Notwithstanding, for general purposes, it is included as one of the twelve tissue remedies. (It would be interesting if our materia medica could have provings of all the substances which compose the body, as remedies. We do have some of the complicated ones. For instance, Lecithin and Cholesterin have been partially proved.)

Calc. Sulph. was mentioned long before Schuessler. Hahnemann stressed the importance of a number of the inorganic cell salts, as he called them, proving Calc. Carb., Natrum Mur. and Kali Mur. Stapf in his *Archives* in 1832 spoke of the great importance of the essential components of the human body as homoeopathic remedies, and Hering and von Grauvogl both spoke of these remedies. In 1873 Schuessler brought out his *Physiological Function Remedies*, as he called them, which is perhaps the best title of all for them.

Calc. Sulph. itself is rather imperfectly proved. It was proved by Hering and by Wittein in 1847, best by Conant in 1873 (*Transactions* of the A.I.H. for that year), subsequently by an unknown lady, and then by an eclectic physician, very recently. Its presence in the body in bile, if one took stock in the Doctrine of Correspondences, might seem to indicate it as a liver remedy. What there is of the provings shows no particular connection there; but it is an interesting point to hold in mind and to check up when it seems to apply to a case.

The relations of this particular double remedy are very interesting. In Hering it appears as compatible after Kali Mur., Natrum Sulph. and Silica, and compares with Calendula and Hepar Sulph. In one other place I found that it was compatible after Belladonna. These are the only relations given for it officially, although Schuessler himself states that it will antidote Mercury and some of its effects and also, in high potency, that it will relieve the effects of gross poisoning by quinine.

Calc. Sulph., according to some, stands mid-way between Hepar Sulph. and Silica; according to others it is even deeper and should be given after Silica. This of course is chiefly in the realm of boils and pus conditions.

Unfortunately not all our homoeopathic vegetable remedies have been analyzed chemically in order to see what their inorganic constituents are, but some few have been. Of those that have, there are four in which calcium sulphate has been found – Ailanthus, Apocynum, Asafoetida and Phytolacca. That seems a strange four, but you remember how excellent Phytolacca is in boils. That may be due to the amount of calcium sulphate in it; Asafoetida contains 6.2%. That is interesting because Calc. Sulph. also has caries of the bones as well as a more marked mental symptomatology than I had thought before I began to study it, which again may go with the Asafoetida.

Calcium sulphate is the same as gypsum, plaster of Paris, another form is alabaster. Hepar Sulph. is the sulphide of lime; Calc. Sulph. is the sulphate.

According to Schuessler, the role of Calc. Sulph. in the liver is to destroy the old red blood cells by abstracting water from them, and when Calc. Sulph. is deficient these clogging dead blood cells stay in the organism; when it is doing its work they are thrown out in catarrhal discharges.

Just as a matter of amusement I took the Kent *Repertory* and went through for all the symptoms of Calc. Sulph. which stood in the third or highest degree, under Mind and Generals. I found that in those two sections in the third degree there were twenty symptoms, and in the second degree there were forty symptoms in our entire Mind and Generals. That shows you how slightly proved the remedy is, and how little is known of those two most important departments of it.

A Tissue Remedy

It is very interesting in any remedy which has two distinct elements – as this one has, the calcium and the sulphur – to see which is dominant and which recessive, and what symptoms can be hitched up with each side of the combination. In this instance I think the honours go to the sulphur. Of the great mentals and generals, more than two-thirds are like sulphur and only one-third like calcium. Some of the chief mentals are irritability, anxiousness, capriciousness, aversion to company, contradictoriness and obstinacy, fear of death and evil and insanity, and other fears, as well as timidity, a craving for stimulants, and mental irresolution, which is a marked feature, a taciturnity, and also a maliciousness. The number of remedies that have a real maliciousness mentally are relatively few, and very interesting to think of. Every now and then we get a patient who we know must have that symptom.

The Generals of Calc. Sulph. are quite interesting. It is both a warm and a cold remedy. In other words, it stands three for heat and two for chilliness in the *Repertory*, and it may swing either way.

One interesting modality in that connection is that it is much better uncovered. This is one of the differentiating points between Calc. Sulph. and Hepar Sulph., because Hepar Sulph. is worse for uncovering. Calc. Sulph., however, has complaints after becoming cold; it also has complaints from washing and complaints from working in water, which you would expect from the Calcarea. It is worse from exertion and particularly averse to motion. It is a lazy, indolent, good-for-nothing remedy in one mental phase. It is also worse from over-heating, and from standing, as you might prognosticate from the Sulphur, worse from the warmth of the bed, and worse from wraps and from a warm room. It has a curious and perfectly definite modality of better from eating, not only at noon, but at all times. It also takes after Sulphur in that it is a great remedy for suppressed perspiration and the evil effects of it. It has a marked craving for acid fruits and pungent vegetables. The symptoms are rather more right-sided than left-sided, although it is not one of the strongly right-sided remedies. One of the main spheres of its action is the respiratory, where it is relatively little known. It has coryza, often inveterate, of the right nostril, slightly acrid and fluid, sometimes alternating, the right nostril being worse in the morning, and the left in the evening, and vice versa, one stopped and one flowing. Also in regard to the respiratory tract, it has one great use which is hard to find in the books but which I have seen demonstrated clinically – it helps close up fistulous openings in the chest after empyema. Calc. Sulph., if the symptoms agree, will do wonders in healing up such a sinus with granulations from the bottom.

There is an interesting thing in regard to Calc. Sulph. in hare lip and cleft palate. Duncan, in his little book *Acid and Alkaline Children*, speaks of a number of cases in which women have borne hare lip and cleft palate children; one case had had four and another eight, in all of whom it had been present. Duncan got to thinking about it, wondering what he could do. He had had these women on what he thought were their constitutional remedies, and still the babies kept coming with hare lips and cleft palates. Finally he went back to embryology and found that that abnormality occurs prior to the third month in gestation; he found it was a bone deficiency, and decided that it must be a lack of some of the calciums. The question was, which one.

In the particular case he then had in hand the mother was very clearly a Sulphur patient. He thought he would try Calc. Sulph. empirically for the mother at her next pregnancy, to see what he could do in the way of obviating hare lip. He gave her Calc. Sulph. over seven months of pregnancy. She bore her fifth baby, the first who had not had the condition. He repeated it in three other cases while the baby was in utero, and each child was born with no hare lip. There are many possibilities of a slip betwixt that cup and lip, but it is an interesting field, and the whole subject of possible prescribing for the development of a child in utero is opened up by it.

Another great sphere is in women's diseases, in bringing back suppressed leucorrhea, in getting rid of menstrual difficulties and in fibroid tumours of the uterus. But the greatest sphere of Calc. Sulph., probably, is upon the skin. Where wounds do not heal, where bruises are neglected, where boils keep coming in crops, where there are abscesses, often painless, in the anal region; where there are fistulae of any kind, Calc. Sulph. is one of the remedies to be particularly considered.

Let us consider Calc. Sulph.'s relation to some of the nosodes. It is given in some of the books, notably in Kent's, as one of the great remedies for those cases where the seemingly indicated remedy does not act, for those cases which need to be followed up with a deeper influence, and is classed with Tuberculinum and Psorinum. The particular nosode to which I want to point out certain resemblances is Pyrogen. At first sight I did not know myself how I could do it, because they are so different in so many ways. But as you go through, comparing the two, you do see certain striking similarities in usefulness.

Calc. Sulph., for instance, is one of the rare remedies which has hilarity in its mental makeup – it is quite refreshing to see one that is not despondent – particularly toward twilight, at 6 p.m.; Pyrogen too, in its first stages, together with loquacity, has great gaiety.

Moreover, of course, Pyrogen has the tendency to septic abscesses, and is a magnificent remedy for crops of boils which can be traced back to prodromes of blood poisoning in the past; also in peritonitis, if one has the temerity to prescribe before sending for the surgeon, Pyrogen will often be called for; as will Calc. Sulph., where there has been a vent for the pus and where it keeps forming and coming in large quantities long beyond the time when healing should be present.

There are also certain respiratory analogies between Pyrogen and Calc. Sulph. For instance, they both have lung abscess and some of the many symptoms agree fairly well. Pyrogen has a strange keynote 'as if the heart pumped cold water', whereas Calc. Sulph. has 'as if the bronchial tubes were pumped full of hot water'. They also have in common a slight symptom of the head – the sensation of a cap on the head.

A word about Pyrogen. It ought to be called the Briareus of remedies (he was the gentleman who had a hundred hands); your Pyrogen patient will lie terribly sick and feel as though he had hands all over the bed. It has been called the Aconite of typhoid; it is Baptisia with a very high fever; it follows Rhus Tox. often and carries through its work in other cases where there is great rattling of the chest; it may follow Antimonium Tartaricum.

Think of these two remedies when you find cases in the spheres of the respiratory or gynaecological or dermatological diseases which have any of these symptoms.

Homoeopathic Equivalents of Endocrinological Remedies in Paediatrics

At the risk of repeating a truism, it is necessary to state that the most active force for the restoration of normal balance between the endocrine glands is the homoeopathic simillimum, whatever that may be, whether or not it has ever before been connected with gland function. Ordinary medicine endeavours to replace the lack of glandular activity by administering extracts of animal glands, and this often means the continuation of such adjuvant treatment indefinitely. Although the symptoms may clear up, there is no tendency to increase the activity of the deficient glands. Indeed, any vitality they have may be atrophied by such pandering to their weakness. The indicated remedy stimulates the vital force and tends to produce increasing and harmonious action of the glandular tissue.

To speak of any definite remedies smacks, as usual, of pathological prescribing, and yet there are certain remedies whose frequency of indication is notable in certain syndromes. For instance, the infant who does not develop, who is late in walking, teething and talking, suggests Calc. Carb., Natrum Mur., Calc. Phos. or Silica. The symptoms in these little ones are mostly objective, and require watching and deliberation. If the fundamental chronic remedies of the parents can be ascertained, they often illuminate the baby's case, as remedies run in families. Also, if the miasmatic trend of the family is known, the suitable nosode may open up the case.

Some fundamental pituitary difficulties cause dwarfism or gigantism. Dwarfs very often need Medorrhinum or Syphilinum and sometimes Mercurius, or if complicated with cretinism, Baryta Carb. Giants run to such remedies as Phosphorus, Calc. Phos. or Sulphur. The fat boy of the comics – adiposa dolorosa – with the piping voice needs Graphites, Calc. Carb. or other remedies.

A boy of nine years was brought to me for extreme weakness and breathlessness on any exertion and for a hysteric disposition. Short, fat, blonde, precocious, craving air, no physical signs except big tonsils and a very rapid heart. Frequent nosebleeds when washing the face, chilliness; Ammonium Carb. 50M, one dose. Within a week, instead of weeping from exhaustion from the least exercise, the boy was asking to play with his peers, and after one repetition four months later was able to practise in the school scrub football team without undue acceleration of the pulse or fatigue. The parents came of a deeply psoric stock, the mother also sycotic, having needed Graphites and Medorrhinum.

Thyroid difficulties are the most frequent. In the hyperthyroid cases homoeopathy is at its best. Iodum, Natrum Mur., Spongia and many others will remove the dangerous symptoms. In hypothyroidism Baryta Carb., Calc. Carb., Calc. Iodatum and Medorrhinum shine. Some of our physicians prescribe Thyroidinum in potency. I have had little experience with it except in slowing the heart. Fucus is very popular among the German homoeopaths and Lycopus is to be considered. Sometimes in low thyroid conditions Sulphur will start the ball rolling.

A girl at puberty was sent by the teacher because of stupidity and poor co-ordination. Father abnormally stout, girl way overweight, excessive jaw, eyebrows meet in the middle, menses very scanty and black, skips months, frequent urging to urination with no results, stool in balls, bites nails, sick from candy which she craves, nightmares, fullness over thyroid gland, thyroid profile low, history of discharging left ear with excoriation and blisters suppressed. Sulphur 1M, one dose. Within a week the teacher reports increased tidiness, child more awake, studying much better, and the family report disposition at home entirely changed, now sunny where she was irritable and egotistic, which I had not known. Calc. Carb. will probably follow.

Girl of six, stout, dry skin, Hutchinson's teeth, protruding ears, narrow high palate, history of psoriasis in the mother and acute syphilis in the father. Thyroid profile low. Pale, listless, peevish, picks nose, itching rectum, stool examination shows worms. Cina 1M, one dose. Several worms passed, child eats better and is less anaemic. Eruptions developed around the mouth with brownish crusts, cracks in the corners of the mouth. Graphites 200c, one dose. Face cleared, rash developd on the forearms, excoriating leucorrhoea (in a child of six). Teeth are black, child will not eat meat, oily perspiration, aggravation from dark until morning. Merc. Viv. 10M, one dose. New teeth coming in sound. After some interval and an attack of chickenpox, I gave her Syphilinum 1M, one dose, with great improvement. This case shows the necessity of shifting remedies in complicated cases. The child has become thinner, brighter, and more biddable. All her symptoms are much improved. Thyroid profile improved markedly.

Ovarian problems are a famous field for homoeopathy. Its success with climacteric symptoms obviates the need for replacement therapy. Apis, Lachesis, Sanguinaria and Sepia are the sheet anchors here.

Boys with undescended testicles often respond to Aurum if the background suggests it, and there is no better gonadal stimulant than Lycopodium.

These fragmentary suggestions are merely to show that the indicated remedy profoundly affects the endocrines, along with the whole constitution, and to recommend its use instead of the substitutional methods of usual endocrinology.

DISCUSSION

Dr Grimmer: Relating to Dr Hubbard's point about the shifting of remedies – in certain chronic cases I think it is justifiable and we have both Hahnemann and Kent to justify it. In the mixture of miasms, where one miasm is improved for a while under a deep remedy, it is usually psoric. Indeed, we sometimes then find the syphilitic or tubercular miasm coming up, which will require a chronic remedy of a different nature, and that must be given for a while.

Dr Kent speaks of that procedure in his *Philosophy of Chronic Disease*. We do sometimes meet cases that require a succession of remedies of an entirely different nature, until the whole economy is brought into a state of harmony, where one remedy is finally found that you can give through a series and lead to cure.

Dr Hubbard: I wonder if Dr Grimmer thinks I would have been better off if I had started that girl with Syphilinum. It did not occur to me, even though she had definitely inherited syphilis, but she did not have the symptoms then.

Dr Grimmer: The doctor's prescription is justified by her results. I thought strongly of Syphilinum, and you have done it.

Dr Wilson: Did you not say that she had Hutchinson's teeth? That was enough. I would surely have given her Syphilinum right away.

Dr Dixon: Speaking of shifting remedies, it is interesting to read Burnett's old book, and know of the really national reputation he attained through alternations of Bacillinum, Tuberculinum and Thuja in those enlarged tonsils in children. I do not know whether he gave a single remedy or alternated them at the same time. I am in a quandary to tell from his case reports, but he really did excellent work with either the combination or the alternation, or the repeating of first one and then the other two remedies. I find that a dose of Tuberculinum, followed with

Thuja later on (I have never alternated them) clear up surprisingly large numbers of those tonsils in children.

Dr Grimmer: There is a point I should like to enquire of the society. I heard it said by some very good men, and have confirmed the observation by experience, that you will rarely cure any case of chronic disease with a nosode. You will have to give other remedies. I should like to hear what others have to say about that.

Dr Charles Boericke: I should like to ask Dr Hubbard if she has ever used endocrines in potency for these endocrinological cases.

Dr Hubbard: With the exception of Thyroidinum, which I have used in the 200c potency and never with very pleasing results to me (although it slowed the heart, but it always seemed rather mechanical), I never have used the others. Perhaps I should. I personally do not like to give Diphtherinum or some of those potentized things from diseases themselves. I do not know why, but I have an instinct – I would rather give some remedy in nature in potentized form if I can, unless it is one of the great nosodes of the miasms.

I am very much interested in Dr Grimmer's remark about not curing a case with a nosode. I was hastily trying to think if I had ever seen one I felt had been cured with a nosode and nothing else, either before or after. The proportion of chronic cases curable with one remedy anyway is relatively small, although sometimes there will be a brilliant one.

I wonder if there is any difference in the nature of the remedies and in the class of remedy they use. For instance, I am of the opinion that often you see a Silica case which is purely and clearly and totally Silica more than almost any other remedy. I have had some chronic cases that cleared up with Silica and nothing else, and I do not know whether that is the case with elements in general, rather than with the mixed salts or the more complicated remedies. I would be interested to hear what anybody would think about that.

Dr Grimmer: I have cured some very chronic cases with Sepia and no other remedy.

Dr Hubbard: But that is a complicated remedy chemically. I am interested in whether the elements as such are more searching.

Dr Underhill, Jr: In my experience the nosodes are essential many times in clearing the field, as Dr Grimmer says, for the remedial action of other drugs, but very seldom or practically never do you find that they actually complete the case.

I think the urge to experiment hits us all at some time. A number of years ago I had a case that I had taken care of for eleven years, up to the time of the patient's death. It was one of the worst cases of rheumatoid arthritis I have ever seen. This woman's knees were the largest I had seen and they were ankylosed, and her fingers and hands were terribly distorted.

I took a specimen of her blood and had it potentized, and ran it to 30c, 200c and 1M. When I hopelessly fell down on some cases of arthritis, I tried that, but with no results whatever – nothing I could detect.

Finally that patient died and the family continued under my care. Her daughter is married and has a daughter of her own around ten or twelve years old. One day she came in with the same kind of appearance of the skin that her mother had – almost like a honeycomb tripe – ichthyosis. It was strikingly similar to that of her mother's condition, and when she began to complain of pains in the joints, the temptation to try her mother's potentized blood on her was too great for me. I gave it, and I got action. It flared up terribly and laid her right up in bed, but I stuck to my guns and did nothing. I did not dare repeat it and I did not dare do anything else, so I let the case ride. After a terrific aggravation she made a beautiful recovery – the ichthyosis cleared up and has never returned; but I have never dared give her another dose.

Her dead mother's blood still had power when it came to her own daughter. The relationship between mother and daughter was what made it take hold, and not the fact of the arthritis.

Dr Hubbard: That case of ichthyosis makes me think of a young man I have had in my practice for three years, who has one of the worst cases of ichthyosis you can imagine. He can never go swimming because he is a sight from his waist to his neck. Luckily, he has none on his hands and face. Otherwise he is an extremely husky boy of twenty-three, and I have given him his chronic remedy as it came out, and this is Phosphorus. Strangely enough, you would never think of Phosphorus in ichthyosis, but that is what his remedy was. He is so much better, although he has had the problem all his life, from babyhood. He is now able to wear a bathing costume without being laughed at and feeling self-conscious.

The Use of Nosodes in Children

The majority of children inherit various tendencies to illness, or at least certain trends of constitution. Constitutional administration of a similar remedy can wipe out these inherited difficulties, and promotes a healthier future for the child and its descendants.

Work for the new-born child should be begun on the parents. Although one may not do the actual obstetrics, the homoeopath should make the mother realize the importance of her receiving proper constitutional treatment during pregnancy. In case there have been grave difficulties with a previous child, the father also should undergo treatment before the conception of the subsequent child. A thorough study of the disease trends, even in grandparents, aunts and uncles as well as in the present generation, gives a picture of the family stream which is especially helpful in guiding towards the most profoundly suitable nosode. In nosodes we have remedies applicable to long-range tendencies, even several generations back.

For example, a little child was brought to me some twenty years ago with ears poorly set, high narrow palate, Hutchinson's teeth – a typical product of a syphilitic taint in her father's family. The parents did not recognize these implications and brought the child for minor annoyances such as catarrh, and because it seemed 'not quite bright', as they said. The opening gambit was a dose of Syphilinum 10M, followed at intervals of several months by Mercurius and other remedies as the symptomatology called for them. The child developed splendidly and is now a healthy and competent nurse.

You all know the list of nosodes in the precious fourth volume of Clarke's *Dictionary*, called the *Clinical Repertory*. Of these, the most basic ones which tie in with the classification of chronic diseases suggested by Hahnemann are Syphilinum, Medorrhinum, Tuberculinum, Bacillinum and Psorinum. No proper practice of homoeopathic paediatrics can develop its best results without the frequent use of these resolvers of the past.

Take the gassy baby who screams with colic frequently during the day, who has a snuffly nose, mucus obstructing the throat, perhaps mucus in the stool. It shows few distinctive symptoms for any remedy chosen according to the law of similars. Then you notice that its colic is immediately eased when it is turned over on its abdomen, and that it does not lie stretched out but draws its knees up under it almost in the knee-chest position. This baby needs a dose of Medorrhinum, even though no immediate history of gonorrhoea be forthcoming or even suspected. The taint may be further back in the family.

Look at the angel infant or small child of whom the friends say, 'It is too beautiful to be long for this world', with alabaster skin and a tendency to frequent colds and coughs. If there is any family history of lung trouble or tuberculosis think of Tuberculinum Bovinum, in a single dose, 200c potency, or higher, according to the vitality of the child. (Bacillinum is used more in actual cases of tuberculosis or where there is secondary infection.) Tuberculinum Bovinum is used in the inherited tendency cases, the listless, weak child or those who have had glandular difficulties. Also those with violent temper tantrums, kicking and screaming on the floor, and those who have no perseverance or concentration.

The child who needs Psorinum may be allergic and, like the Medorrhinum baby, have a tendency to asthma. But in the Psorinum infant this is usually combined with, or alternates with, skin difficulties; dirty, smelly, itchy, sweating, whining little darlings!

In all constitutional homoeopathic work, one selects not only the similar remedy at the moment but jots down the top-ranging half-dozen remedies, their acute collaterals, and the nosode or nosodes most strongly permeating the case. Get your nosode in early in children. They are the 'stitch in time that saves nine'.

It is also necessary to remember one of the graver aspects of what usual medicine does for children. The idea is to prevent the infant having what used to be considered normal childhood diseases, the exanthemata. The baby is shot full of 'anti' everything, from smallpox vaccines through diphtheria, whooping cough, scarlatina, measles and even colds. Basically, children *should* have the childhood diseases. These throw off certain inherited impurities and clarify the constitution. Cases properly handled should leave the child with no sequelae and in better health. Patients who come to the doctor in adulthood or in middle life, saying they had never been ill and boasting how they had no childhood diseases, are often those with serious or incurable troubles. For instance, many cancer patients, and many who die suddenly from heart ailments although they were apparently in vigorous health, give no history of childhood diseases. Aside from the fact that one should have the childhood diseases, another point is that, if skipped in childhood, they often occur later on in a far more serious form, such as mumps in grown men involving the testicles. Furthermore, these preventives, given in good faith in the name of perfect health, introduce elements through the normal protective skin covering that are completely foreign to the human body.

As so many of these so-called protective measures are now legally required, homoeopathy has also developed, from and for each of these diseases, certain nosodes which contain no gross foreign animal matter, and which should do for the body what the disease itself would do if it were undergone. By this I mean such substances as Diphtherinum, Morbillinum, Pertussin (Coqueluchin), Scarlatinum, Variolinum and others.

Whether or not you use these nosodes with your children is relatively unimportant, compared to the primary need of helping clear up the health of the race with the basic miasmatic nosodes. Train your patients to bring even relatively healthy children at least four times a year for a constitutional remedy. Remember somehow to give every child who comes under your care, however briefly, its suitable nosode, in high potency, at least once. For example, if you are called for an earache and give the acute remedy, take the time to find the symptoms which will lead you to the choice of a nosode; if you know that the family are not likely to bring the child back for a chronic check-up, leave the nosode to be given at the end of the illness and ask the parent at least to telephone you after having done so.

Remember, too, that in many infants and small children symptoms are far to seek, at least those of a constitutional nature, but that if you give the correct nosode, it will bring out chronic symptoms for further prescribing.

If several nosodes are perceptibly indicated in the family stream, you will have to choose which one to give first, and should be guided by the most recent symptoms. When that layer is cleared away, you can give the nosodes for the deeper latent tendencies.

If all children could have constitutional prescribing, the race could be notably improved in two or three generations. Proper homoeopathic paediatrics can be the hope of the future.

Some Unusual Uses
for the Nosodes

The dictionary defines a nosode as 'a disease product used as a remedy'. Many of our homoeopathic doctors would describe nosodes in opprobrious terms; some prescribers give nosodes where the miasmatic history is clear and the symptoms are mixed or obscure; others put them in as 'intercurrents'; the French school combine or alternate the suitable miasmatic nosode with the most similar remedy for the top layer, or recent symptoms. In cases where no remedy stands out, after patient questioning and repertorizing, some give the nosode of the main miasm in order to stir up the depths and throw out indications for a curative prescription. We hear much of the role of the nosode when seemingly well chosen remedies fail to act or hold, and in the clearing up of recalcitrant relapses. The strict homoeopath uses the exanthem nosodes for immunization often, although Merc. Cy., Belladonna and Drosera prevail, too.

The list of nosodes in current usage in homoeopathy is sizable. In Clarke's *Clinical Repertory* we find mention of twenty-two, including such a well-known remedy as Secale. Bach in Great Britain developed a new group, mostly of the intestinal variety. Certain ones from the exanthemata have been added, such as Scarlatinum and Pertussin. Some are rare to many, as Melitagrinum, Skinner's nosode from eczema capitis, or Nectrianinum, the tree cancer remedy. The big three, corresponding to Hahnemann's miasms – Psorinum, Medorrhinum and Syphilinum – are well known to all, as is Tuberculinum or Bacillinum. H. C. Allen's book, *The Nosodes*, is a classic on these; but an adequate knowledge of them must be built up by study of J. H. Allen's books on two of the three miasms, as well as modern sources such as H. A. Roberts' masterly lectures to the American Foundation for Homoeopathy Summer School.

The best practice, I believe, gives the nosodes by their definite symptomatology, like any other remedy; and this truism has led me to make some brilliant results in acute cases. While driving on your rounds, ask yourselves the acute uses of Syphilinum or Psorinum.

As an example, let us take the case of Miss X, who was beside herself with agony at receiving an enema from a skilful nurse. Sensation of unbearable constriction at rectum, with pushing down pain and actual prolapse of anus, clusters of hard tender piles with fissures and burning; history of obstinate constipation for years; habitually took an enema twice a week and dreaded the ordeal to the point of hysteria. Luetic family history. Fears the night, when she is worse, and the exhaustion of waking, and insanity. Such remedies as Aesculus and even Lachesis had been given without relief. Syphilinum 1M, one dose; relaxation of the rectal spasm in a few minutes, followed by almost normal bowel action for the first time in her memory, with relief of depression, etc.

Or again, Mrs M., in the knee-chest position, cyanosed, gasping and wheezing, her coarse unruly hair standing out in all directions, muttering, 'If I could get to the seashore – if I only could.' Medorrhinum 10M, one dose, with relief in five minutes while I watched. Previous adrenalin in other attacks had given no help.

An eleven-year-old boy in bed with fever of 39°C, room stifling but a woolly muffler wrapped around his head, pale, dirty skin, drenched in foetid sweat, slight thin discharge from ear which could be smelled on entering the room. No pain whatever unless his head was raised on a pillow, as I discovered on asking why the pillow was on the floor. History of running ear on and off since scarlet fever at four years of age. Psorinum 10M, one dose. Fever dropped in two hours, ear discharged violently for a week; chilliness, sweat and odour gone. Three weeks later his mother said he had never been so well; no ear discharge for ten months, at which point it became necessary to repeat dose.

DISCUSSION

Dr Baker: I agree that you get your best results using the nosodes where you can prescribe them as a regular homoeopathic remedy on the symptoms, only you cannot always get the symptoms. Then you have to use them until you do get the symptoms – especially that case of the knee-chest position and the Medorrhinum. I have seen that work like a charm.

Dr Grimmer: I agree that the most logical thing to do in using nosodes is to get their symptoms and history. There are cases with a very great paucity of symptoms where, with a family history and the personal history of the specific miasm to which they related, you will sometimes get a brilliant unlocking of the case, if not a cure.

I can remember very few real cures by the nosodes. My experience has been that they have helped, but I know of only one case I really cured, which was a case with Tuberculinum, a very bad case of migratory pneumonia in a child six years old. I went two thousand miles to put a powder of Tuberculinum on this child's tongue when he was just about moribund. He had had three well-regarded doctors in the city, and they said there was no hope. The child had a few symptoms when I got there. He had had about two weeks of this, with a very high temperature and violent chills. Every time there would be a new area of infection and he would have a chill followed by high temperature, little spots all through the lungs, pneumonic spots, a chain of the glands of the neck swollen and hard, bird-like claws, extreme weakness.

I got into the case with the doctors' consent. They removed their medication. (They were giving him expectorants.) I gave him Tuberculinum 10M, and in twelve hours that case ended by crisis, not by lysis. He had a coughing spell and spat up about a pint of pus, and then went down from a temperature of 41°C to about 36°C. He had a drenching, very profuse sweat. The other doctors came in at the family's solicitation, and said he was dying. I said, 'No, he is not dying.'

He had a good pulse in spite of all this. I said, 'It is merely reaction. He will be all right in a short time.' He made a brilliant cure and a perfect recovery without any further medication.

Dr Lewandowski: The totality of symptoms, as we all understand, is the deciding factor in the selection of the remedy. However, in the repertorizaton of any case it is very rare that a nosode comes out. When you do recognize a nosode, use it with caution, since we all understand that it is a very powerful missile.

Dr Waffensmith: One point that has been very valuable in my experience is the euthanasia power of Tuberculinum. Very often after prescribing for an incurable acute condition one will find that the remedies, as indicated in series, fail to hold. That of course is a positive diagnosis of incurability. As the patient progresses toward the final stage the family is restless, and something is expected to be done to neutralize the ultimate agony of death.

If you find that there are symptoms in the case pointing to Tuberculinum, or a family history of tuberculosis, it is here that you will often get a remarkable pre-death improvement. The patient, where previously he had been unable even to swallow the medicine you have given, or liquids, may for a very limited period of time ask for nourishment and be able to swallow it. But do not allow that to deceive you, as it is the pre-death euthanasia which comes from any simillimum, but particularly from the nosode Tuberculinum.

Some Unusual Uses for the Nosodes

Dr Farrington: It is true that we seldom get a nosode in repertory work, but that may be because the knowledge of the particular symptoms of these diseased products is deficient and the repertories contain comparatively few of them.

If you look deeply at H. C. Allen's *Nosodes* you will see that there is a wealth of symptoms, especially for Psorinum and Medorrhinum, and some of them which cannot be found under any other remedy. That is especially true of Medorrhinum. If you have ever used his slip repertory you will have nosodes coming out more frequently. Many of the symptoms that are recorded in the other repertories are marked in his in high degree.

Dr Allen has been accused of abusing the nosodes, but I do not believe it. He knew more than any other person about them, and like Guernsey with his keynotes and others who have had some special method of prescribing, they knew so much that with one or two symptoms they saw other things, and perhaps without realizing it themselves they really did prescribe on the totality.

I have seen a number of cures with nosodes, especially with Tuberculinum, where it was the only remedy in the case. However, as a rule the nosodes carried the case to a certain point and other remedies had to be given to complete the cure.

Have you had many aggravations from nosodes? – I have never had any. In Dr Grimmer's case, where he gave Tuberculinum, he said the patient got well by crisis. Is it not possibly true that although under good homoeopathic prescribing lobar pneumonia gets well by lysis, if there is a hyperpyrexia that is not possible. I can think of one case of 'blue' pneumonia (which is not supposed to be pneumonia, I understand), where a temperature of 41°C came tumbling down in two hours to 38°C after a dose of Phosphorus, and the patient got cold and sweaty and almost collapsed. It was a young woman of twenty-six who had just recovered from tuberculosis after a long period of homoeopathic prescribing. I do not know in this case whether it was galloping consumption or pneumonia. She recovered, but her hair fell out and she became bald as an egg. Then the hair came in curly and my oldest son fell in love with her and married her.

Dr John Panos: Recently the wife of one of the best homoeopaths in Dayton suffered from what was termed colitis and, as usual, one went to the symptoms. For two years he prescribed to the best of his ability and finally asked me if I would help in taking care of her. He told me he had been giving Arsenic, Lachesis, Carbo Veg. and a few others.

We decided on Arsenic, which brought some relief. We waited for two months but there was no further progress. Then she got a cold, and the doctor prescribed, hurriedly, Aconite and Bryonia. Then we decided a dose of Sepia might clear up something. Sepia was given with no results. The sweat and the characteristics of Psorinum were present and we gave a dose of Psorinum. There was an aggravation for a week and then she came back with the previous line and stayed there for four weeks, when Lachesis became very nicely indicated. One dose of 10M cleared the case up beautifully and she is very well today.

Dr Wilson: One interesting aspect of the nosodes is their use against some of the prevailing diseases.

When I was a student at Hahnemann College the seniors had the privilege of going to the municipal hospital and seeing smallpox. I wanted to see smallpox, because I thought I would never see it when I got into practice.

We went up to see diphtheria, scarlet fever and then smallpox at two-day intervals. The first day we went in to see either diphtheria or scarlet fever, and the intern asked to see our own vaccinations. I happened to be the oldest person in the class and he looked at them all and passed me by. I finally said, 'Don't you want to look at mine?' (I had one that was done way back in the 'eighties). He asked how long ago was it done.

I said, 'Twenty or twenty-five years ago', and he replied, 'I would have one or two scratches made if I were you.'

Some of the other students were vaccinated. Some of them did not go into the wards when the critical time came, but I began taking Variolinum, and took it for a period before I went in, and also after I came from seeing the case of smallpox.

They insist in New Jersey that all children are Schick tested, and there was one little one in my practice. My attitude toward vaccination has always been that the more healthy the child, the less fit he is to be vaccinated. As a consequence I never have vaccinated anyone, and would not be vaccinated myself if I could help it, so I sent some powders of a CM of Diphtherinum to the mother of this child in place of having her Schicked by injection.

The health authorities telephoned me and wanted to know about it. I did not tell them what I had done, but simply said that in my estimation the child was thoroughly inoculated against diphtheria.

So I have used Variolinum as well as Typhoid and Diphtherinum in that way. As Dr Hubbard says, we have all used them where we think there lies tuberculosis, some syphilis or some gonorrhoea (and some of these lie under all of us). We cannot help it. It is somewhere around, and many times an intercurrent of one of those nosodes helps a lot.

Dr Van Norden: Dr Allen used to tell us that when people were weak they got tired easily, and where you could not get results with other remedies, Tuberculinum would often do the work. I have followed that out many times in practice and have almost invariably found it to work.

Dr McLaren: Variolinum will cure smallpox, and it will prevent you from getting smallpox – I have tried it out. I was called to see a man suffering from smallpox who had three children, and they all lived in a very small house. The three children had never been vaccinated and were exposed to the disease. I gave them all Variolinum. The eldest child had smallpox pustules without any pus in them, and only one day of fever; the second child had one day of fever and one or two fleeting nodules or pink spots, and the third child had nothing at all.

Dr Knerr: I have always used Variolinum to prevent smallpox. I had the peculiar case of a woman of about fifty to whom I gave it and she promptly developed a beautiful pustule on her right arm. It was during an epidemic, and she never had any further symptoms.

Separate to this, it is known that the constituents of saliva include the sulphur cyanide of potassium. It was discovered in an epidemic in Philadelphia that where silver plating was done, where they used the cyanide of potassium, no cases of smallpox occurred at all among the workers. This started Dr Hering to investigate the cases in the smallpox hospital in Philadelphia. He examined their saliva, and found that the cyanide had left the saliva, but he found it in the pustules. As soon as the patients got better the cyanide left the pustules and went back to the saliva.

This led him to use the sulphur cyanide of potassium in liquid form. When sprinkled around on the sheets in the sick rooms, it had the effect that there never was another case that did that.

Then Dr Hering wished to find a remedy from a plant. He thought a plant that contained the sulphur cyanide of potassium would yield the remedy, and he found it in the black mustard, *Sinapis nigra*.

Dr Hubbard: I agree with Dr Lewandowski that the remedies which come out sixth or seventh in the repertory, if they are rare ones that stand high, are extremely important. I am more likely to give the one that comes out No. 3 than the one that comes out No. 1.

I personally hope we take every case according to Dr Spalding's wonderful method, in that we should consider which of the nosodes of the fundamental miasms are most closely related to that case. We know that the remedies are grouped around the miasmatic divisions, and we should have a care to remember that in our selection of the remedy.

Dr Farrington was right when he said that my cases were chronic rather than acute, but they were in the acute stage at the moment. After all, I suppose every case is really chronic, no matter how acute it seems.

Remedies in the Cure of Common Colds

Nature cures a cold in a fortnight, a good doctor can cure it in fourteen days. This old adage represents the attitude of our 'regular' colleagues. To be sure, a few of their specifics, such as quinine, soda bicarbonate, silver nitrate, ammonium chloride, potassium iodide, aid at least in suppressing the manifestations, but we realize that these five remedies are homoeopathic to certain types of colds. They are known to us respectively as China, Natrum Carb., Argentum Nitricum, Ammonium Muriaticum and Kali Iodatum. At a 'regular' medical congress in Boston I heard the Dean of the Harvard Medical School remark that it was inexplicable how remedies sometimes work for what he called the same condition, and sometimes, more frequently, fail utterly in other types of patients.

Unconscious homoeopathy!

The old wives who gathered herbs knew more of the true lore of cure. Who cannot remember the use of onion poultices in certain colds, and the not unfounded idea, at least in the sense of correspondences, of putting a bit of coral about the baby's neck to ward them off?

Through our handling of the common cold we homoeopaths can do much to impress upon our regular colleagues the principle of case individualization. Give your inquiring medical friends a case of thirty-six remedies in, say, the 30th potency. Invite one to make your rounds during a season when there are many colds. He will be impressed and intrigued by the results that even he as a novice can obtain through your painting of the picture of the different remedies.

Will you come briefly with me now on my visits as an old-fashioned family doctor?

It is spring. We find a baby with watery eyes, clear water running from the tip of its nose, its left nostril excoriated, red and swollen. We watch it. It takes a long breath, and then sneezes. It cries for food (like Sulphuric Acid and Hepar Sulph.). The mother tells us she took the baby out yesterday despite the damp north-east wind. She apologizes for the coolness of the room but says, 'Baby is better outdoors if she dared to take him.' Last night, she tells us, he was much worse; even now we can hear the profuse mucus in his tubes. Suddenly he crouches with pain and

123

holds on to his larynx, while splitting coughs rend him. You do not need to be told that this is the Allium Cepa baby. Farrington says that this remedy will often drive a cold down on to the chest, and we may then need Phosphorus.

Our next visit is indeed a contrast. The room is stuffy, hermetically sealed, the shades half down, there is even an electric heater, by the side of which sits a hypersensitive, apprehensive gentleman in a flowered dressing gown. We note that although he looks thoroughly prostrated, with a pinched, white face, he is neatly shaven and has a cheerful handkerchief in his pocket. He tells us that this April he has been down in a malarial region and had some quinine dosing. He has used considerable alcohol and tobacco. Yesterday he got overheated and felt chilled afterwards, and about midnight was wakened with sneezing, which, strangely enough, did not relieve him. He felt a stoppage at the bridge of his nose, with burning, and this morning when the acrid watery discharge started running from his right nostril, like tap water, it did not relieve the burning. His upper lip was fairly scalded by the slimy discharge, but in spite of that his nose feels totally stopped up, so that he cannot lie down. By him is a glass of hot water from which he sips frequently, which relieves him, for his throat burns between the swallows (Aconite, Capsicum). He aches all over. This morning he tried to go up to the next floor but was much worse ascending. Nearly every April one of these colds catches him, he says. You do not need to be told that this case calls for Arsenicum.

Our third visit is to a portly gentleman who has lived not wisely but too well. Carbo Vegetabilis is sitting by the open window, fanning himself diligently with the newspaper while tucking in the blanket about his knees. He tells us in a rough, deep voice, which fails on use, that he has not been well since an acute infection a year ago.

The day before yesterday he got his feet wet, which started the trouble, and then hurried to an appointment and got chilled and sweaty. Last night he could hardly speak, but it did not hurt him. (He stops to cough three times in succession and then sneezes.) Cough ends in a sneeze (Agaricus, Anacardium, Badiaga, Belladonna, Senega). 'I am a great sneezer', he said, and stopped to belch a bit. 'But lots of the time I'm ineffectual at it. This warm, moist weather I cough night and day, but worst about midnight. I am sorry it is so cold for you here, doctor. Too bad this 'glowing coals' in my chest can't warm up my knees!'

We shall have two visits at our next call. Mrs Hepar Sulphuricum and her neighbour, Mr Kali Iodatum. 'I rode on a bus in that high west wind yesterday, doctor, with my niece, Aconite. She got a violent cold from it.

I hoped to escape because I was so well bundled up as usual, but I took off my glove to find my money; you know I never can uncover, even a hand or foot, without catching cold. Or it may have been when my hat blew off I got it, for my head is so sensitive, like Aunt Psorinum. I have been all in a sweat since, and so irritable from the pain I am on the point of fainting. And I am hungry, yet worse if I eat. When I swallow, pains like splinters go into my ears (Nitric Acid). But hot drinks help, especially lemonade or anything acid. Early this morning I coughed horribly. They say I moaned before every one for fear of the pain, and though it rattled I couldn't seem to bring anything up. Oh, don't press the bones of my face, doctor, or feel the sore throat glands; I do hate being touched, and before you go, do look in on K. I.'

He is one of these open-air people, yet his cold is worse from it. He runs a subnormal temperature, has drenching night sweats, and is emaciating. He has had that obstinate cough ever since his pneumonia. He raises copious green, salty sputum, or a sort of soapsuds, and keeps trying to sneeze, but when he does it is like a convulsion and his eyes get puffy as a toad. The discharge, mostly from his right nostril, is copious, though the head feels stuffy (Arsenicum) and is cold (how hot his half brother Iodum is!). The cold has stopped the discharge and I fear sinusitis or antrum trouble. His headache is awful at 3 a.m.

We have time for only one more visit to the arch enemy of Hepar and K. I. He has succumbed to the wet weather. 'It doesn't matter whether it is hot or cold', he says, 'or it may have been a draft. Last night I was sick, creeping chills, cold, sticky sweat which did not relieve me, pain in the limbs, stiff neck, couldn't bear the heat of the bed, nor to lie on my right side. I got up and tried to sit by the radiator, but that was worse than ever (Antimonium Crud. and Pulsatilla). No, doctor, my slimy, acrid discharge is not watery this time, but yellowish. My throat stings worse on swallowing, which I have to do continually, there is so much saliva. Don't come near to look at my tongue – my breath is so offensive. I feel as though my mouth was made of metal and I could not stop my racking cough until I smoked. Indeed, my wife said I kept on coughing while asleep. I wish I could ward off a cold like my daughter, Biniodide.'

Let me add a briefer outline of a dozen of my favourite remedies in colds. Ammonium Carb. for plump, nervous blondes or old people, with its winter catarrhs, aversion to water, worse at the menses, acrid watery coryza with its dry mouth which suffocates by night, with its waking in a sneezing spell in the morning, and its violent coughing at 3 a.m. Not to mention its septic sore throat with bluish offensive mucus. Remember it in colds that go down to the bronchi. Then Capsicum again, a blonde, obese and chilly, with peppery, smarting pharynx (Caladium, Senega); drinking makes her shiver between the shoulderblades; when she coughs, her head would fly to pieces if she did not grasp it. Urine spurts with the cough (Ambrosia, Bromium, Cantharis, Causticum, Phosphorus, Natrum Mur., Pulsatilla, Staphysagria). Carboneum Sulph., common lamp-black, you must not forget, nor Corallium Rub., with its longing for acids, its mucus like melted tallow which spots the linen, its violence and 'minute gun' cough with suspension of breathing.

In the early stages of colds remember not only Camphor, Aconite, Ferrum, Phosphorus, Nux Vomica, Bryonia and Gelsemium (which, strangely enough, is not mentioned in the third degree in all Kent's repertory on coryza), but also Dioscorea, which begins with dry smarting throats into the ears, hacking cough and abdominal cramps with the cold, worse doubling up, better straightening out. In the last stages comes Pulsatilla for the ripe cold, often needing Kali Sulph. to finish it off; Kali Iod. or Kali Mur. or Sanguinaria or Sulphur or one of the nosodes will finish it off. If a cough persists, especially a dry one, remember Agaricus, Conium, Cuprum, Drosera, Hyoscyamus, Ignatia.

Another on my list is Lac Caninum. It alternates in the nose as well as the throat, with thick, white acrid discharge, worse at night, worse resting. Its colds often begin and end with menses, as do Graphites, Mag. Carb. and Zinc, also Ammonium Carb., Kali Carb. and Hyoscyamus. The nocturnal nasal discharge of Lac Caninum stains the pillow yellow-green.

Two metals should be more used than they are – Manganum (coryza worse in the evening, better lying on the back, with marked hoarseness); Zinc, also left-sided and worse in the afternoon or evening, with sudden attacks and intolerable pain at the nose root. Staphysagria you will know. Bland, one-sided thick discharge. The patient is humiliated by his cold, and vice versa catches cold from the effects of emotion. In stuffy colds with great dryness, nothing surpasses Sticta. Headaches before discharge comes, constant blowing of the nose (Teucrium) but no discharge, and in infants Sambuca, dry snuffles with sweat on waking and suffocating cough, worse from fruit and light. Remember also what Chelidonium will do for cold. Bromium in protracted colds. Iodum, Calcarea Sulph., Sabadilla, Sanguinaria, Chlorine are all wonderful remedies.

Let me suggest a few remedies to be further tried out. Aralia Racemosa (*Homoeopathic Recorder*, 1921, Dr Hutchinson): keynote, expectoration difficult to detach but comes up easily. Chromico-kali-sulph. (*New, Old and Forgotten Remedies*): chronic rhinitis. Quillaya Saponaria (Dewey, *Practical Homoeopathic Therapeutics*, page 57, also

Lilienthal). For beginning colds with very sore throat: Penthorum Sedoides (*New, Old and Forgotten Remedies*, page 444, also Dewey). Plantago Major, Selenium and Tellurium need further verification.

Cough and Company

I was educated by Pierre Schmidt. He used to say, 'When you do the Kent *Repertory*, study mind first, generals second, and cough third.' I was a young thing – that was many years ago – and I thought, 'Why cough third?', but now I know why.

The most handy thing, aside from the repertories and one's own knowledge of the materia medica, is that little gem, Lee and Clark's little repertory on *Cough*. It is what Bell's *Diarrhoea* is to diarrhoea. Also, if you are a user of Boger's *Card Repertory*, you will find one-third of the cards in his box are pertinent to cough. That is amazing – cough is quite a subject.

Every remedy in the materia medica, practically, has cough, so how are you going to know what kind of cough? What symptoms do you need to guide you?

I have a British husband and he came to me the other day and said, 'Woman, I have a cough. Give me something for it or I shall go to the allopath.' I said, 'What kind of cough have you, dear?' and he replied, 'Begging your pardon, a hell of a cough.'

You cannot find that in the repertory, and yet there are certain remedies which have a hell of a cough, and I never want to go out on an acute house visit without them. It is really beginning at the end to tell you what I consider those few remedies to be, but certainly one of them is Belladonna.

I can think of two cases in which the coughing was so dreadful I really thought one old lady, who had a little aneurysm, would burst something if we did not stop it. She had been coughing for hours before she called for me, and when I finally got there she was in such a continuous spasm of coughing, I think an allopath would have given her chloroform. I did not even look at her. I went into the bag – I could tell by the sound – and got Belladonna 50M, and two minutes later she said, 'Oh, well, that is the first time I haven't coughed like that in six hours.' So you want always to carry Belladonna for some of these perfectly frightful coughs.

Then I had a small boy whose family telephoned me one morning. Literally he had coughed every sixty seconds all night, and the whole house had been up – just 'Bing, bing, bing, bing, bing, bing!' You know what that is the minute they begin to cough, and there were practically no symptoms of consequence except the sound of that sharp repeating. He had no cold or fever, felt perfectly well, could not get his breath, and just kept on coughing and coughing – dry and unproductive.

I looked at him and asked, 'What did you want to eat today?'

His mother laughed and said, 'He has been impossible. He won't eat anything. He went into the pantry and grabbed a jar of anchovies, which we don't let him eat, and ate them, and then went and got a box of salt crackers and ate them in between his 'Bing, bing, bing'.

The homoeopath knows that Corallium Rubrum 'craves salty things'. The poor child had one other symptom that I got out of him, and which is in the book: 'Sensation as though a draught of air goes through your head and chills your air passages when you breathe'. That child, again inside of ten minutes after a 10M dose of Corallium Rubrum, stopped his dreadful 'Bing, bing, bing!' This is another remedy to carry around with you.

Some of the worst coughs I have ever seen, curiously enough, needed Ignatia. I had a charming French lady patient, of most uncertain age, daintily dressed and so delightful, and I found her children had spoiled her. She told me that she coughed every night, chiefly, but pretty much also all the day, and that it had such a spasm.

She never coughed when she came to my office, and I couldn't make her cough. I said, 'Please, madam, will you cough?' She replied, 'But I can't.' 'Do you really cough as badly as you think you do?' The daughter-in-law said, 'It is just terrible how she coughs.'

I tried to get out of her something about herself, and said, 'Why don't you cough when you come to my office?' 'I don't know', she said, 'I don't want you to see me at a disadvantage.'

And I thought, 'My goodness, she doesn't have to cough. How foolish – I should have given it right away, but I didn't,' for she had said, 'The cough simply strangles me and I almost vomit.' I was in a hurry and did a little 'rapid-firing', and gave a dose of Cuprum. That has 'Lovely spoiled ladies and spasmodic coughs', and I sent her home feeling proud of myself. The next day the family said, 'Mama is terrible! She coughed all night again.'

Then I remembered she did not cough when she came to see me because she did not want to make a bad impression, and I sent her Ignatia 50M, one dose. She had been coughing like this for nearly two weeks, but never coughed again.

Then of course there are the coughs that are quite desperate, that bark and choke, and want to have three or four pillows, and crave hot drinks, and that sound like sawing through a board. Spongia will often bring peace in the household with those. That is another of my "hell of a remedy"s.

But my good husband did not need any of those. As he would not tell me any symptoms, I stuck around and listened to him, and he sounded like somebody ringing a bronze gong when he coughed, a most terrific metallic noise. How a human chest can make it, I do not know. He said he had no other symptoms whatsoever. He loves beer, and I said, 'For you, Kali Bichromicum.' He took it and his cough went away, so he did not have to go to the allopath!

Now, to come back from these 'terrific remedies', what is it really we want to know about coughs in order to be able to prescribe for them?

I have many suburban patients who write or telephone in and expect me to perform a little miracle out of the case they have at home. I say, 'Get the patient to the phone. Let me hear her cough.' The one thing I want with a cough is to hear it, and over the phone you can often get an instant reaction to something from the sound of that cough.

I should like to mention the sound of certain coughs I know. I wish I could imitate them. There are the people that go 'H-h-h-e-ah-he-he-ah' – so feeble they have not got enough pep to cough. You say, 'For goodness sake, come across and cough', and they do it and do it and do it, and you worry about them. I worry about them much more than the people who need Cuprum and Spongia. Those mean little 'Aheh-heh' coughs – they often just vanish with a dose of Tuberculinum or Bacillinum. Those little coughs are very nasty, and I do not know any so-called acute remedies which will reach them as well as those nosodes will.

Then there are the terrible barks for which you give Aconite – croupy barks, a different sound, again, from Spongia; they sound almost animal. Belladonna or Aconite for the croupy or metallic sounds. Spongia sounds woody, like a woodwind, instead of like an animal – to me, that is. I suppose everybody hears things differently, but you get a perfectly definite sense as you do in the realm of smell. Some doctors come into a house and can smell diphtheria. They do not have to see the patient. Certain diseases do smell like that.

I was called one day to a tonsillitis, got that smell and took a throat culture. The Board of Health said it was negative, but the patient got a remedy which is great for diphtheria.

Have you heard Ipecacuanha patients cough? They cough with a wheeze mixed in, a kind of tension or tightness. In contrast, Antimony coughs with a rattling and feeble cough and can do nothing about it. One cough I like to hear is the Iodine cough. It is as hard as Phosphorus and as violent sometimes. All the Iodine things are violent – as violent almost as Corallium and yet it has a roughness, like somebody playing badly. Take Bromium – that is a curious combination of the hardness of Phosphorus and the roughness of the halogens. It is a very distinctive cough – 'concussed' is the word I would use for it.

If you get those things into your soul, it saves you a lot of time and you do not have to repertorize. So, I like to hear the patient cough, if I can. Then what do I want to know if I cannot hear the patient cough? Usually patients will just hand it to you, if you say, 'Tell me about your cough.' They come out in the most charming way and tell you the symptoms you need to repertorize, or what you need to know – if you are blessed with good homoeopathic patients. You have to work much harder when you get an allopathically-trained patient. They tell you everything you do not want to know and nothing that you do want to know. With them I ask 'What is queer and strange about your cough?', and they look at me as though I were crazy, and begin to think what is queer about it and tell me some little trifle. One said, 'I cough chiefly when I laugh. It is perfectly silly. I can't go in company, I can't go anywhere socially. I laugh and go into one of these awful coughs.' That was helpful. It was interesting even though the patient had not realized it.

Then we need to know the modalities. A strong modality is a great comfort, and very often you can get quite a few very distinct modalities from patients, once you have taught them what it is you want to know.

Another thing that particularly helps me in prescribing for coughs are the concomitants of the cough. Very often patients have some little thing they do not connect with the nature of their cough. A child will get a fit of coughing in your office and not cry but shed some tears while coughing, or get red in the face while coughing. A woman will tell you that she spurts a little urine when she coughs. Those concomitants are priceless rubrics for picking a really exact remedy.

Then there are some very troublesome coughs, which I call terminal coughs, and which come after you have cleared up some sort of illness. I find I usually do not need a specific remedy for these. They need the patient's constitutional, if you know what it is or if you can determine it, or one of the nosodes. Tuberculinum, Bacillinum, Medorrhinum, or even sometimes – if you know the cause – Influenzinum, will clear a terminal cough long after an influenza.

I could make a much longer list of the remedies for coughs. Instead I will tell you what remedies I would put in my cough kit, if I carried one. I would include Antimonium Tart. Every homoeopath knows why.

Alumina for the horrid little dry hacks, where they have a wad of phlegm low down and have uvulas that are too long. Belladonna, and of course Bryonia. Everybody thinks of it first for coughs, yet Bryonia does not get cough alone – only those going in pneumonia. For just a plain cough, Bryonia is not much good to me. Bromium if it has hoarseness and a feeling of fumes in the throat. Have you ever smelled hydrocyanic acid? It hits you in the back – that is, in the nasopharynx, and Bromium does that, burns and hurts. Of course, Carbo Veg. and Causticum. You can hear the Causticum – you hear it scrape the trachea, the way you hear something scrape along a pipe. Cina – how I love Cina in the naughty children. Rub the end of their nose and they fly in a tantrum and will not let you examine them, and cough their heads off, and throw up about it.

Coccus Cacti – I rarely have any success with this. Corallium, of course; Chromium – beautiful cases of Chromium. Cuprum – you could not do without it; Drosera, Hepar Sulph., Hyoscyamus, Ignatia, Iodum, Ipecac. Kali Carb. – my cough kit would not have Kali Carb. in it; for pneumonia, yes, cough with asthma, yes, but not just plain cough. Kreosotum, sometimes. I have had a couple of cases in men of a syphilitic background with a great deal of catarrh, in whom Kreosotum was brilliant, but I have not personally seen it often.

Strangely enough, Lachesis has cured many a tough cough for me and so has Arsenicum, although one does not connect either of them particularly with that. Mercurius, sometimes, though I think I see less than some people do; Phosphorus, very often; Pulsatilla, universally – no one would believe the number that yield to that. Rumex and Sanguinaria are among the big polychrests and constitutionals. I would say I had cured more coughs with Lycopodium and Sepia than with any of the other big constitutional remedies; and finally Spongia, Stannum, Squilla, not often, but when you want it, how beautiful it is! Dr Roberts said he never went out without Cantharides and Squilla.

Finally, Sulphur, the old standby, which has cured many an old, stubborn cough after I have tried to prescribe for it and have not succeeded.

Thuja Occidentalis

Thuja, one of Hahnemann's favourite discoveries, is one of the most difficult remedies for the beginner to learn. Its symptoms are more mixed and scattered than most of the remedies, and its personality only emerges after long delving and experience. The remedy Thuja is made from the *Arbor vitae*, the Tree of Life. Its common name is the white cedar and it belongs to the Coniferae, closely related to the Euphorbiaceae. The other members of its tribe which are used in homoeopathy are *Sabina juniperus*, *Abies* of two varieties, *Pinus sylvestris* and *Pix liquida* and *terebinthina*. *Taxus baccata*, the yew, is a close ally.

The dark, conical silhouette of the *Arbor vitae* is to be seen in swamps and along rocky banks and through the stone pastures of New England. You will find it in Italy, and elsewhere, surrounding pools, and in formal gardens like the Villa d'Este. It often looks into water narcissistically. The cypress (*Cupressus*), which is so closely allied to it, is connected in our minds with stately grief and might be called the Tree of the Dead. Such cosmic gamut from life to death is indeed within the range of this great evergreen.

Its form is conical, its buds are ovoid. Along its stem are resinous callosities which look like oozing warts, and when Thuja is needed as a remedy the patient will be all curves. The grossly fat suggest its use, those with pendulous abdomens and heavy breasts, triple chins and piano legs. Those with low thyroid, lymphatic constitutions, given to troubles of the skin, hair and nails, and of all oval organs like the glands, ovaries, prostate, testicles, spleen, etc. It has sway over similar tumours, polyps, papillomata and spongy or fig warts (not the flat and smooth warts of Sepia or Dulcamara). It is characterized, like the tree itself, by oozing and greenness and odours, and by an exuberance of proliferation. The one word characterizing Thuja is *excess*, a surplus of life, badly organized and badly edited.

To understand Thuja one must study Hahnemann's theory of chronic disease and his three much-maligned miasms. Thuja, as one of the greatest polychrests from the vegetable sphere, includes in its nature all three of the miasms. As Mercury is to the syphilitic or ulcerative trend, and as

Sulphur is to the psoric or nervous-functional trend (commonly called scrofulous), so Thuja is to the sycotic or proliferative-inflammatory diathesis. With the sycotic nosode Medorrhinum it is called the Mother of Pus and Catarrh. It is essentially a left-sided remedy and hence a feminine one, although of course it is also frequently indicated in the male. It typifies the hydrogenoid constitution of von Grauvogl.

The word sycosis comes from the Greek word for fig. In Hahnemann's time, more than now, the after-effects of suppressed gonorrhoea were characterized by fig warts, and Thuja is our great remedy for the effects of suppression of gonorrhoea, whether in the individual or from generations back. It has power to correct states of the system which obstruct the curative action of other remedies, especially in conditions where warts are a concomitant symptom. It has power over the dissolution of fluids caused by perverted lymphatic secretions. In this lies the secret of its sphere in connection with vaccinosis, since the smallpox vaccine is prepared by using the calf, the product of calf lymph being introduced beneath the protective human skin. Thuja is not only similar to the effects of vaccination, but also to many cases of smallpox itself. It is, however, especially suitable when repeated vaccinations by the usual method have not taken, and for the bad results of vaccination appearing long afterward in the form of neuralgias, skin trouble, intestinal troubles and growths. It has a special fitness where there is a history of animal poisonings of any kind, particularly if these are not recent. The Thuja patient, like all sycotics, tends to die suddenly, on the golf course or at work, or after a 'successful' operation. They do not linger, as do the psorics.

Thuja shares with other sycotic remedies the hurry and the worry so characteristic of Medorrhinum, Argentum Nitricum, etc. However, even though it is excessive, it is also quiet and furtive. It desires to be alone and is averse to being touched or approached. It is slow in speech and confused in mind, the latter being relieved by sitting up, and it has a long thoughtfulness about trifles, which is reminiscent of Zincum. As so often in our remedies, it also has extreme talkativeness with shifting from one thing to another, like Lachesis. Mental embroidery and proliferation is ever the enemy of continuity. The Thuja patient has too much matter and too little form, the opposite of Silica. The Thuja patient is oversensitive, not to pain, but weeps from music, like Natrum Mur. He is scrupulous about trifles, though grossly oblivious to larger things. He is discontented and dissatisfied, as are all those who have not order in their mentality. She may be ugly to her husband or her mother, especially during pelvic pain. She is quarrelsome and sulky and very jealous. Thuja is angry at jests. Salacity runs through the remedy, not with the exhibitionistic tendencies of

Hyoscyamus but with a kind of impotent delight in the lascivious. Like all sycotic remedies, there is an element of deception, cheating and lying in our Thuja.

Many mentally handicapped people of a fat, lax, slobbering type need Thuja (the violently insane and murderous run to the syphilitic remedies; the neuroses to the psoric; but the perversions and imbecilities to the sycotic). Thuja, even when not insane, has curious fixed ideas, such as that she is brittle, her limbs made of glass which would easily break, or that a leg or an arm are wooden, or that she is pregnant, when she is not, or that something is alive and moving in her abdomen (like Crocus). She feels as though the soul and body were separated; this feeling is relieved in the open air; as if she were under the influence of a superior power (compare Lachesis and Anacardium), or as if another were thinking for her. She has a sense of floating or levitation, as if she were not wholly in her body (indeed, the excess of etheric leaves little room or access for the ego). She is apprehensive for the future, dreams of the dead and dead bodies, of flying and falling and dying, and of amorous adventure.

In appearance the Thuja patient is fleshy and rounded (or ovoid), with lax musculature and large glands, dark predominantly but may be light-haired; the hair is strong and dry (not wiry like Medorrhinum), splits easily and falls from the head and brows uniformly (real baldness comes under the syphilitic remedies). There is an excess of hair on the face and body. This remedy is, in my opinion, the best for the removing of excess hair where it should not be. The nails are brittle or thick, deformed, tough. Thuja has the power to soften abnormally hard things. The Thuja patient is exhausted and soft, has a waxy, greasy, shiny face, a cachectic look, a greyish complexion, dark under the eyes, spidery veins, pimples between the brows, freckles and blotches, a spotted, dirty appearance, de-pigmented or over-pigmented areas (chloasmata of pregnancy), hair on the skin of the face, dilated or contracted pupils, naevi, warts, epitheliomata, broad, fleshy noses (the psoric nose is long and pointed, the syphilitic retroussé or pug). There is a sensation of heat in the face without redness, sweat or thirst.

In general, Thuja suits patients who have never been well since they were vaccinated, who lose consciousness temporarily on sitting up, who are chilly but not cold, who have pulsations all over the body and a tendency to neuralgia. Their pains are wandering or tearing and tend to extend, they radiate upward and backward, with frequent urination during pain. These patients tend to proud flesh, scars, livid red spots left over after injuries, their pain is in the muscles and not in the tendons, they have lipomas and tumours, especially those that bleed when touched.

Their discharges are green (but thinner than Pulsatilla, who have a tendency to chronic catarrh after exanthems). Their discharges have odours like fish brine or herring brine, or garlic, or honey, or sweet and pungent, or smell like burnt horn, feathers or sponge.

The main modalities are as follows. *Aggravation:* 3 a.m. and 3 p.m., early morning, night, overheating, sun, light, closing the eyes, warmth, afternoon, narcotics, walking, extending the limbs, letting the limbs hang down, lying on the left side, touch, sometimes motion, damp, cold air, the waxing moon, the heat of the bed, warm rooms, uncovering, draft, ascending, riding, coition, change of position, eating, excessive use of tea, after breakfast, sours, fats, onions, tobacco, during menses and also before. *Relief:* from being alone, open air, head backward or looking up, pressure, cold, rubbing and scratching, drawing the limbs up, and sometimes motion, sometimes local heat.

Some of the principal particular symptoms are as follows.

Vertigo
Worse closing the eyes (Lachesis, Theridion).

Headache
As of a nail, in small spots (Ignatia, Anacardium); as of a tight hoop; worse in left temple; tearing over left brow; from sex excess and overheating; better for pressure, air, head back; worse for warmth, one-sided; from malar region back to occiput (opposite of Spigelia); numb head.

Eyes
Myopia; lid tumours; styes; objects tremble; floating black spots, or green stripes; as if cold air were blowing through eye; tearing pain in left eye better by heat; sclerotitis.

Nose
Warts; eruptions on wings; green, bloody coryza.

Ears
Hum in left ear and brain; cramping pain in the ear; polyps.

Face
Boring in left zygoma, better for touch.

Mouth
Twitching left upper lip; visible papillae on tongue; warts on tongue; ranula; varicosities of the throat; tartar; sensitive teeth; teeth break at the gum; black mark at the gum line; caries of sides, not roots or crowns.

Gastrointestinal
Desires cold drink before eating; thirsty in afternoon; big spleen; sore, red, pouting navel; stool recedes; torpid constipation; hard black balls or large stool habitually; several loose stools a day (Pulsatilla). Diarrhoea from vaccination, coffee or onions; gurgling like water from bung of barrel; grass-green stools; ileus knotty, lumps protruding from abdomen; watery diarrhoea after breakfast; left hernia; piles worse sitting; fissured anus; condylomata; pain in rectum during stool.

Genito-urinary
Urinary complaints; gonococcal prostatitis; chancroid; retracted testicle; knotty prostate; thin, green, scalding discharge during urination; gleet (last drop); hydrocele; orchitis with squeezing in the left testicle; left kidney pain extending to bladder; retention of urine with painful urge, with sensation as if the urine passed; trickling and dribbling; sensitive vagina; inner thighs red and excoriated; bloody, watery or green gonorrhoeal discharge, better by motion; tearing pain in left ovary extending to the thighs, worse during menses; burning, bursting in the ovary; menses early, short, scanty; foetus too active; nipples retracted.

Chest
Asthmas in sycotic children (Medorrhinum, Natrum Sulph.); bronchitis chronic, or after acute disease, with oppression of the chest, loose cough, copious green or white morning sputum; persistent, dry hacking cough from throat irritation (Thuja cleans up more chronic bronchitis than any other remedy I know); breast lumps after vaccination.

Back
Stiff from the left nape to the ear.

Extremities
Post-gonococcal rheumatism relieved by cold and motion; cracking of joints; restless knees; painful soles; myositis ossificans; elephantiasis; fingertips cold, as if dead; flesh as if beaten from bones; tingling of the left middle finger; sciatica; left paralysis; brown mottling of the dorsa of the hands; hang nails; offensive foot sweat.

Sleep
Insomnia, worse after 3 a.m.; takes long time to wake up.

Chill

Fever and sweat. Chilly in the morning; chill starts in thigh; chill with yawning; shuddering on uncovering; copious sweat on falling asleep; sweat on undressing; sweat on all but the head (opposite of Silica); sweat only on uncovered parts; sweat during sleep; sweat stains yellow; one-sided sweat; thirst before sweat stage.

Skin

Eruptions on covered parts only; livid spots remain after eruptions; absorbs proud flesh and scars; blisters worse for uncovering; zona worse on labia or prepuce; cephalomata; cauliflower or coxcomb excrescences; pale polypi; lipomas; annular, scaly blotches. (Thuja prevents pitting in acne or smallpox.) Warts: fig, seed, jagged, pedunculated, divided into parts with broad base, burning, spongy, soft, bleeding. Strawberry marks, birth marks, angiomas.

Relationships

Complementary to Arsenicum Alb., Medorrhinum, Natrum Mur., Natrum Sulph., Sabina, Silica. Goes in series: Pulsatilla, Silica, Fluoric Acid, Thuja; or Arsenicum Alb., Thuja, Tarentula.

Related to Nitric Acid, Pulsatilla, Staphysagria, Agaricus and, according to Boger, also Mercurius. Compare with Castor – the beaver who lives on the bark of resinous trees. Follows Cannabis Sativa and Staphysagria. (Note that Arsenicum Alb. is syphilitic and psoric, but not sycotic.)

Teste groups Thuja with Platinum, Bismuth, Castor and Squilla.

Such is a glimpse of the *Arbor vitae*, which is supposed to have specific antibacterial action. It is not used nearly enough in those of its spheres which are not directly related to genito-urinary troubles. It is to be thought of with the nosodes for frequent and fundamental cure.

Remedies in Hypotension

Why is it that the world belongs to the chilly? If one person in a room minds the draught the other ninety-nine must swelter. Similarly, what a dither there is about hypertension, and how few really pay attention to the low blood pressure cases.

What are the symptoms of low blood pressure? Exhaustion, easy fatigability, fainting, dizziness, the feeling of being weak in the knees, numbness, pallor, chilliness, inability to concentrate.

What does orthodox medicine offer for this often-neglected complaint? Vitamins, tonics, liver in various forms, salt, coffee and stimulants, food, especially meat. Even strychnine, or adrenal extract.

Differential diagnosis including laboratory work is essential. Has the patient Addison's disease, is he anaemic, has he heart trouble, is he diabetic, has she dieted herself into a decline, is she pre-tubercular, has she thyroid or liver disturbance? Is some psychic or human relations factor at the bottom of it? Has she been depleted by long loss of vital fluids?

Common sense and a wholesome regimen will solve a certain percentage of such difficulties. We all use rest, hydrotherapy, diet and exercise.

The most powerful stimulant to the human body, however, is that exact but puissant imponderable: the simillimum. Take the hypotensive's 'chronic case' and give him the indicated constitutional remedy. Unfortunately, many of these patients show few distinctive symptoms, and mainly only common ones. However, the persistent use of the two most valuable words in homoeopathy – 'What else?' – will elicit some salient trifles.

A few grand remedies will deal with many of these cases. Lycopodium – when the patient is irritable, of a uric acid diathesis, with a liverish hue or discoloured brownish patches on the skin, with craving for sweets, rumbling flatulence, 4–6 p.m. or a.m. aggravations, relief from motion, a mental giant who is slipping into innocuous desuetude. Natrum Mur. – if she eats salt out of the salt-cellar, faints in the hot sun, keeps everything in, weeps in secret, has headaches at 10 a.m. China – where there is dizziness, fainting, a skipping heart, everything eaten turns to gas which will not go up or down, a finicky appetite, noises in the ears, a history of loss of vital fluids. Sepia – when there is a yellowish tint with dark circles under the eyes, a general dragged-down feeling, pulsation throughout the body, desire for sour things, relief from violent exercise (to their own surprise), an empty, all-gone feeling in the epigastrium before lunch, liver spots, indifference to life and loved ones.

Of the nosodes, Tuberculinum and Psorinum are the most helpful. Calc. Phos. in exhausted, fast-growing young people, or Kali. Phos. in neurotic older women. Picric Acid, or indeed many of the acids when indicated. Stannum, if there be catarrh and neuralgias with midday aggravation. Even our frequent friend Gelsemium or its rival Cocculus, or Causticum, despite being an ammonium, may serve.

Study the blood chemistry of your low tension patients. Often their chlorides will be out, their cholesterols low; their nitrogen metabolism may be disturbed, contrary to what one might have supposed.

At all events, in a field where little is known or done, the homoeopathic remedy can vitalize the patient to a remarkable degree and fit him to lose, more or less joyously, another button in life's wringer!

Remedies in Backache

A bone specialist came to me and said, 'You know, there is something in this homoeopathy, but I haven't the time to study it. I am just going out of business if somebody doesn't teach me how to cope with backaches. For some reason, doctors refer their backaches to me, because I am a bone specialist, and I am fed up with it.'

I kidded him and tried to get him to come to the homoeopathic summer school, and he said, 'My Lord, I am second in the department at the hospital and busy as can be. I have no time to go. Why don't you write me out an epitome of the symptoms calling for the best remedies for different kinds of backaches?' We had a good laugh and then I said, 'All right, I will write you a paper on backaches, and you can tell me how you get on with it.'

If you are going to treat backache, you have got to know whether the backache is caused by fallen metatarsal arches; or some deep varicose vein trouble; or pure posture (or rather, impure posture), or whether it is caused by a slipped sacroiliac; or whether it is caused by a fibroid; or a tipped womb; or whether it is caused by kidney trouble; or whether it is caused by referred pain from any of a number of possible conditions, such as kidney stones, gallstones, stomach cancer of the posterior wall, colon cancer, or tumour, or terrific mucous colitis, because colon pain definitely refers up higher, which is very bewildering sometimes; or by heart pain, which often goes through the back without pain in the front – they come to you with a heck of a pain in the back, and if you are not smart, you will think it is something else; or backache from a leftover shingles several years ago – an unsuspected cause.

And of course there is pleurisy, and there are pneumonic backaches, which usually are of a different type. These are usually so sharp that they cannot be classed as backaches. They are violent pain, and you can probably think up many other possible differential diagnoses.

Of the actual types of backache, lumbago is possibly the commonest one, whatever that means. It may come from a wetting, or a strain, or a chilling, or over-exercise. It makes old men of young ones!

Then there are the various sacroiliac backaches. There are backaches according to location, some of the most troublesome ones, of the nape of the neck with extension into the shoulders, which may or may not be due to displacement of the cervical vertebrae, or to sheer nerve tension at the back of the neck.

Then there are the dorsal backaches; the intrascapular distresses; the tight, burning intraneuro-subscapular.

Then we have the big muscle, the big latissimus dorsi and the lumbar ones, the sacral ones, and last but not least, the coccygeal pains.

Now, the main remedies. If anybody asked me to make up a little kit of the most frequently needed backache remedies I should put in the following, which I regard as indispensable: Bryonia, Kali Carb., Natrum Mur., Nux Vomica, Rhus Tox., Sepia, and Sulphur. These seven will cover a wide proportion of backaches.

In my secondary list I would put Aesculus Hippocastanum. In the old days they put coral around the baby's neck to keep it from coughing at night, and a bit of amber around to keep it from crouping, and you carried a horse chestnut in your pocket to prevent the piles. Farmers will also tell you that the horse chestnut is very good for what ails you in the back when you have been 'spadin too hard'. Aesculus is a wonderful remedy for sacroiliac strain – which you may think is Rhus Tox. or Sepia, but which is not right-sided, or sacroiliac backache which is relieved by standing. Aesculus, of course, also has a concomitant of piles. If you can find that, that points you to it.

Another remedy that would go in the subsidiary list is Antimonium Tart. You all know the story of the smallpoxes. They have a backache with a capital B; and some of the worst backaches, particularly in acute diseases, are Antimonium Tart.

In the second category you would want to have Calc. Phos. In my haste I have missed many back troubles, sacroiliacs, neuralgics and sciatics that should have been Calc. Phos., and which I did not spot until the second prescription. So never forget Calc. Phos. in the nape of the neck and cervical regions, as well as in the sacroiliac regions.

Also in acute things, the queen of backaches, Eupatorium. When grippe cases do not complain of muscular aches, do not complain primarily of headaches, but of backaches and eye aches, and you later find that they also have terrific thirst while chilling, and pains in the bones rather than the muscles, there is Eupatorium on a silver platter.

One that may be unexpected in my supernumerary list is Magnesia Carb. for some of these back things. It is one of my pet remedies. We all know the Mag. Carb. patient – the typical orphanage kid whom nobody loves, who is really pitiful, weak, emaciated, restless, has no place to hang his or her spiritual hat, and they have all sorts of back troubles relieved by motion. When you see back troubles relieved by motion, do not go leaping for the Rhus bottle. Look and see whether it may not be Magnesia Carb.

Also, curiously enough, in the intrascapular backaches, Phosphorus.

Sometimes when it is more a weakness, and the pains of weakness, if the other symptoms agree, particularly if there are leucorrhoeas or neuralgias, Stannum, where you cannot hold yourself up. And never forget the backache of Variolinum, which comes under the same category as the backache of Antimonium Tart.

Now just a few things about our main big seven. You all know a Bryonia lumbago when you see one. They take to their bed. They cannot move. They want pressure, something hard under the back and preferably cold, and they are thirsty and grumpy, and worse at nine or at three by the clock.

The Kali Carb. backaches are lower. They are sacral, and often go with menstrual difficulties. They are the kind where the patient says, 'My back is broken in two.' The pain goes down the back of the legs, with the typical Kali Carb. symptoms, the whimsical, difficult, fussy, fat, chilly, rather ticklish patient in both sexes, ticklish both in the soles of the feet and in the disposition.

Cimicifuga is terrific for pains in the nape of the neck going down into the shoulders; curiously, Natrum Mur. also has that distress in the back of the neck.

Natrum Mur. is a great standby for backache. They want pressure. They want to put a book behind them in the chair, a hard thing under them in the bed. They go around sitting in chairs with the backs of their hands flat on the sacrum, and you all know the Natrum Mur. characteristics that may well go with that.

Nux Vomica has the backache of the big muscles, all up and down the back, the latissimus dorsi and so on, usually from chilling; often, though, from overexertion followed by chilling, with the crankiness and the aggravation in the morning, until they get limbered up. Although motion does not help, getting going in the morning does. The relief from heat, the constipation, the impatience, the irritability, all come in here.

Then remember Bellis Perennis for what they call 'railroad spine'. The patient has been in an accident, was jolted and grabbed for something, stopping quickly, as in a near collision, and has pain all up and down the back. Bellis Perennis will do a lot for that, and sometimes it will help where a disc has been pressed upon – the compression fractures.

I would also mention that Zincum is a great pet for coccygeal pain, and often Hypericum.

I had a beautiful case of a terrible lumbago in an insurance agent who showed me such a picture of Nux Vomica that it was unbelievable. Nux Vomica 10M helped him handsomely and quickly over the lumbago, which he had had untreated for about two months.

Rhus Tox., of course. Do not forget that although Rhus Tox. is left-sided, a right-sided sacroiliac will respond brilliantly to it.

I once had a backache from falling off a horse, and went to an osteopath. It did not work. I went to a chiropractor. Nor did that. I got a belt. No help and an awful lot of expense. Finally, I went to my beloved Dr Stanton in New York, and he gave me Rhus Tox. 20M. No soap. I was getting a little fed up, so at the summer school I asked Dr Roberts, 'What do you do when Rhus Tox. is indicated and it doesn't help you?'

Old Dr Roberts looked at me in his slow way and said, 'You change the potency.' So I said, 'All right, Stanton gave me 20M. What do you give me?'

He gave me the 200c, and having had a sacroiliac for ten weeks, after two hours I did not have another one for about five years. That is very interesting. Your lovely high 20M to no effect, and a 200c of the same thing – quick!

Then there are the dreadful Sepia backaches from visceroptosis, with the bearing down, the washerwoman's backache, the ironer's backache, worse from using the arms, with all the symptoms of Sepia.

And our prize friend, Sulphur, who cannot get out of a chair without pushing and standing and waiting. I think more backaches in my practice have been helped by Sulphur than by any other remedy, but those are perhaps the pre-arthritic backaches, where an X-ray of the back would show you a certain amount of osteo-arthritis of the spine. Of course, we all have it as we get older, but Rhus Tox. is not the only remedy for the creaky rusty hinge. When they cannot get up out of the chair, and when they try to sit down and get within four inches and fall into the chair, think about Sulphur.

Remedies for the Relief of Pain and Muscle Spasm

In one sense this title is a profoundly unhomoeopathic one, but like many mistaken things it provides an opportunity to clarify a prevalent misunderstanding. The use of the law of similars is, like that of all true laws, cooperative with nature, a means to helping the whole man. Many people, both professional and lay, think that homoeopathy 'cures' or abolishes or acts upon single symptoms. This would be a strictly unhomoeopathic procedure and purely a palliative one, which orthodox medicine regularly employs, mostly according to the law of contraries. The law of similars takes account of the biological element in man, the susceptibility and reactive power of a living organism, as opposed to chemical reactions in a test-tube or laboratory. The totality of symptoms, expressing the individual patient's need for a specific remedial substance, is different from one or two symptoms. Only on a *totality* can curative prescribing be done.

The homoeopathic materia medica does contain remedies which act as pain killers, but never in the sense of dulling the patient's consciousness of pain, as do sedative or physiologically analgesic drugs. We all know that Hepar Sulph. relieves the excruciating hypersensitivity of a throbbing felon, if the modalities of Hepar are present; that Aconite, Coffea, Platina or Verbascum help neuralgia; that Colocynth or Magnesia Phos. will abate intestinal colic; that Belladonna or Lycopodium can ease renal colic, and that Chelidonium, Dioscorea or Nux Vomica allay the agony of gall stones when, and only when, the symptoms agree.

The only proper answer to the question, 'What remedies relieve pain and muscle spasm in arthritis?', is 'The *indicated* remedy'. It is not my purpose here to show how one may arrive at the most similar and hence indicated remedy. In chronic arthritis the constitutional remedy may be the best. In certain instances a nosode may be the opening gambit: Medorrhinum, if it is sub-acute, in the thick-set, robust, hurried, worried patients who suffer all day, can sleep all night, and are relieved by ice; or Tuberculinum, if there is great rigidity, even in sleep, aggravation after excertion, desire for change and novelty (even in their doctors), a family history of Tuberculosis, love of wind, craving for smoked things and the other symptoms peculiar to that remedy. In advanced cases where there has been a succession of remedies, such as cortisone, one may have to start with Sulphur or Nux Vomica, preferably in the 30c potency, to clear the field. Whatever remedies the patient has been taking must be stopped. If he cannot be persuaded to have fortitude, one can temporarily use a different anodyne.

The remedies most frequently useful for arthritic pain and muscle spasm are a somewhat unusual and surprising list. In incipient or early chronic arthritis, the statistics of my practice have shown that Natrum Muriaticum leads the list. This is interesting from many viewpoints. Arthritis is a disease characterized by looking backward, as well as rigidity, frustration and resentment. Lot's wife, you recall, looked back and was turned into a pillar of salt! I have found the second most frequent remedy in early arthritis to be Sulphur. Perhaps the third remedy in frequency is Rhus Toxicodendron, characterized by its fourfold modality: worse on first motion, relieved by motion after it gets going, until tired, when it is again aggravated, and the necessary rest (fourth stage) aggravates again from rest.

One of the great remedies in many homoeopaths' minds for arthritis is Kali Carbonica. This is one of the perilous remedies that can give shocking aggravations. Its whimsy, sensitivity to draft, ticklishness, concomitant constipation and indigestion, stitching pains and general cantankerousness identify it. The halogens, Fluoric Acid and Iodine, are salient remedies for the hot, restless arthritic patient of longer standing, when the symptoms agree. Lycopodium, that prince of polychrests, suits many arthritics: right-sided, warm, better by motion, worse 4 to 8 p.m., craving sweets, bilious and hypochondriac. One must never forget Calcarea Phosphorica, especially in arthritis of the neck and shoulder girdle, and Calcarea Fluorica. Iodum and Fluoric Acid are not alone in their relief from cold. Ledum and Guaiacum are to be considered here, and Kalmia after exposure to cold, where the pains go upward like Ledum, yet shift like Pulsatilla, and where there is heart involvement. In arthritis of the small joints, spindle fingers, think of Caulophyllum. Cimicifuga, (the black snake root, *Actea racemosa*) with its pains like electric shocks, its dreams of evil, its agitation, loquacity, its pain from hip to hip, and in the tendo Achilles, and its lumbago, should be remembered.

In connection with arthritis of the spine and the large muscles of the back, Nux Vomica leads in spasm. Bryonia and Aesculus need comparative study.

Colchicum, so frequently used in orthodox medicine, presents the specific picture of tender joints, shifting pain, worse by motion, small joints involved, averse to be approached or touched (like Arnica), usually with concomitant bloating of the abdomen like a drum.

Formica Rufa has pain in the joints accompanied with sweat (like Oxalic Acid), and with its pain in small spots with numbness, worse thinking of it, should be considered more often than it is.

In the dread arthritis deformans, Causticum leads, with its aggravations in good weather, its relief in bed, its restless legs, its facial warts, its undue sympathy and complaints from grief.

No proper monographs have been written on arthritis treated homoeopathically. The references to it in our literature are strange and confusing. Boger in his Synoptic Key, under arthritis deformans, gives eight remedies: Arsenicum Alb., Aurum, Causticum, Guaiacum, Hepar Sulph., Mercurius, Pulsatilla, Radium.

One great remedy noted for its sclerotic tendency, slow and stubborn pace, dour disposition and great desire to be stretched, which should perhaps be thought of more often in chronic arthritis, is Plumbum.

Lastly, may I say that in almost no disease are psychotherapy and diet more important than in arthritis, this disease of rigidity and despair.

Remedies in the Elderly

What is it to be old? There are two sides to this picture, as to all others. The physician does not need to cope with those who, wise with the wisdom of the decades, are mellow, serene, contented and still fascinated by the changing panorama of events. It is the less fortunate or less astute that are our problem – people who lose resistance, elasticity, speed and endurance, who become rigid, set and slow. Their bodies settle like a building; their senses dim, except that of taste; they become querulous, disapproving of the new and looking backward. The technical term is senility; the kinder and truer term is 'second childhood'. Let me suggest certain remedies which are also useful in the first, authentic childhood: Antimonium Tartaricum, Baryta Carbonica, Graphites, Lycopodium, Magnesia Carbonica, Sulphur and Zincum.

Many of the aged become careless of their appearance – the spotted vest, the soiled linen, the aversion to bathing, the stale odour. They sleep less and wake early; they become dry in skin; blemishes develop – moth patches, warts, naevi, little veins marble their sagging flesh, ridged and thickened, distorted and crumbling. They itch, sometimes without eruption – 'senile pruritis'. In men, sexual power may dwindle, with consequent loss of confidence. Women, after the climacteric, become stronger in health. The world, alas, is to the widows! Men develop prostatic symptoms: delay in urination, an inability which in ordinary medicine can require catheterization. Some folk become emaciated, with loss of subcutaneous fat (Kent, p. 1358 – Ambra Grisea, Baryta Carb., Iodum, Lycopodium, Secale, Silica). Others become unduly stout, either with fat deposited in muscles and omentum, or from water in the tissues – oedema. The teeth, like those of an old horse, show the aging process. Arteriosclerosis sets in, causing lack of memory ('In the aged', Kent, p. 40 – Ambra Grisea, Baryta Carb., Lycopodium, Phosphoric Ac.). Delusions are sometimes troublesome: Phosphorus does wonders for these. Dizziness is frequent ('In old people', Kent, p. 102 – Ambra Grisea, Baryta Carb., Phosphorus, Cuprum, Rhus Tox., Sinapis Nig.). The poor liver does its best to detoxify and store what cannot be eliminated by bowel or kidney, in faithful silence. The aged rarely remember to spare it extra burdens. There is poor oxidation

(Ammonium Carb., Carbo Veg., Sulphur). Premature aging has a special rubric (Kent, p. 1376 – Ambra Grisea, Ammonium Carb., Argentum Nit., Kali Carb., Lycopodium, Selenium).

The depletion remedies apply to the aged, notably the *acids*: Benzoic Acid, Formic Acid, Muriatic Acid, Nitric Acid, Oxalic Acid, Phosphoric Acid, Picric Acid, Sulphuric Acid. The plant world is a world of growth forces, and we should look to certain of the plant remedies for aid in the frail conditions towards the end of life. For instance, Arnica, Crataegus, Hydrastis, Lycopodium, Opium, Secale, Senega, Thuja.

Among the nosodes there are those which are especially good for infancy, such as Medorrhinum; and Tuberculinum Bovinum for adolescence and on up to twenty-five years of age; Psorinum in young adulthood; Medorrhinum again in middle life; and in the time of induration, contraction, ulceration and insufficiency comes Syphilinum. This nosode is a real bonanza in the sleeplessness of the aged, as well as in their depressions and frequent rectal difficulties: haemorrhoids, fissures and obstinate constipation.

In the aging process there is less oxygen and less hydrogen, and the carbon and nitrogen processes become more prominent. Hence our carbon remedies – Carbo Animalis, Carbo Vegetabilis, Graphites, Kreosotum and Petroleum – are often indicated. Petroleum when the old person is thin and over-active, walks miles every day, and has vertigo of the type where things go up and down instead of around, and where eczema – especially of a dry, cracking, bleeding variety – is present. Where the nitrogen process is awry, one thinks of Ammonium Carbonicum, Causticum, Kali Nitricum and Nitric Acid.

One remedy predominant in sclerosis is Plumbum – lead, the metal of Saturn, which slows down and holds back. Other great remedies for the slowness of the aged are Conium, Phosphorus, Zincum. For weakness, especially in the chest and back with inability to keep from slumping, and for weak voice as a sign of lack of vitality, we think of Stannum, the metal of Jupiter, subtly connected with the liver.

Another ailment of the aging is trembling, in which Mercurius and Alumina join in efficiency with Phosphorus and Zincum.

Itching without eruption, owing to dryness of skin and fat deprivation, often yields to Alumina or Arsenicum, Graphites or Sulphur.

In the distresses of men, Causticum and Staphysagria lead with Thuja in prostatic difficulties. Loss of potency finds help in Lycopodium, Phosporus, Picric Acid, Selenium, Sulphur, Thuja.

Sphincter relaxation is often a problem. Here we think of Aloe, Apis, Phosphorus, Podophyllum and Sulphur for the bowel, and Causticum,

Remedies

Natrum Muriaticum, Pulsatilla, Staphysagria and Thuja for the urine.

In paralysis, particularly with bowel incontinence and some heart damage, do not forget Oleander.

In spite of these remedy suggestions, the constitutional remedy is always the most helpful in the long run. I again particularly stress the need for the nitrogen remedies, Ammonium Carbonicum, Causticum and Nitric Acid. In cases of depression, where the patient does not find life worth living, Kali Phosphoricum and Selenium will do yeoman service.

Above all, we must treat the aging with affection and high regard, and make them feel that their continuance on earth can be a benediction. We must urge them to moderation, to care in diet as well as variety, and ensure proper vitamins. Most homoeopathic patients live to a ripe old age and die painlessly, clear and content. Homoeopathy is indeed an Arethusan fountain of youth!

Ten Remedies in Scarlet Fever

Ten remedies for a single disease – what a luxury that would be to the allopathic physician! But to the homoeopath, what paucity! Homoeopathy, like psychiatry, has elements of science in it, but fundamentally it is an art. We go to the bedside not with a preconceived treatment for whatever diagnosis we may decide upon, but rather in a state of receptivity. We have stored within us, according to our training, industry and genius, the pictures of a whole gamut of remedies. Each is alive and vivid to us – they are our intimate, professional friends.

When we come to the patient, with mind relaxed, we first get an intuitive picture of his condition; of who this patient, in his present diseased state, really is. As Kent said, there is always something to tell the story. The more we have befriended our remedies the fewer questions we will have to ask, and the more certain will be our instinctive recognition of the simillimum. To quote Kent again: 'We must let the appearance of the patient bring to mind the remedies that appear like the patient, regardless of whether they are associated with scarlet fever or not.' Moreover, we dare not prescribe only on the picture before us, but must give the remedy that *corresponds to the sequence of events in the illness*. If we do not see the remedy we must not get panicky. As P. P. Wells said in his article on 'Latent Medication', 'The original sin is not being able to wait for a thing.' Wait until you see the remedy, and having seen and given it, wait until it has finished acting before giving any other dose.

Let me give an outline of what follows. We will consider:
1) The obvious Belladonna, together with prophylaxis and the deliria related to that remedy.
2) Arum Triphyllum and the anginal remedies.
3) Ailanthus and the minor septic remedies, followed by
4) Lachesis, with Crotalus and
5) Ammonium Carbonicum.
6) Apis with Hellebore and the remedies for kidney complications.
7) Cuprum contrasted with Zincum and the other convulsive remedies, as well as those connected with suppressed eruption.

151

8) Rhus Tox. with its adynamic correlates Arnica and Baptisia.
9) Lycopodium and the glandular sequelae remedies.
10) Nitric Acid with Muriatic, Carbolic and the other acids, and the treatment of ear complaints.

I need not give you any picture of the indications for Belladonna, which every one associates with scarlet fever. Like Aconite in colds, Belladonna in scarlatina is too frequently depended on. Rather let me list the *"Don'ts"* for Belladonna:

Don't depend on Belladonna as a prophylactic in every scarlatina epidemic. It is suitable only for those epidemics where it would cure the prevalent form of the disease. Individualize each epidemic from the first few cases. Sulphur is an admirable general preventive, as it raises the resistance of psoric constitutions. Hale and Blackwood recommended Eucalyptus as a great protective. The nosode Scarlatinum should be tried out as a prophylactic on the same principle as we give Diphtherinum. Allen considered Rhus Tox. a more suitable prophylactic than Belladonna for the more modern scarlets.

Don't give Belladonna unless it is a Sydenham scarlatina with clear Belladonna symptoms; in plethoric, phlegmatic people who are unusually well when they are well and overbearing and intolerable when sick. Unless the rash is smooth, with headache and cerebral congestion, Belladonna will impede your case. It is useless where there is an irregular eruption.

Don't forget the globular pulse like buck-shot under the finger.

Don't forget that there is pain under the rash in Belladonna.

Don't forget that Rhus Tox. or Lachesis will often carry through what Belladonna has begun.

Don't forget that the Belladonna child wants to be covered snugly even though he is burning up.

Belladonna cases will often go into delirium, calling for Hyoscyamus. Hyoscyamus is as stupid as Opium, more so than Rhus, Baptisia, Lachesis or Phosphoric Acid. Its motions in delirium are angular; it has less inflammation and congestion than Belladonna or Stramonium. This latter has graceful spasms, gyratory, not jerky, with coppery rash and great loquacity and the typical wild Stramonium mania.

The typical Arum Triphyllum child is intensely restless, not with the anguish of Arsenic, the fidgets of Apis, the nervousness better by motion of Rhus, but because of the terrible itching of the scanty, patchy rash. All the force of the disease seems concentrated in the throat and nose. The child cannot drink, its mouth is so sore. The buccal cavity looks like raw beefsteak, and the child cringes with pain and puts its hand to its throat. The lips are swollen and streaked with the acrid discharge from the itching nose, especially on the left side. The one thing that the exquisitely tender throat and almost denuded strawberry tongue can tolerate is milk. The child screams if you stop it boring into the side of its nose and picking the nostrils and lips, and it screams with the pain while it is doing it. It also picks its fingers until they bleed, but they do not ulcerate. The child, like the Apis patient, is worse from too many clothes. It is not a terribly sick child but it is a very distressing one to the eye, although not to the nose. Toward the end of the disease the desquamation comes in great flakes and the Arum child will often peel two or three times.

Other remedies which especially emphasize *throat* aspects are Phytolacca, Lachesis, the Acids (especially Carbolic Acid), and two other remedies often overlooked. These are, first, Capsicum with its capriciousness in rotund, chilly children of over-stimulated men, its disproportionately burning face, its throat pain between swallows, its craving for pungent things, its gooseflesh from a cold drink, and its sluggish circulation where the skin and mucous membrane, if pinched, stay raised a long time; and second, Cinnabar with its stringy mucus, bloated neck and mercurial breath.

Whoever has smelled the stench of the 'Tree of Heaven' in June, or seen the canaries hung near it die, will appreciate the baneful power of this next remedy. You do not need it very often in scarlet fever, but when you need it you need it badly. It is one of the few remedies in which the exanthem is malignant from the start, like Crotalus and Hydrochloric Acid.

The Ailanthus child shows a sudden early prostration and a stoical torpor which rapidly changes to stupor in the first stage. It lies supine in the bed with violent vomiting, dilated pupils, and red face which turns to a mahogany colour that is almost pathognomonic of the remedy. There may be a chill; red mottled spots, roseola-like, appear here and there on the body. The skin looks more like little dark patches of measles rash. The background of the skin becomes livid, and the eruption is miliary, even with real vesicles interspersed. It remains worst on the brow, neck and chest. When you press with the finger there is a white mark which is very slow to fill up, slower than in any other remedy, and this is so even on the parts of the skin where the rash is not out. The slowness of the return of colour measures the malignancy of the disease, according to Kent. To the touch, the skin is not hot but very dry. The rash may be almost carmine, or more plentiful and bluish, sometimes violent and scaly.

There is nothing bright about this remedy – neither the rash, nor the mental state nor the prognosis! The sicker the case gets, the more brown does the mahogany face become. Petechiae develop and there is an amazing tendency to rapid ulceration. Blebs form and fill with claret-coloured fluid. The ends of the fingers blister and ulcerate. Black blood oozes from the ulcers with a cadaveric odour like stinking meat. Putridity runs all through it, but it is not as penetrating as in a Baptisia case. The throat is not as marked a feature as in Arum, though it is tumefied with purplish patches; copious, thin, excoriating, bloody fluid comes from the throat and nose. The poison seems to concentrate on the nervous system, not to arouse it but to overwhelm by toxaemia. (Ammonium Carb. is overpowered, too, but there the heart rather than the nervous system is hit.) The Ailanthus child has not the restlessness of Arum, it lies benumbed, what consciousness there is seems like a dream, it sighs and occasionally mutters that it sees rats and snakes, or feels them crawling up a limb. The stupefaction is so profound that this hardly terrifies. There is involuntary stool and urine. After a dose of Ailanthus in high potency the malignant scarlet fever will often change to a mild one. There may be critical, offensive, bloody diarrhoea. Not all Ailanthus cases begin malignant, occasionally a child with a 'light' scarlet fever will take cold followed by suppression of the rash and sudden zymosis within twenty-four hours. As Lilienthal says: 'There is no such thing as a light case of scarlet fever.' Often, as in diphtheria, the apparently light cases develop the most complications and sequelae.

In Ailanthus-like states study: Echinacea, especially where there is marked sepsis; Pyrogen and Phosphorus where there is suppuration about the neck and extremities, with hacking, shaking cough and a desire for a stream of ice water running down the throat all the time, where the rash is purple and the petechiae brownish. Hughes quotes P. P. Wells in favour of Tabacum in such malignant states. The Ophidia are the closest analogues to this condition.

Lachesis is one of the grand remedies in scarlet fever. Kent classes it among the nine chief ones in the *Repertory*, the others being Ailanthus, Ammonicum Carbonicum, Apis, Belladonna, Lycopodium, Mercurius, Nitric Acid and Rhus Tox., with Carbolic Acid and Zincum for special phases. The indications for its use are those for Lachesis in general: a constitutional septic condition greater than the local manifestations would indicate; diseases settling in the throat, with purplish colour, usually going from left to right (as the snake coils); worse from hot drinks, more difficulty in swallowing liquids than solids, marked loquacity, sensitive to pressure even of the bed clothes, aggravation after sleep, etc. It is needed in 'Black Scarlet', with black or bluish miliary rash which develops slowly, with delayed desquamation; in spring rather than winter scarlets; when there is swelling of the part of the body covered by the rash.

Closely allied is Crotalus Horridus, especially in scarlatina with jaundice or yellow splotches and streaks, with oozing haemorrhages from all orifices and even from the pores, of dark fluid blood which does not clot, and tendency to ecchymoses. It differs from Lachesis in being more right-sided, swallowing solids with more difficulty than liquids; and mumbling and stumbling in its loquacity rather than wildly interrupting. It is indicated in cases which are very malignant from the beginning (like Ailanthus and Hydrochloric Acid), and where there is little fever. Its complaints are general rather than localized.

Kent says when you need a big remedy in a scarlet fever, study Ammonium Carbonicum. 'It has in its nature all that there is of the nature of things grave and serious.' It was suggested by Dr Thorer, of Germany, as a specific for scarlet fever. It is more suitable to our nervous modern civilization than Belladonna. You need Ammonium Carb., I think, in complicated natures, in scarlet fevers of older people, which are occasioned by psychic shock or conflict. The whole psyche of the case calling for Ammonium Carb. needs revision and re-integration. Think of it when the economy cannot keep the rash out; when it is overpowered by toxaemia (like Ailanthus, or even Zinc); when the rash comes to the surface but the patient is not relieved as he should be; when the rash recedes too early from weakness and brain trouble threatens; when the rash stays out longer than usual; when the rash recedes with nosebleed, cramps, weak heart and sudden collapse; when there is heart weakness and failure; when there is a lack of response to remedies and few symptoms to prescribe on; when there is defective reaction at the close of scarlet fever; when Lachesis has been wrongly given; when the patient shuns water, and water on the face and indeed the whole body mottles the skin, and nosebleed follows washing the face and hands; when the patient cannot sleep at night because he cannot breathe, i.e. stoppage of the nose at night necessitating mouth breathing; when the throat is gangrenous, bluish-red, with terrible acridity and sticky, adhesive, profuse saliva; when the rash is bright red but miliary, or scanty and bluish-red; in patients with brown liver spots and freckles; when there is marked desquamation, especially of the trunk, arms and thighs, with heart prostration; when the patient is chilly, better by external heat, but needs air; when a naturally stout person emaciates very rapidly during the exanthem; in stubborn patients and confirmed bachelors.

Will you come with me on a hurry call? The mother has told me over the telephone that Johnny broke out with a rosy rash yesterday about 5 p.m., which was so rough to the touch it felt pointed, but as he had no fever, was not thirsty or restless and had an unimportant sore throat, and did not seem particularly sick, she did not call me, but put him into a rousing hot bath and then he had convulsions. When we arrive we find Johnny lying fairly quietly in bed, fidgeting with his feet and trying to kick off the bed clothes that his mother has heaped on him, although he is shivering. We notice that he does not seem to mind when she tucks them in around his neck. His face is puffy with purplish-white bloated lids, his upper lip swollen. He is muttering but with a curious, happy look on his face. We sniff in vain as we stand and watch him. His mother offers him a hot drink, the child pushes it away with an awkward gesture which nearly spills it, whining, and starts to tumble about the bed like a kitten. We ask her to offer him cold water, but despite his oedema he is not thirsty. We uncover him, which calms him, but he jumps violently when we touch the sharp rash, it is so sensitive. There is even rash on the palms of his hands, but there it is smooth. Parts of his body are hot and others are cold, and transient, partial sweat which smells like musk breaks out and dries up. Before we can stop her, his mother has moved the electric heater nearer the bed as we uncovered him, and Johnny nearly suffocates from the whiff of radiating heat. We throw up the windows, to his evident relief.

His mother tells us that yesterday before the rash came out nothing suited him. He was fickle and changeable and screamed whenever she paid any attention to the other children. After the hot bath she says he had several convulsions, preceded by a piercing cry, and he has passed no urine since. His feet are swollen and his genitals tremendously so. She thinks one eye seems crooked. We look in Johnny's throat; it is bright red and beefy, with glazed tonsils, and a sore tongue with a red, triangular tip like Rhus. Yesterday it was the right side of his throat which was most sore, but today it seems to be the left. The mother cannot understand how Johnny can get so sick so fast. We remind her of the phrase 'making a bee line', and explain the correspondence of this attack to the remedy you have guessed by now to be Apis Mellifica. We give Johnny one dose of Apis 1M. You can almost see it work, and we go home confident that the remedy will save Johnny from nephritis and hydrocephalus.

Johnny's case reminds us of the case of the Hellebore boy, who lingered on with passive brain trouble, a 'say-nothing', 'do-nothing' delirium. He bored his head into the pillows, grinding his teeth and chewing (not the lateral jaw wagging of Bryonia), and lay on his back with his limbs up making slow, vague automatic motions. We remember his wrinkled face with its sooty nostrils so different from happy Apis. Young Hellebore was stubbornly silent and had a fixed idea of death without any fear of it, but a dread and fear of water, though his tongue was like dry leather. After his dose there was no such swift satisfactory relief as Apis got, but two days of vomiting, diarrhoea and dreadful tingling in his limbs, which we dared not stay and watch lest we nervously give another remedy and spoil the chances of recovery. If he had had dropsy it would have been a sudden one of chest or abdomen from acute nephritis in a so-called 'light' case of scarlatina, with suppression of urine or a coffee-ground sediment in the scanty amount passed.

Here let me mention some of the other main remedies in kidney complications of scarlet fever. After Apis and Hellebore in importance comes Arsenicum and then Colchicum, whose dropsy is accompanied by great prostration, constant sweat and nervous trembling with tenesmus, and smoky, albuminous urine. It is oversensitive, especially to odours, and violently worse from motion. If there is scanty urine and saliva there will be copious stool, and vice versa. Terebinthina fits acute Bright's disease with much blood though few casts in the urine, with dropsy chiefly of the upper parts, suppressed urine, twitching and even convulsions, often with burning tympanites and glossy, smooth red tongue. One is not in danger of forgetting Cantharis if there is a burning, cutting pain, nor Apocynum in dropsy with great thirst and worse from cold (opposite of Apis), the thirst being for cold water which nauseates while hot relieves. A valuable remedy for acute Bright's disease after scarlet fever from catching cold or bathing is Dulcamara, which Hartmann especially stresses. Do not forget Lycopodium when the rash pales suddenly and bloating and dropsy ensue. Asclepias Cornuti, Helonias, Squilla and Eucalyptus are also useful. Hepar is said to be a preventive of nephritis afer scarlet fever, as is Kali Mur.

Cuprum has one outstanding use in scarlet fever. When the rash is suppressed by an outward cause, such as chill, exposure to wind, or catching cold from a draft after a hot bath, the patient goes into convulsions owing to the suppression of the rash – that is, any form of discharge into or through the skin. (*Remember Cuprum in any discharge which has been stopped by outside means.* Shut safety valves call for Cuprum.) In Bryonia we have a remedy for convulsions because the rash fails to come out, and in Zincum for brain trouble because the child is too weak to throw out an eruption, or to keep it out once it has appeared. Dulcamara will have suppression of the rash from taking cold or injudicious bathing, but it will not show the convulsive picture of Cuprum.

The Cuprum child will go suddenly blind, its thumbs will turn in and its fists clench, it will shriek or bellow – not the pitiful, piercing, single cry of Apis, but more vociferous and varied. It grimaces and hides under the covers; it may lie on its face, breech upward, getting black in the face; it will alternately flex and extend the limbs (like Tabacum). Terrible cramps attack the calves of its legs and its chest, and it may have choreiform twitchings. These attacks are likely to come at night, especially after midnight. The child is maniacal, wants to fly, to hide, to be held down. The convulsions are better from pressure and bandaging the limbs. Between convulsions the Cuprum child will lie as if dead or in ecstasy, every muscle quietly quivering, with its eyes turned up; if it speaks, its voice is cracked and squeaking, and it gets relief from a drink of cold water, which is swallowed with a gurgling sound like water being poured from a bottle. A knife-like pain from the xyphoid to the back may transfix the child as if impaled. Diarrhoea often accompanies the convulsions, and is relieved by hot drinks and hot water bottle, and especially from binding up the abdomen in a tight bandage. Complaints change suddenly and completely from one part of the body to another, with alternation of physical and mental conditions, for example diarrhoea and mania. The Cuprum patient has little if any fever. When uraemia sets in with suppression of urine, Cuprum Acetate or Cuprum Arsenicosum may be indicated.

In contrast to the activity of Cuprum we have the passive brain conditions of Zincum. The patient is incredibly weak; he does not look so bad, but when you question him he stares, and after an interval says, 'Oh!' and then answers. His reflexes are abolished, he lies at death's door with moving jaw, rolling head and fidgeting feet. He is excitable in a frail way. His face during the convulsions is pale (not blue like Cuprum, nor red like Belladonna). He has not even the strength to perspire, or if he does it does not relieve, and he wants to be wrapped up during it. You cannot give your Zincum patient even wine jelly without his face becoming flushed. His cold, sleepy, fixed collapse may give way to remarkably high temperature without inflammation. Do not forget that he is worse at 3 p.m. He will even get a sort of passive meningitis from non-development or recession of the rash, with strabismus. It is, like Cuprum, one of the best remedies for long, persistent strabismus after scarlet fever, and it covers cachectic neuralgias. Cuprum and Zincum in conditions like these are indeed the heavenly twins.

In connection with the above, we may remember a few other

remedies. When convulsions are brought on by covering up the child, or by a hot bath (like Apis), and it lies in a sort of snoring coma with a very red face and convulsive twitching, we think of Opium. If this child is conscious it may have a kind of restlessness, not from nervousness or pain but because the bed itself feels so hot he cannot lie in it, and must move in search of a cool place. When the head sweats profusely and the child is moaning and turning its head from side to side, especially if there is an icteric tinge to the skin and acute hydrocephalus is impending, Mercurius may save. When the repelled eruption brings on dyspnoea with rattling, cyanotic face, thirstless passivity, pungent odour, amelioration from cold and unwillingness to be touched or looked at, to the point where the child howls or goes into convulsions, Antimonium Tart. is indicated. In sudden disappearance of the rash without apparent cause, think of Phosphorus. In some severe cases where the rash will not come out and the child flickers in and out of stupor, if the symptoms agree, Arsenicum may aid. Undeveloped or receding rash with alarming chest symptoms brings to mind Calc. Carb.; or with gastric symptoms, Ipecacuanha. In any suppression, especially where the orifices are burning red, think of Sulphur, as also where there is coma at the onset and the child looks like a boiled lobster, or as though the skin were a red cloth, when there is too much rash; also in slowly progressing cases in psoric children, and in a large number of cases at the desquamating time to ward off sequelae (Kali Sulph.).

Next, let us look at a triumvirate of remedies for adynamic scarlet fevers, typhoid forms. First Rhus Tox., which is the least alarming and most normal of the three, and often supplants Belladonna. The mental symptoms of Rhus are helpful. He is a mild patient, aristocratic, especially about his eating, craving oysters and dainties. He fears poison in the medicine or in the cold milk that he craves. He is freaky without being petulant. The rash is true scarlet red, the abdomen particularly so, and the eruption may be millet-seed in form with violent itching (often better by applications of scalding water, despite the general aggravation of Rhus from bathing), or vesicular and even erysipeloid. The rash is coarser than in Belladonna and may increase like urticaria, passing off in the sweat. It is the first remedy to think of when the glands are involved in scarlet fever, especially if they are affected first on the left and then on the right. It has enlargement of the left parotid, and cellulitis of the neck (like Phosphorus); it has swelling of the axillary glands with suppression of the rash. It goes into a typhoidal state with gentle delirium and picking at flocks. It is a safe remedy to give when the typhoidal state comes on in scarlatina and no special drug is indicated. It is especially helpful where the perspiration has been checked. There are liquid yellow stools and the urine often leaves a red stain. The characteristic Rhus restlessness is present.

When Rhus fails and the typhoidal state merges into sepsis with aching and rigors, and a varnished, fiery tongue replaces the triangular tip of Rhus, when the pulse rate increases much faster than the temperature (or pulse and temperature are out of rhythm either way), especially if there is fighting delirium with semi-clairvoyance and threatening heart failure with a carrion-like sweat and loquacity, Pyrogen will be the remedy to follow Rhus.

If your typhoidal scarlet fever case is in a full-blooded, not debilitated person, self-opinionated, obstinate, with overwhelming fear of being hurt, both mentally and physically, think of Arnica. He is apathetic and lies drawn up in a heap, though he, too, is restless – not from the internal nervousness of Rhus, but because the bed feels so hard and he is sore from lying. He is so weak he must change position little by little. Black and blue spots and small boils come on the parts lain on. He is chilly, like Rhus, but uncovers. He is morose and sullen, does not want to talk or be touched, thinks he will mortify, dreams of muddy water, wakes with distress in the heart at night with horror of instant death, and wants the doctor sent for at once. But when the doctor comes he says: 'Go home, I don't need you.' The typhoidal states of Rhus and Arnica come on slowly.

When they come with amazing rapidity, a low septic state in seventy-two hours, accompanied by such a pungent stench that even burnt rags do not relieve it, and the nurse gags and retches, you have a Baptisia state. He is besotted, purplish, as though he had been drinking heavily. He lies curled up like a dog, muttering: 'I can't do it, I can't do it', meaning that he cannot gather together the parts of himself which he thinks are scattered all over the bed. He is maudlin, stupid, putrid, with a typical Baptisia mouth and sordes. He can swallow only liquids. The darker his throat the more it is Baptisia. His complaints are remarkably painless. He develops bed sores. He, too, when high fever and loquacity ensue, may need Pyrogen.

Lycopodium will help many abnormal, peculiar cases. It has deep blood poisoning. Secondary eruptions and blotches come out on the hands, face, thighs and back. It is suitable in neglected cases (like Nitric Acid) and in diphtheria, complicating scarlet fever. Malignant cases where the child wakes screaming and knows no one, and wrinkles his face if a door slams or a bell rings. One foot is often cold and the other hot. In many ways it is similar to Arum, picks its nose and has the very sore throat, which here goes from right to left. It is mainly a remedy for the late stages, and has been advised frequently during desquamation. It has colic with constipation at the time of the peeling. In convalescence the child emaciates, the hair falls out, there is thick, yellow, offensive discharge from the ear with deafness. In dropsy it develops ulcers on the leg and has strangury, better from hot drinks. It has swellings and suppuration of the glands of the neck.

After Rhus, Arsenicum, Calc. Carb. or Kali Carb., Lycopodium will finish off gland sequelae, or Baryta Carb. may be needed to follow on. Phytolacca is often suitable where glandular swelling is marked, and Anthracinum may be needed if the glands under the chin are stony hard, especially if the joints are painful. Hempel and Jahr stress Conium for hard, big submaxillaries and especially parotitis during desquamation, particularly if accompanied by rectal affections with diarrhoea, tenesmus and strangury. Ammonium Carb. for the right parotid, Rhus for the left parotid, and Lac Caninum often aid. In passing it is interesting to note the frequency of parotitis in scarlet fever.

Finally, let us consider the Acids as a group. Nitric Acid is valuable in neglected scarlets, where the throat inflammation extends to the nose with excoriating ichorous discharge, and ulcers stud the inner cheeks and sides of the tongue, with acrid saliva which is not ropy. There may be a leathery, gristly false membrane. The Nitric Acid patient cannot bear anyone to walk across the floor, because of the jarring, not the noise. It is useful in subsequent ear discharges and deafness. Muriatic Acid is one of our sickest looking cases. A brunette, disposed to anger and chagrin, who lies slumped down in the bed groaning and moaning deeply, with restless arms, though quiet feet, better uncovered. The rash is rough, scarlet and irregular, with petechiae, and is especially marked at the nape of the neck. There is disproportionate muscular weakness and great malignancy, although the mind is fairly clear. Blackish, sloughing ulcers and bed sores develop. Sulphuric Acid has much to do with this picture but without the relief from uncovering, and the rash is darker. Phosphoric Acid has mental prostration and weakness with relative muscular strength (opposite of Muriatic Acid), a vast indifference, and milky urine. Carbolic Acid has the typical dusky face with white circles around the mouth, a sensation of a rubber band around the forehead, miliary rash all over the body (never vesicular), and one of the most gangrenous of throats; putridity without pain.

Hydrocyanic Acid is perhaps our most desperate remedy. Hopeless cases from the start, with a livid rash and many petechiae, coldness of the feet with paralysis of the oesophagus and often long fainting spells.

Scarlet fever in its malignant forms is a great sphere for the acids.

One of the most frequent and troublesome sequelae of scarlatina is ear trouble. Here also Nitric Acid is a leader. You will naturally think of such remedies as Hepar Sulph. Mercurius, Pulsatilla, Silica, Calc. Carb., Lycopodium, and Sulphur. More especially valuable in the otorrhoeas after scarlet are Bovista, where the discharge is profuse, excoriating and of long standing, Aurum, and the metal associated with it in nature – and also, as often, in disease – Tellurium. When new abscesses keep forming in the middle ear, Kino is advocated by German authors. If mastoid is threatening, Capsicum will do yeoman service. Terebinthina has ear as well as kidney complications, and H. C. Allen stresses Teucrium.

Dr Hubbard closed by inviting the reader to consider the following questions. — Ed.

Will Belladonna suppress a scarlatina? (Deschere quotes a case where Belladonna apparently stopped the prodrome, the child seemed well, and after three weeks the rash came without prodome or illness and was followed by desquamation.)

What data do you have on the effects of homoeopathic remedies given prophylactically in altering the Dick test reactions?

Have you experienced the alleged dissolving powers of alcohol on membrane in the throat in scarlatina or diphtheria, as suggested by Farrington?

What, if any, is the value of lard inunctions as preventives of anascara, as suggested by Jahr?

What experiences have you had with Eucalyptus globules, Mancinella, or Ammonium Muriaticum in scarlet fever?

The Planets

Our materia medica gives a horde of symptoms for each of the well-proven remedies, on an empiric basis. This is practical if we can synthesize and remember the welter of detail. But our crying need in materia medica is to *deepen* it, to study the substances in themselves, in their relation to the cosmos and the natural sciences. Then a sense of the inevitability of the remedy picture grows in us. Instead of a feat of the memory, it becomes a growing power in the prescriber's soul. New implications arise which painstaking research and vigorous thought can carry through from hypothesis to science. That which Hahnemann made into homoeopathy had its source in the ancient mysteries. He himself acknowledged his great debt to Paracelsus, and some of our best homoeopaths have been deep students of alchemy, like the late Dr Emil Schlegel of Germany. The Doctrine of Signatures and the Correspondences of Swedenborg hold much light for those into whom they can penetrate.

In ancient wisdom the elements, and particularly the metals, have a special place, being connected with the planets. Many of these metals we use and stress – Aurum, Argentum, Mercury, Ferrum and Cuprum. There are some which theoretically should be as important, but which do not come into their own in our knowledge and prescribing. For instance, consider Stannum, or tin. This is the Jupiter of the alchemists, one of the seven most important metals, each being allied to one of the seven major planets. (Aurum to the Sun, Argentum to the Moon, Plumbum to Saturn, Stannum to Jupiter, Cuprum to Venus, Ferrum to Mars and Mercurius to Mercury.) The more recently discovered planets, such as Uranus, Neptune and Pluto, are not yet assigned to metallic correspondences. Some of the metals are intermediary, a combination of forces – for example, Zinc of Plumbum and Stannum, Magnesium of Ferrum and Cuprum.

In the alchemist's view these metals influence or represent different planes of the human economy: Aurum the Ego, Cuprum and Ferrum the astral (emotional), Stannum and Mercurius the etheric (vital), Plumbum and Argentum the realm between the etheric and the physical. With the exception of the Ego, each plane has two chief metallic influencers. The

163

one increases the forces and the other diminishes them. If you check this abstruse concept by our knowledge of homoeopathic medicaments, and even by orthodox physiology, it is surprising how they all fit in. For instance, copper (astral) is connected with Venus and is the element which frees the astral that has too strong a hold. When emotionality is excessive we have hysteria and cramps, which are of the essence of our homoeopathic Cuprum and Ferrum; the other astral aspect (Mars) strengthens the astral grip. In other words, the anaemic flabby Ferrum patient needs more of the defining, rigid, astral influence. Again, Stannum (etheric), connected with Jupiter, is the forming force – ideals realized in the physical – whereas Mercurius, connected with Mercury, represents the dissolving forces of healing. For the etheric plane is the plane where healing takes place. We know, homoeopathically, how Mercurius will resolve the clogged antrum, the hard swollen gland and so on (the glandular is etheric). We also know how Stannum will build up and strengthen vital (etheric) weakness. To follow, Plumbum, related to Saturn, frees the etheric from the physical, thereby tending toward the isolation of the physical, which means death. We know how slow, devitalized, chronic, emaciated and near dissolution is the Plumbum patient. Argentum, corresponding to the Moon, permeates the physical with the etheric, thereby vitalizing, warming and fluidifying the solid.

In the Ego realm (corresponding to the Sun and warmth) Aurum brings the Ego in, strengthens the spirit. We know the warm powerful Aurum personality, with its despairs in the higher realms of the Ego, and with its action on bones (bones belong to the Ego sphere). Although I have not found it in the literature, I feel that the other metal acting on the Ego must be Platinum, the false Ego, as it were, when the Ego is too strong and needs releasing, just the opposite of Aurum, where it needs fortifying.

Metals for Healing

Observe a piece of manganese. It is without doubt the deadest-looking of all the metals. It is famous for a disease which, though not prematurely fatal, makes the patient who has it look gradually more and more dead – namely Parkinson's disease, in which one becomes progressively expressionless. Women with vacant faces, spastic gait, trembling; who feel well when lying down and wish they could spend the rest of their lives in bed; people who are a complete monotone, except for trembling and paralysis; festinating gait, increase of reflexes, tense soreness, excessive prostration, hysteria, inclination to walk backwards or sidewise like a crab; vertigo and falling backward; writes backward; frequent nystagmus; sad, anxious, fretful; full of hate; chronic hoarseness, dry cough, completely relieved by lying down. Everything affects the ears, deafness in damp weather; asthma, aggravated by feathers. The Manganum patient is worse from motion, worse at night, from jar, from talking, before thunderstorms, and from bending backward. Relief from lying down, bending double, and eating. It has slow healing, diagonal pains, paralyses which extend upward, joint distresses which go crosswise. The menses of Manganum are frequent and scanty; there is intermenstrual bleeding, and the first menses may be as late as age twenty in pale chlorotic subjects. It is related to the syphilitic miasm, certain chronic skin diseases like pityriasis and lichen, erythema nodosum, and periosteal arthritis. It is a sovereign remedy for the results of encephalitis.

Antimony is in many ways like Arsenicum, but more drowsy; whereas Arsenicum wants to hold your hand, Antimony is averse to being touched or even looked at. Debility, fainting, pitiful whimpering, not relieved by rest. Children weep when angry; chilly and cold sweat, but worse by warmth; worse for lying down, sour things and milk; sooty wings of the nose; so short of breath they must sit up, or lie with the head thrown back; worse lying. They cling and want to be carried; the head trembles after coughing, the tongue is white and pasty with red edges. They may be bold, wild, mirthful and quarrelsome, and will bite. They have a shocking lumbosacral backache with a feeling of weight on the coccyx. No thirst. Quivering chin and jaws, craving for apples and acid fruit. The perfect remedy for pulmonary oedema and for exanthematous diseases with deficient eruptions. There must always be a careful differential diagnosis between Arsenic and Antimony.

Combined with Sulphur instead of Tartrate, Antimonium Crudum shows a different picture: warm-blooded, complaints from overheating. Resembles a pig; gross feeder, greedy, obese; solid, stout children who object to being looked at or questioned, who are angry at any kind attention, who are sulky, cross, and contradict. Worse for radiant heat, cold bathing, full moon, sun, the evening, sour wine, water, washing, and the acid which they love. Tongue as if whitewashed; cracks and fissures in the corners of the mouth and eyes, brittle deformed nails, horny warts and calluses, gout with gastric symptoms.

Ferrum Metallicum, the metal of Mars, one of the three basic remedies of Rademacher (the others being Cuprum and Kali Nitricum). Ferrum is one of the charming debutantes of homoeopathy, and can be found at any Junior League party together with her friends Cuprum, Ignatia and Pulsatilla. She gets no credit for being sick, for she has a pretty flush – false plethora. She is the sanguine temperament. She blushes and flushes from emotion or pain. It is a great remedy for puberty and weeps and laughs immoderately. Its face alternates between pale and red. These girls are delicate and chlorotic. They are self-centred, haughty, proud and vehement. They quarrel easily and are worse from contradiction. Complaints from anger. They have no endurance. They have anxiety, worse from noise, even the crackling of paper, like Asarum. Dread of air, complaints from loss of fluids, like China, which is closely related. They have thoughts of death and are full of despair. They have complaints *while* eating, such as cough, vomiting in whooping cough, epistaxis, diarrhoea. Their vomiting is without nausea, like a leather bag emptying. They are relieved by slow walking, like Pulsatilla. Their aggravation is at twelve midnight and noon, like Sulphur. They are worse sitting, like Sepia. Aggravated in the winter, by rest, from sour things, and markedly from eggs; also from drafts and cold bathing.

There is an interesting aggravation from descending – Borax and Stannum are not the only remedies for this. Their pulse is full and yielding, and their muscles flabby. Their bones are soft. It is a great remedy for haemorrhage, especially from the lungs, which is bright and clots easily like Ipecacuanha and Phosphorus. Ferrum also has vicarious haemorrhages. It is among the remedies for the most violent headaches, pulsating, without respite, for three days. It has vertigo looking at water, as when crossing a log over a brook, dizziness on sudden motion, descending, and from walking. It has the curious keynote of red face and thirst during chill. It is one of the profoundly constipated remedies, and very short of breath, a leading medicine in exophthalmic goitre, and in deltoid rheumatism and bursitis.

Stannum – tin – the major ingredient of pewter, sometimes called *Plumbum candidum*, white lead, and sometimes *Diabolus metallorum*, metal of the devil, because it is so brittle and makes such a great noise when bent. It resists decomposition and does not rust. It is not affected by the atmosphere. Its atomic weight is 118, close to Antimony, which is 120. It is chemically related to Silica, the complement of Pulsatilla, and is often needed in Pulsatilla cases. Astrologically it is the remedy of Jupiter, and the ancients felt it controlled the liver. Its homoeopathic nickname is 'the dromedary' – slow and sure. Its symptoms begin in the morning and very gradually get worse until the middle of the day, and then gradually recede. It is related to the pituitary gland; it is one of the hydrogenoid remedies of Grauvogel. It is supposed to make the etheric forces receptive to the ego, and like Phosphorus, make it possible for the ego to come more deeply in.

In looks the Stannum patient has the Jovian high brow, like Sir Walter Scott and indeed Hahnemann himself. Weakness is perhaps its predominant symptom. The voice (which shows the ego) is so weak; the back is so feeble that the Stannum patient falls into a chair. She is emaciated and has enteroptosis. She is worse talking and especially worse laughing, and better with motion. Better also from hard pressure and better during menses. She is worse at noon or at 10 a.m. like Natrum Mur. Worse from touch and descending, also from drafts, change of weather, and cold. Sudden onset, as in Belladonna, is a contraindication for Stannum, which is gradual and slow, both increasing and decreasing in its pains and symptoms. It has a marked periodicity. Mentally it is a sad remedy, with aversion to men, unwillingness to answer questions, sadness before menses. It is a great remedy for neuralgias after the suppression of leucorrhea. It has complaints on Saturday or Monday, 'Monday constipation'. Its all-gone feeling is not relieved by eating. Cramps around the navel and colic are better from hard pressure, from lying on the abdomen, from doubling up and from walking, and are accompanied by colic with hunger. It has glassy leucorrhea, monthly periods early and profuse with concomitant malar pain. Prolapse, aggravated by stool. Knotty stool or urge to soft stool which it cannot expel, like Alumina. Its discharges are green, sweet-tasting and bland. Alternation of leucorrhea and neuralgia. It is magical in haemorrhage from the stomach. It has emptiness in the chest, feeble hacking coughs, three or four in paroxysm; worse at night, from warm drinks, from sunrise to sunset. Singers find expiring difficult. Exhausting coughs with knife-like pain in the upper sternum brought on by laughing, and relieved by bending double.

All the mentals of Stannum are relieved during the menstrual period. It is in general better lying on the back and lying on something hard. Lying on the stomach makes it sleepless. Stannum will often sleep with one leg bent up and the other stretched out and the head flexed. It has hemiplegia with constant sweat of the paralyzed part. It has musty sweats, worse at 4 or 5 a.m. and a green sweat, worse morning and evening. It is worse before the changing of the moon. It has convulsions with the thumbs in, like Cuprum, and drops things from fatigue or weakness, not haste. It is a great remedy for worms. Its discharges are debilitating, like China. It is a safe and useful remedy for tuberculosis and bronchiectasis. Particularly is it helpful in the despondent tubercular.

Mercurius, the human thermometer, is lax, blond, alkaline. A volatile chameleon, elusive as quicksilver, which it is. We are told not to give Mercury in psoric cases. The Mercury patient has two sides, one brutal, ugly, cruel; murderers, suicides by shooting or knifing. Stupid, chronically ill, disgusted, morose, mistrustful, weary of life, treacherous. The other aspect is like the mythological god Mercury, the messenger and prankster among the gods. Mischievous, overbright without character, hasty, ineffective, timid, hurried. Averse to company, cannot talk well, slow to answer, poor will and memory, uncoordinated angular movements, drowsy, talks or groans in sleep. An important remedy for tremors; desires stimulants; frequent colds; slow to heal, ulceration plus swollen glands, mostly small and hard. Worse sunset to sunrise, especially worse from change of temperature. Sticky sweat without relief. Very thirsty for cold drinks, though with a wet mouth. Discharges are slimy, bloody, with pus, acrid. Worse lying on the right, worse in the warmth of the bed, worse from dampness, touch, pressure and motion. Exostoses and bone pains.

The tongue is typical, flabby, showing the imprint of the teeth, scalloped edges, metallic odour, mucous patches, decay of the crowns of the teeth, not near the roots like Thuja. Stomatitis, sneezing in the sun, iritis, photophobia, running ears, quinsy. The remedy for 'foundryman's glare'. Vertigo lying on the back; alternate hot and cold, alternate constipation and diarrhoea; bowel trouble, especially caecum, colon, appendix. Mucous colitis. Tenesmus, 'never-get-done' feeling. Bloody, shreddy dysentery. Nephritis. Sweat of the genitals, chancroid, secondary syphilis, menses excessive with swollen labia and acrid leucorrhoea. The ancients used to say 'salivation is salvation'; Mercury is full of excess saliva, drooling at night and spraying when you speak. Red coppery skin eruptions, eczema, itching in bed, toxic trembling, paralysis agitans, bone sequestrae, sinuses, osteomyelitis, rheumatic fever, anaemias which do not respond to iron or transfusions. High sedimentation rate. Fainting. There is a whole family of Mercuries of great value – Merc. Cor., Merc. Cyan., Merc. Dulc., Merc. Iod. Flav. (proto-iodide), Merc. Iod. Rub. (biniodide) and Cinnabar (red iodide of mercury). Compare with Podophyllum, called the 'vegetable mercury'. Everything in Mercury is worse from sunset to sunrise, it being a profound syphilitic miasmatic remedy.

One of the seven great planetary metals used relatively infrequently in homoeopathy is Plumbum – lead – related to the eldest planet, Saturn. It is a sclerotic, emaciated slow personality, atomic weight 207 – 'heavy as lead'. Mentally Plumbum is a thief, full of deceit, father of lies; a timid, anxious, restless, amnesic, demented person. Desperate anaemias, contraction of the spirit and body, relief by *stretching*. Backward or epileptic children; trembling paralyses, tendency to abortion, boring pains, fear of assassination, odd positions in sleep. One of our greatest remedies for intestinal obstruction. Give your remedy, whether it be Plumbum, Cuprum, Nux Vomica or whatever, summon the ambulance and the surgeon, call the hospital, and by the time the patient arrives there, in my experience, the obstruction or intussusception is resolved and no surgery is needed; it is also often the same with strangulated hernia.

One of the leading keynotes of lead is as though the abdomen is attached to the spine with a string. Whereas the Belladonna abdomen is puffy and distended, the Plumbum one is retracted and concave; there is a cold sweat during stool and a singularly severe constipation, with a constriction of the anus and an unsuccessful urge; only small black lumps pass, like sheep dung. Lead is one of the greatest remedies for hiccup and *the* remedy for aluminium poisoning, as Alumina is for lead poisoning. Plumbum is one of the remedies for the 'ball sensation' – from the throat to the brain (compare Anacardium, Asafoetida, Ignatia, Sepia, etc.). Lead has a greasy face, like Natrum Mur. and Thuja, and colic with constipation, neuralgia and spasm of the rectum, neuralgia alternating with colic. Slipped discs and stubborn sacroiliacs and sciaticas, worse at night, better by exertion, like Rhus Tox., but better from pressure and worse from motion; also worse from company. Cramps in peripheral arteries; paralysis of single parts, mainly extensor, preceded by headache, blindness or spasms; heavy limbs; swollen tongue; partial epilepsy ending in sleep. Radiating pains. Contracted pupils; as if a string through to the rectum; hyperaesthesias and anaesthesias; the patient is worse at 8–9 a.m., and faints on entering a room full of people. This is a remedy of the deepest and most serious conditions; multiple sclerosis, progressive muscular atrophy, uraemia, gangrene, stinking foot sweat, faecal vomiting, brown tongue with red edges. The patient feels cold from exertion in the open air. Plumbum is altogether one of the least attractive remedies.

Argentum – silver – the moon metal, is best represented homoeopathically in the nitrate, which is one of the three greatest geriatric drugs (the others being Lycopodium and Conium). Silver is the great rationalizer and has an excuse for everything; it is an exhibitionist; they buck up at once if someone keeps an eye on them. In order for this remedy to be needed, the mentals must be paramount (must really hit you in the face). It is a highly superstitious remedy – touches every lamp-post and steps on every crack. They escape into alcohol; they are spare, dyspeptic, shaky, off-balance, uncoordinated; they are the prize loud belchers, and enjoy it. There is fear of failure, and they often do fail (unlike Silica).

There are errors of perception, as if one eye were enlarged; sensation as if the head were enlarged or empty. Headache relieved by tight bandaging of the head, like Silica, though in Silica it is the warmth that is wanted. Argentum Nit. has the nitrogen sticking pains; it has complaints from anticipation, especially diarrhoea, which is called firebell diarrhoea, and the stool is noisy, green, shreddy, and worse from eating and drinking, like Croton Tig. It has the chronic gastritis of alcoholics. The remedy is worse from warmth in any form, like Apis, Iodum, Lachesis, Ledum, Pulsatilla, Secale and Sulphur; worse on the right side, worse eating. It is full of throat and larynx symptoms, and is one of the three greatest remedies for peptic ulcer (together with Kali Bich. and Uranium Nit.); in abdominal gas it vies with China, Colchicum and Lycopodium. It loves cheese and salt almost as much as Phosphorus, but its major passion (in fact, it has binges) is sweets, which aggravate. Six lumps of sugar in the coffee and a loud belch, and you think of Argentum Nitricum.

Strontium Carbonicum

The predominant characteristic of Strontium Carbonicum is vehemence. The subject is impetuous, violent, passionate, beats everything that gets in his way. He is quarrelsome and this mood lasts a long time. Ill-humoured and irascible, he has a bad conscience. He is apprehensive, anxious, fretful. He is taciturn, averse to talk, and extremely forgetful. He is an emaciated patient, most of whose complaints are right-sided. He is chilly, hypersensitive to draught, relieved in the sun and by warmth and by wrapping up the affected part; worse from uncovering. His pains wax and wane gradually. He is worse in the evening, at night, and from 2 a.m. to 3 a.m. Worse by walking, motion, rising after lying, lying with the head low and by touch, rubbing and scratching.

Strontium is a great remedy for surgical shock after a severe operation, and for the chronic effect of oozing blood loss. It has debility, languor, phantom pains, changing and difficult to locate, felt least in the open air and worse on uncovering the part. His dreams are mortifying, of fire, of grief, or else maybe vividly joyous. He has involuntary starting on falling asleep, is restless and wakes smothering. He is weak in the morning. When half asleep, he awakens trembling in the evening with heavy chest and apprehension. The face is flushed, especially on walking. He is an arterio-sclerotic; apoplexy threatens. His mouth and nose give off heat. He is full of twitching and jerking, pulsation of the arteries and fullness of the veins. It is a great remedy for the climacteric. He falls asleep late, wakes after a short sleep. There is jerking of the upper body from violent dreams, often of fire.

It is a great headache remedy, from the nape up over the head, better wrapping the head warmly, like Silica and Magnesia Mur. Worse with the head low. Violent sticking pain in the left frontal region. Supra-orbital neuralgia. Worse from cold and in the evening. Tension from vertex to jaw, as if the head expanded. Tight, chilly scalp. Headache better in the sun. Vertigo at noon. Tearing or violent boring in the right antrum; numb mouth on waking. Worse from water and washing. Has more pain than Calcium or Barium; pain alternating with itching, sore pain with numbness. Pain with oedema (left sciatica with swelling of the left ankle). Hot flashes with aversion to uncovering.

Curious eye symptoms; sees green spots, sees blue and red edges; jerking of the left upper lid. Twitch of the upper lid and left zygoma.

Cracked lips, twitching of one side of the nose, bloody crusts, tearing in the roots of the teeth preceded by salivation. Spasmodic pain in the head through the eyeballs. Corroded tip of the tongue. Severe pain in the stomach during digestion; violent hiccoughs; violent thirst for beer, craves rye or brown bread; cutting colic, with diarrhoea and chill; watery, yellow stool with pinching pain, tenesmus and burning anus during and after stool. Nausea with burning hot face. Stitches in the groin; large, lumpy knotty stool. Periodic exhausting night diarrhoeas. Stomach pressure better eating, worse walking; constricted or burrowing pain with watery eructation. Faints with hard stool. Must lie down after stool. Urine smells of iodine or ammonia.

Menses early, like meat washings, later clotted; delayed puberty; short menses; constant slight show of menses. Enuresis.

Oppression of the chest; drawing pectoral pain; sternum pains to touch; stitches on inspiration. Burning in the sternum extending upward, like lightning. Coronary sclerosis; sticking pain in the heart during climaxis so cannot stay still. Angina worse walking. Distress around the heart as if pressed upon, with uncomfortable fullness and swelling of the abdomen. Lowers blood pressure and decalcifies aneurysm. Stenosis of the oesophagus.

Bruised pain in the back, worse for touch and stooping. Bone pain especially in femur, deep in marrow, burning, boring, gnawing. Tearing of the limbs in bed. Exostoses, osteoporosis, caries in children with diarrhoea. Chronic sprains of the ankle with oedema, icy feet with cramps of calf and sole. Complaints of tendons and ligaments. Bone tumours. Profuse night sweats with pain in the limbs as soon as uncovered. Sweat of the affected part. Fistulous tumours. Trembling in the evening; trembling hands on getting wet. Weary legs worse at rest. Burning pain in the right shoulder; right arm as if paralyzed, yet warm. Numb right thumb. Cold spots on the calves. Joints worse hanging the limb down. Numb right heel. Hot hands and cold feet.

Strontium tends to loosen adherent skin on scars, and rids the body of urates. It helps avert post-operative pneumonia and has an analgesic action. It alters bones in growing animals, such as sclerosis from chronic phosphorus poisoning.

This searching remedy forms 0.02% of the earth's crust, regardless of man's atomic activities. More and more patients each year are showing Strontium symptoms, and as homoeopaths we must be aware of this and counteract them constructively.

Mental Portraits of Remedies Familiar and Unfamiliar

To the honoured science of medicine, homoeopathy adds an especial human artistry – the perception of who the person to be healed really is, and the recognition of his unique individuality in the roster of the proven instruments of healing. This similarity between patients and remedy follows the venerable law of correspondences, even the Doctrine of Signatures. The nature of substances must be apprehended intuitively by the use, not only of our six senses but of other more delicate and deep accords with the human being. There is a special genius which can know human nature, which can enter into the unspoken, which can perceive the process behind the pathology or the functional disharmony that eventuates in organic illness. Medical students use acrostics, often ribald, to fix dull facts in their memory. The homoeopath knows the remedy like the friends of his spirit.

What does Fluoric Acid mean to you? An essential for proper teeth? A question of water supply? A substance which gives an El Greco-ish cast to your skin? A strange light on the avenue? Not so to the homoeopath. To him it is Casanova. A charming, fickle butterfly, the man about town who ogles women in the street, the 'one-night stand' young man with a yen for variety and a great love of strangers. It is a male remedy, or one for mannish women; debauched, always trying to prove his manhood through lecherousness and variety. Sudden aversion to his wife and children, which he fights against. Elated, buoyant, happy, as only Phosphorus or Tuberculinum can be, yet more vital than them. All his geese are swans. Compelled to move about energetically, to walk fast, fearless of misfortune, flickering like a fluorescent light. Hasty, craving cold, and actually ill from warmth and warm drinks. Hungry to the point of gluttony, relieved by discharges which are thin, foul and acrid. Compulsion for long walks to let off steam. His hair is bristly, tousled, dry, his nails have longitudinal furrows, and both grow abnormally fast. Telangiectases, naevi, exostoses. Nails too thick, or thin and irregular; brilliant redness of the palms of the hands.

What does the substance magnesium mean to you? A ribbon to make a flash of light? A toothpaste? Or cathartic? Actually it is light, fragile, brilliant, brittle, swift to be consumed, a flash in the pan. It cannot resist,

173

it flames and peters out with a faintly sour, metallic odour. If Sulphur is the great unwashed, Magnesia Carb. is the great unloved, the illegitimate child, the droopy yet tense orphanage kid, anxious, silent, insecure, with twitching face and fingers and reproachful eyes. With sunken neck and temples, always nibbling for comfort, craving meat, a veritable Oliver Twist. Marasmus, inanition, unwanted. Magnesium in the human body occurs pre-eminently in the sperm; in the vegetable kingdom, in seeds. The child needing magnesium lacks creativity. It has great trouble with wisdom teeth; it is for people who come hard by what wisdom they have. Puny, sickly, sour babies who refuse milk, pitifully sensitive to noise and touch. Children of a tubercular background who are going into a decline. Spare, thin, dark, irritable, exhausted, unattractive children whom nobody loves. People who need soothing. Worn-out women who cannot even keep house properly; restless, chilly, listless shadow-wives of exigent males. Magnesia Carb. is to exhausted nerves what China is to loss of blood or fluid, a replenisher, a sustainer. Deficient vitality, too tired when sitting, relieved by walking and motion, sudden crumpling up without loss of consciousness. It is the chronic of Chamomilla. The thymus gland and the cerebrospinal fluid are also rich in magnesium. Magnesium deficiency causes lack of mother-love in animals. Magnesium is to chlorophyll as iron is to haemoglobin. A magnesium deficiency in the diet is said to favour cancer.

Another defective vitality remedy is Zincum, sometimes called the mineral Opium. It appears in molluscs. It is preternaturally calm, especially in regard to death, which it loves. Speaks of death with pleasure, though not suicidal, lies with eyes closed as if in a coma, and when questioned, hesitates, repeats the question to gain time and finally slowly gives a rational answer. Brain fag, a 'punch drunk' Nux Vomica. Too weak to bring out an exanthematous rash. Effusion into the ventricles with rolling eyeballs and half-open eyes. Starting at noise, jerking in sleep, constant fidgeting of the feet, feeling as if she had committed a crime, complaints from fright. Complete inability to sleep. Hangs the head down over the bed. Flushed with the least sip of wine. Energetic during menses. Zincum is a sovereign remedy in post-measles encephalitis.

Almost anyone with blonde daughters will recognize the whimsical, changeable, weepy, flirtatious Pulsatilla, with their late menses and corpus luteum deficiency, their religious streak in puberty, their jealousy and love of sympathy, their suggestibility, selfishness, self-pity and sanctimoniousness. Sullen, slow, sedentary, self-conscious, always wanting to make a good impression and to blame things on somebody else. Every big family of girls has one. The anemone *Pulsatilla* has been called the Tears of Venus. It wilts easily and blows in any wind. Homosexual women, dreading men and averse to marriage; easily discouraged and touchy; unexpectedly stubborn; avaricious. Fears ghosts and the dark. Even the ovum is superficially implanted and does not take hold. Aborts easily and early (fifth week).

Many a blonde charmer, however, is of the type of Cuprum, the metal of Venus; the hysterical blonde who has never been crossed; a spoiled brat who needs a spanking, and craves one. 'Off the handle'; loquacious, sullen, headstrong, malicious, morose, with fixed ideas, terror of death, complaints from fright. Tricky and spoiled. Disorderly, changeable, dissatisfied. Maniacal rage; cramps of spirit as well as body. Wild-eyed; mad fits. They stage scenes; bellow like a calf; lie like someone dead, blue and alarming and rigid. Ecstasy with quivering. Greed, malice, desire to injure, to run away and scream, to escape. Shrinks from people. Mimicry. Emotional nausea more than any remedy; nervous prostration in the young. Brain metastases; delirium with distorted face ending in sweat. Chorea, convulsions, epilepsy worse before menses; worse at noon. Uraemia.

Who knows the dried-up old maid of homoeopathy? Spare, dry, dark, timorous, staggery, hopelessly depressed. Confused, cannot believe that they have said what they say. Do not think they are themselves. Craving dried food, tea grounds, chalk. Fears insanity. Peevish and puckery. Illusions of being larger, numb, smooth, etc. Suicidal at the sight of a knife or blood. Uses up rolls of toilet paper because of her adhesive, soft stool, for which she must strain. Cannot speak for hoarseness. All the sap dried out of her. Did you recognize Alumina?

Every now and then a real neurotic will challenge you. Perhaps they came because they cannot meet any engagement, however pleasant, without diarrhoea. She will tell you that her complaints are worse from mental exertion. There is a lack of balance between the mental and the physical; she is withered by intellect. She is full of whims and superstitions, for example, never stepping on a crack in a sidewalk. She hurries, almost running in the street because she thinks someone is following her; houses seem to crush her in the street. Time goes too slowly. She has strange impulses and notions, and fears that she will fail at everything. She is the prize rationalizer. Her memory is one of her chief complaints. Predicts the time of death. Dreams of snakes and sex. Fears crowds. She is an exhibitionist and will buck up if someone is keeping an eye on her. She is off-balance and uncoordinated. She makes errors in perception, especially of size. Enlarged sensation. She has a fear of high places and is inclined to jump. Fear of fainting and disease. Indisposed to talk, which makes her nervous. She goes on sweet binges which aggravate, and escapes to alcohol. She is a prize belcher and enjoys it. She wants the room icy and all her food cold, and is aggravated from warmth in any form. Especially worse in the sun. She is a moon child. This is the actor's remedy, full of hoarseness, painful throat, faltering speech from panic, failure and nerves – 'Alibi Ike': Argentum Nitricum.

'If I rest I'll go mad' is the keynote to Iodum. Never can stay in bed, even with 105°F fever. Must have cold air, always much too hot. Compulsions to violence without cause. Wants to hurt her child. Dark, thin, tawny-skinned, shrivelled, withering; shuns company; melancholy, suspicious, suicidal. Always eating and never full, yet emaciates. The glands enlarge at the expense of the rest of the body. She burns the candle at both ends and is cross and anxious.

Among the bees the queen is paramount, the drones and workers serve her. Apis is a jealous widow, deprived though not depraved, amorous, vain and hard to please. She is bossy and wants to run the world, a breaker of rules; absent-minded, apathetic, awkward, drops things and breaks things (whereas Natrum Mur. stumbles). There is a sting in her gossip; direct malice, not devious. She is impatient, dictatorial, whiney, fidgety; averse to constriction, upset by trifles, irked by small talk, procrastinating, worse after sleep and violently aggravated by anything hot.

If Rhus Tox. is the human barometer, Mercurius is the human thermometer, suited by neither heat nor cold, alternately hot and chilly. Many criminals need Mercurius. It may be a brutal, ugly, cruel type – the murderer's remedy. Suicide by shooting. Like the substance mercury it is elusive. Like Mercury, the messenger of the gods, it is glib, tricky, mischievous, mistrustful. Weary of life. Hasty and ineffective. Quicksilver is called the chameleon mineral and is volatile. The typical Mercury patient is chronically ill, disgusted and morose. He may be stupid and slow to answer, or over-bright without character. He is averse to company, timid, with feeble will and poor memory, worse from sunset to sunrise. He is bald and slimy, uncoordinated, tremulous, irregular in his movements. He is embarrassed, homesick, absent-minded, even imbecile. He has impulses he fears to follow. Mercurius acts on the lymphatic system as Aconite acts on the circulatory. In olden times mercurialization was almost universal, witness the slogan – 'Salivation is salvation'. Mankind has been thoroughly poisoned by this substance.

What does the stately cedar make you think of? The Villa d'Este?

Moth protection? Indeed, the *Arbor vitae* was the secret of Egyptian embalming, dissolving tissue and flushing out the cavities. *Thuja occidentalis* is oval in its shape, in its buds, and those who need the remedy are elliptical, all curves. It is the great remedy for the Japanese people; for drinkers of tea, for those prone to excess. It is the former of tumours, lipomas, cysts, papillomas; warts, dark as the cypress and canalized. It has strange odours of fish-brine, of garlic, of honey. The Thuja patient has too much hair. Women with moustaches and coarse, black hair on the limbs. It is waxy and greasy-looking and pallid like the buds of the cedar. Extremely sensitive to people, to music, which makes it weep. Worse in the moonlight; sensation of being separated from oneself, of floating; dreams of falling, the dead and levitation. Salacious; hasty, yet often slow in speech, mistakes in reading and writing. Fixed ideas; thinks she is pregnant, that the legs are made of wood or elongated. Heavy trunk, short neck and thin limbs. Small bones, short children with irregular teeth which decay early. Pituitary dysfunction; mentally handicapped children, ugly-looking people. Chronic ill-effect of animal poisons such as snake bites or serums, and especially of vaccinations which do not take. Feels he is under the dominion of a superior power, or as if a stranger were at his side. Exhausted and soft. Dissolves tumours. Excess of mucous discharges. The most vesicular remedy.

The most precious of metals – gold, or Aurum Metallicum – represents the sun, the ego, the blood. Paracelsus and Avicenna spoke of it. It is usually thought of as the masculine ego, the feminine or false ego being Platina. In the modern world the Aurum patient is a solid businessman, a good father. He tends to be robust, earthy, ruddy and bald. His distresses in the mental sphere have to do with perversions of the affections. He is turbulent, uncommunicative, angry, worse from contradiction. He broods, feels guilty and inferior. He is concerned about his salvation. He is taciturn, melancholy, and even suicidal by jumping. Having had a jolly night with the boys the evening after the financial crash, he is the one who jumps off the roof or out of his office window. He is especially oriented toward money (the gold standard again). He has an insanity of the will, and although he is very able, nothing succeeds, or so he thinks. He is full of self-criticism, angry at trifles, restless and always in a hurry. In your office he will pace the floor and say nothing, whereas Natrum Mur. will just say nothing. He craves the wide open spaces. Music is a great relief to him. He is one of the few remedies that goes into despair from severe pain. Like Belladonna, he will hit his head against the wall. He is always too warm, craves air as violently as Lachesis. He fears people. He is warm-blooded, better in cold weather and from cold bathing; often olive-skinned and dark-haired. He has a relationship with the dead, like Thuja and Zincum, dreams of them, of falling and robbers. He is markedly aggravated at night, sunset to sunrise, and may sob in his sleep. It is the most deeply syphilitic and suicidal remedy. He craves alcohol. He tends to complaints of the heart and bones. Although superficially flexible, he is basically extremely stubborn.

The nickname for Arsenicum is the 'gold-headed cane' patient. Though so weak that he is almost dying, he will remember to want his flowered dressing gown, and will really suffer if the pictures are crooked on the wall. The keynote of the Arsenicum patient is irritable weakness, restlessness without relief from motion, drives him from bed to bed; prostration out of all proportion. Burning relieved by heat, including stuffy rooms, hot drinks and foods. Aggravation after midnight, especially at 1 or 2 a.m. Chilly, right-sided, wants someone constantly to hold his hand. He is vain, mean, avaricious, malicious. In fact, to the homoeopath the Nitric Acid and Arsenicum patients are the ones most to be dreaded – except for the prize pest (who does not mean to be) Psorinum. Arsenicum actually means every nasty thing it says or does. They are full of fears: of being alone, of death; are fastidious and exacting. Even their secretions are scanty, like their kindness: acrid, thin and cadaveric in odour. The great remedy for shortness of breath and for improving the skin and hair. The Stygian island arsenic eaters can do great feats of mountain climbing. The Arsenicum patient is cowardly, vicious; he curses like Anacardium. He cannot live – from anxiety rather than from pain. A great remedy for racehorses to improve their wind and coats.

Then there are the fat, flabby, red-faced, strawberry-blond Capsicum children, who are quietly homesick and want to be let alone and sleep. Refractory, stubborn, slow in all their reactions, alternate pale and red faces, lazy beyond belief, they dread the open air. Children of overindulgent parents (the opposite of Magnesia Carb.). They are suspicious and take offence easily; obstinate, contrary, clumsy and awkward. They do not have desires – they have impulses; persistent suicidal thoughts, although they do not wish to do it; now jovial, now angry at trifles. Cannot learn at school for emotional reasons. Lack of reaction, craves stimulants, in a class with Nux Vomica for delirium tremens. It is a sort of degenerated Belladonna. The headaches of Capsicum, however, are accompanied by a *cold*, red face, by rigors and shivering on drinking. Pain in distant parts on coughing, like Causticum. Gloomy Gus – Natrum Carb. – is one of the sad, sensitive Natrums. 'Brain fag', the bookkeeper who can no longer add correctly. This Sodium is as lean, dyspeptic, excitable and stooped as a Sulphur, but he is greatly aggravated by mental exertion, which gives him a headache. He is not only sad but oversensitive; he starts violently at noise, at music. His taste is overdeveloped, he is irritable after eating. His nose is red, like many dyspeptics, and the tip of his nose is puffy and pimply – the so-called red cabbage nose. His mind is acid as well as his stomach. He worries over trifles and has total debility in the summer heat. Withered infants with weak digestions and diarrhoea from milk. Headaches from the sun and light.

Nitric Acid is one of the most disagreeable patients. As infants they desire pica, indigestible things, salt or earth, and are relieved, as in later life, by riding in an automobile – in other words, by jar. Like Arsenicum they are malicious and exigent. They are also vindictive and ungrateful. They have complaints *after*, for instance, stool or urinating, or vomiting. It is the great remedy for diarrhoea after the use of the mycins. The Nitric Acid patient waxes his moustache, which does not conceal the deep lines of suffering from nose to mouth. He has cracked lip corners, mapped tongue, bleeding, jagged warts, piles, and rectal prolapse. He is miserable at both ends. It is most suitable for people past middle age, thin, dark-haired, diarrhoeic people, well enough but full of woe. Very much alive, but hypochondriac. Anxious over his illness, thinks he will die soon; cantankerous, taciturn, joyless, sad in the evening, lives in the past, headstrong, peevish, obstinate; inveterate ill-will. Do not bother to apologize to Nitric Acid – he will be unmoved by it. His mood is worse on alternate days. They have pain in the bones where they come near the skin, such as the shin. One of our greatest homoeopaths claims that since nitrogen is a main element in organic life, Nitric Acid should be one of our most powerful and most frequently needed remedies.

Phosphorus – think of phosphorescence, a gleam, a glitter, a fitful light, but no warmth. The sanguine temperament, sensitive, sudden, euphoric, creative; new interests; wonderful beginners and poor finishers. Young people, cultists, one of the few remedies for ecstasy (compare Fluoric Acid). Phosphorus will counteract the effects of anaesthesia, especially those of chloroform. It is also the remedy of choice for people who have been struck by lightning or have had an electric shock. The Phosphorus patient is fey, very psychic, like Aconite and Belladonna. The nation most like the Phosphorus temperament are the Irish, and the background of Phosphorus people is usually tuber-cular, rather than syphilitic like Nitric Acid and Aurum. They are usually slender or emaciated, strawberry-blond, or with blue-black hair and blue eyes. Very subject to freckles; stoop-shouldered, clairvoyant. Incredibly incautious (opposite of Causticum). Full of fear, mainly of disease, the dark, thunderstorms, water, death. Chilly, left-sided, better eating and sleeping; always tired, bruises easily; wounds heal and break open again, loves being mesmerized and massaged gently. Delirium of the body being in fragments. Grandiose mania. People who grow too fast. The Phosphorus patient has alabaster skin, long silky eyelashes, mental speed and physical slowness. Is often the result of inbreeding or consanguinity in the ancestry. They are vehement, superficial, destructive, intellectual, immodest, amative, mental and physical exhibitionists; it is the most frequent homosexual remedy in men. Somnambulism, insanity with exaggeration of the ego, vain, loquacious, worse alone, averse to children, sympathetic, susceptible and easily influenced.

Silica – quartz, crystal, flint, sand. The Nordic type: angel children, neat as dolls, clean, orderly, alabaster skin, flaxen or tow hair, blue eyes, transparent look with veins showing, hair too fine, nails poor, big square heads, late-closing fontanelles. They lack grit, they are too delicate, their bones too small, they are too tall and too slender, like the grasses and the grains, which are mostly Silica. They are oversensitive, mild and weepy, but unlike Pulsatilla are averse to being consoled. Sensitive to beauty, will not be pushed around, resent interference. They are timid, shy, fearful of the dark and thunderstorms, yielding and faint-hearted, status lymphaticus, thymus cases. Poor endurance. Professional folk, lack of self-confidence; adults fear failure when they are *not* slipping (Lyco-podium when they are). Silica children eat sand. They are intelligent, touchy, self-willed. Imperfect assimilation, aversion to responsibility, fixed ideas. They are the albinos of the spirit, often shirkers, cry when spoken to, cling to mother's skirt, need stamina, dread the public. They are brittle, not torpid or flabby. Precise, high-strung, over-conscientious, accurate, impatient, searches for pins. Badly insulated to life, washed-out but will not give in. Transparent and not murky. Homesick, cries when scolded; somnambulism. Students who continue studying because they fear to start on their own. Sensitive to the full or new moon.

Sepia is the animated carbon, from the cuttlefish, cousin to the octopus, from whence we derive sepia ink. Have you ever watched the cuttlefish hiding among the rocks in an aquarium? You can hardly find it, and suddenly it swoops out, exuding a murky cloud of brown liquid, and as quickly retires again. So the Sepia patient, inactive and uninterested one moment and violent the next. They are unable to feel emotion, although anxious to do so. Tall women, mustachioed ladies with narrow hips (vice versa, men who rarely have to shave and who have the typical feminine pelvis). They are easily offended, slow in speech and usually dark, but may be a delicate blond or even redhead. Subject to sudden excitement, but in general indifferent to everything – life, their loved ones, their homes. Women who have worked hard and had too many children and resent it, and drag around the house (compare Magnesia Carb., who long for the affection they do not get). Sepia is nervous among strangers, though they have turned against their own family (opposite of Fluoric Acid, who has a great love of strangers). Sepia is the great remedy between puberty and the climacteric. Its motto is 'I don't care'. Aversion to work, weak memory, morbidity, dreads to be alone; avarice (like Arsenicum and Lycopodium). Sepia women seek relief in operations. They cause bachelors to thank God they are still single and gynaecologists to be very busy. Passive, vehement, aggravated by consolation. Tea-drinkers, like Thuja. Dark circles under the eyes, or yellow saddle across the nose. Brown moles. Always wants to have the last word. Apprehensive of the future and fears starving (like Bryonia, Psorinum). Sensitive to odours. Better by violent exercise. Puffy, flabby, venous people who faint. Sepia can be more insulting than any other remedy. They lack the realization of love. Affection does not register. They seem never happy unless annoying someone. They are greedy as well as miserly. They make gaffes and tactless breaks, are estranged from their loved ones, cold, stoical, spiteful, sarcastic, peevish, averse to opposition, everything seems strange to them; no joy.

Graphites or black lead, plumbago as it is called, a member of the carbon family (Carbo An., Carbo Veg., Carboneum Sulph., Petroleum), is one of the great remedies for the climacteric. A middle-aged woman, fat or recently emaciating, chilly, costive, dry – inability to sweat, itchy, fissures or cracks over the knuckles, near the nails, on the ball of the thumb, behind the ears (salt rheum), in the perineum; moist, smelly eruptions where two folds of skin meet, as under the breast; wens and keloids. Not sensitive physically but exceedingly so emotionally. Irresolute and wavering, depressed and sad, changing moods, flippant. Children laugh at reprimands and adults laugh in the wrong place. Weep at music. Aversion to mental work. Thoughts of death and salvation. Cautious, fidgety, hurried, critical, fretting, impudent, teasing, irritable at trifles, startles easily. Averse to coition, almost like Sepia, anxious grief. Nash said, 'As Pulsatilla is to puberty, so is Graphites to the climacteric.'

The yellow jasmine, Gelsemium, reminds one of a high-strung, delicate Southern lady. Complaints with the coming of warm weather in the spring; summer colds; distress in warm countries. Mental confusion, drowsiness, stage fright, fear of falling, neurotic lassitude from bad news, complaints from ordeals, grief or embarrassment. Fearless as Opium or Belladonna, worse thinking of ailments. It increases the memory. It is improved by alcohol. It relieves the trembling of tobacco and helps to cut down smoking. Aggravated by bad news. Nerve exhaustion, tremors, even paralysis. Better by urinating. Hysterical blindness from sex deprivation or shock. Awkward and clumsy, ineffectual labour pains. A remedy which was proved to raise the opsonic index. It averts many influenzas.

The homoeopath is familiar with the precious metal, gold, the homoeopathic remedy of the male ego. There is a feminine counterpart, the other precious metal, platinum, which we call in our specialty the false or feminine ego. This is one of our more striking and fascinating remedy personalities. Prim old maids, respectable, high-born, snobbish with dirty minds. Nymphomaniacs, paranoid folk – the leading symptom is not only pride but contempt for the world. To them, even physical objects seem smaller than they are, as though looked at through the wrong end of opera glasses. They have a disordered sense of proportion. They love to be alone, are exceedingly erotic to the point where it is almost impossible to do even an ordinary physical examination on a Platina patient, not to mention a pelvic.

The Platina patient kills the loved one, either actually by homicide or through withering with contempt and contumely. It is aggravated by chagrin, as is Staphysagria, although it is likely to be more vocal about it. It has the curious range from hilarity to anger, reminding us of certain other remedies like Fluoric Acid. It has a fear of death to a marked degree, and guilt sensations, and it is always washing, almost like Syphilinum. Like Lycopodium, it is constipated when travelling, and also has that bowel difficulty when pregnant. It is aggravated in the twilight and greatly relieved by walking in cool air. Pains come and go gradually, like Stannum. It is aggravated both sitting and standing and in the evening. It is a chilly one and is notable for coldness of single parts. It is one of the great remedies for pain with numbness, like Gnaphalium, especially neuralgias, and tic douloureux. It also abounds in constriction sensations as if bandaged, like Mancinella. Its numbness goes almost to the point of anaesthesia, despite the marked hyperaesthesia of the genitals. It is one of the greatest remedies for onanism. It is one of the remedies that is worse from fasting, like Sulphur or Phosphorus. Its stools may be as soft and sticky as Alumina, though difficult to pass, or hard and black like Plumbum (it is sometimes a remedy for lead colic). Its menses are early, profuse, black, thick, even clotted. It has burning in the ovaries, worse in the left, and stitching in the ovaries, worse in the right. Abdominal colic extends to the back. Sensations as if the navel were tied with a string to the spine, reminding again of Plumbum, as if squeezed in a vice. Colic extending to the back, even paralysis, in general right-sided, should be compared with Palladium, which is almost as haughty, and Cuprum, Plumbum and Stannum.

Plumbum Metallicum, the remedy connected with ancient Saturn, and with both ego and etheric, is one of the heavy metals. If one must define it in one word, it would be 'sclerosis'. Another S connected with it is stretching, which relieves, and slowness, sweat, spasms, sleep peculiarities such as odd positions, single part paralyses, sensation of a string to the spine. It is not a pleasant person, our Plumbum, deceitful, lying, thieving, anxious, restless, timid, emaciated, atrophied, anaemic, trembling, and paralyzed. Fear of assassination, greasy face, idiot epileptic children, contractions, boring pains, impaction of the bowels, constricted anus with urge followed by bloody lumps, intussusception, strangulated hernia, miscarriage, wandering pain, like Kali Bich., Pulsatilla and Tuberculinum, extensor paralyses of single parts, blindness in connection with headache, relief of pain by pressure and exertion, neurological diseases, alternations of neuralgia with colic, stubborn sciatica, sacroiliac pain, urinary retention with tenesmus and nephritis. A slow, desperate remedy, good in aluminium poisoning, often the chronic complement of Rhus Tox. and related to Opium.

We know from the Classics of Socrates drinking the hemlock, Conium Maculatum, a curious remedy for old maids and bachelors, singularly painless. A remedy for the celibate who suffers from the lack of normal relationships, but not consciously, like Apis. Domineering, averse to contradiction, scolding and nagging, easily angered, imbecile rather than insane, dreading to be alone, yet unsocial, passive. One of our greatest remedies for vertigo, turning the head or eyes, and for seasickness where dizziness is the outstanding feature. Photophobia, ptosis, worse standing than at rest, turning, touch, jar, pressure, and alcohol. Many urinary symptoms, slow stream, inability, stopping and starting, headache with suppression of urine, teasing dry cough, worse at night and lying down. Rheumatism and periostitis of the leg, better hanging the leg down. Yellow nails, sweat on closing the eyes, lumps of the breast, stony, heavy tumours, the stitching pain in breast cancer, faints at stool, constipation on alternate days. Great desire with impotence, large hard testicles, prostatic discharge with faeces; dysmenorrhoea with drawing pain in the thighs; painful foetal movements; must sit up to cough out mucus; railroad spine like Bellis Perennis; numb, weak legs like Cocculus. A remedy full of hidden grief, passive.

The Kalis are plump, heavy, chilly, feverless, brutal people. The most frequently used one in homoeopathy is the Bichromicum. The insensitive beer-drinker; rheumatoid diathesis. They are known for alternations, for instance of bowel and throat complaints, for wandering pain and distress in small spots. They have stringy, yellow, tough phlegm, in fact all the discharges, whether from the conjuctiva, the vagina or wherever, tend to be ropy and golden. Punched-out ulcers, headaches from suppressed coryza, with sinus trouble; migraines, preceded by blindness; loss of smell and taste, typical follicular tonsillitis, sensation of hair in the fauces; snuffles, glazed glistening tongue with raised papillae. Metallic or brassy cough, with pain to the shoulders. Better lying down. Hoarseness, post-nasal crust, casts of the bronchi; duodenal ulcer pains extending through to the back, and pains from the sternum to the back (opposite of Cuprum – pains from the back to the front). Kali Bich. wants hot drinks and has a seasickness relieved at the bouillon hour. Pains at the root of the nose, difficulty in digesting starches, alternations of spring and autumn complaints. Although this remedy appears not to have many mental symptoms, it is one of the group of brutal, stoical remedies related to the syphilitic miasm.

Far more sensitive is its fellow Kali, the Carbonate. The ticklish Ts – plump, chilly, asthmatic, full of indigestion and gas, malicious, spiteful, timid, whimsical, one of the difficult patients. Marked aggravation at 3 a.m. One of the most susceptible to drafts. Kali Carb. is not the captain of its soul. It is slack and has no will; it fears illness, death, and the future, and craves company. Defeatism combined with much ado about nothing. A vagotonic, peevish, fatty degeneration; fainting, usually low blood pressure; startles easily; puffy over the eyes like Apis; stitching pains in the right chest like Bryonia. Shortness of breath prevents eating. One of the few remedies whose expectoration flies out of the mouth in a cold ball. The asthmatic sits bent forward for relief, opposite of Spongia. Dyspepsia of the aged, distension with cold abdomen; constipation during menses; desires sweets and sours; gouty, foamy urine, craves hot drinks, violent backache as if broken, sacral. The Kali Carb. patient is not one who interests you nor stirs your pity. They are averse to being touched, feel as though something were loose in the brain, as though a fishbone in the throat; a partial sweat, and pains have changed location. They are of low sexuality and worse after coition; cardiac insufficiency, sleepy after eating. Their menses are pale and scanty. Has sweat of painful part. Often anaemic. It is a difficult remedy to prescribe, and one of those which gives the most trying aggravations.

These few examples of the inner nature and usefulness of remedies according to the homoeopathic law should inspire you to undertake the adventure of getting acquainted with the different substances, as though they were people whom you wish to make your friends. When you come into a party, look around and see how many constitutional remedies you can identify. As you strap-hang in the subway, peer over the newspaper into the nature of the travellers. Get so that you can recognize a remedy through accurate and swift observation, even as they walk past you in the street or enter your office. It will reward you and the patient every day.

Such are the fascinating faces of some of our helpful remedies; but as La Fontaine said, 'Gardez-vous de juger les gens sur la mine!' Sulphur may be clean, Silica angry, Pulsatilla thirsty and Arsenicum left-sided. Especially in acute diseases, remember that your familiar types, such as the above brief portraits, are not the safe criterion. The physical generals are the best lifeline. Paradox is of the essence!

Oleum Animale

Man of fifty-eight, a heart case, now back at work and relatively well. He complains of a numbness of the left upper lip, of coldness of the feet and hands, falling hair, and of a pulling sensation upward in the left upper lip. Also of unwanted nightly erections, although impotent when attempting coition.

Kent, under 'Face, numbness, left' gives us one remedy only – Graphites. This also has the incomplete erection problem (page 695); the patient also has a dryness and a curious sense of humour, now teasing, now rather out of place, all of which suggests Graphites. However, he has already had this remedy, and although it helped him as a person some time ago, it was useless in this curious pulling up of the left upper lip. As so often, I had recourse to Robert's *Sensations As If*, and there on page 386, under 'Pulling', appeared one remedy – Oleum Animale (Dippel's oil, from stag's horn). It is obtained in the preparation of bone black, says our *Pharmacopoeia*. The patient has dark smudges under his eyes, and a whole appearance suggesting Graphites and the carbons. This was the first time in forty years of my practice that this remedy has ever been indicated. The fascination of homoeopathy never ceases!

CASES

Elizabeth Wright Hubbard insisted on treating patients as body, mind and soul. She had a superior way of individualizing a patient's needs and a deep knowledge of the substances to fill those needs. She treated the patient who had the disease rather than the disease itself. Why did she choose Natrum Mur. 10M when the Repertory called for Phosphorus? In her words, 'This is a singularly interesting perception of the personality of the patient.' She considered the sensations 'as if' indispensable, especially in the case of a woman with complaints of violent pain in her left eye.

To listen, to ask, to observe. With the right remedy, many cases will clear without surgery, including breast lumps, duodenal ulcer, varicose veins and even some appendix upsets. — Ed.

Homoeopathy as an
Instrument of Precision

Modern medicine is proud of its instruments of precision; but as with many inventions, these often supplant the use of our natural faculties. An instrument, according to the dictionary, is a furtherance, an agency, a means to an end, and comes from the Latin *instruere*, meaning *to prepare*, from the same root as instruct. A secondary meaning is that of tool, which is really an extension of the human hand. The old-fashioned physicians could smell diphtheria or scarlet fever or typhoid upon entering the house, and even today many of us know the odour of cancer and of approaching death. But even those doctors whose senses are keenly alive, and who combine vivid perceptions with the assiduous use of modern scientific technique, are at a loss for a large part of the time, and feel that their work in therapeutics is vague and only partially satisfactory.

Conventional medicine (and much of so-called homoeopathy) give drugs on the basis of diagnosis or pathology or organs affected, or at best on what we call common symptoms, such as vomiting, purging and so on. Its practitioners are oblivious to the fine distinctions between cases of similar classification. The secret of precision is in *individualization* and not in trying to put the parts in place of the whole. The homoeopath who is worthy of the name knows that only by being an artist can you arrive at exactitude. To give Bryonia for pneumonia, Rhus Tox. for rheumatism, Sulphur for eczema or Nux Vomica for indigestion, is not real homoeopathy. The more exact the similarity between the patient's symptoms and the single remedy given, the fuller and more salient the totality of the symptoms elicited, the more swift and brilliant the cure, because of the precision of the prescription.

Over and above all usual medical lore, the homoeopathic specialist has unusual and specific knowledge: of general symptoms pertaining to the patient himself as a whole; of aggravations and ameliorations as applied to each complaint; of discharges, those most revealing vents of the inner man; of repercussing suppressions and their devious sequelae. In chronic work he elicits the health trends from childhood, and even in the parents. From this welter of detail he arrives at a totality of the symptoms. This does not mean that he retains for final analysis every least item, although in confused cases a careful compilation is needed as a background. Then follows elimination and emphasis – the evaluation of symptoms. The final choice of remedy may be based on a mere five or six striking points which characterize the person in different spheres, in somewhat the way that a caricaturist, in half a dozen lines, shows up the inner and outer nature of his subject. Many fine prescribers claim that their grasp of a similar remedy is intuitive, but probably in addition to a sixth sense, they are using a vast unconscious store of wisdom, information and experience. The editing of our case-taking is perhaps the most important point in homoeopathy – to be able to sense what is germane, what is primordial and what is poignant in a case.

Doctors need to study botany, zoology and mineralogy, learning to enter into a substance, take on its life, pulse with its currents, read the signatures and correspondences, and keep unsealed the eye of ancient knowledge. The signs are there that he who runs may read, but he must run, not halt or stumble. As an illustration, let us take the octopus in the aquarium with its apparent apathy, its swift rages making murky the whole ambience with its ink; its womb-like shape; its flabby, sucking tentacles. What a compelling entity is Sepia!

The true homoeopath may not merely be accurate with the most common hundred or so remedies, but must enlarge his knowledge systematically by daily study of the materia medica in myriad books and magazines. He must search into remedy relationships and let his mind play on the free association principle. How revealing to realize that Opium, Chelidonium and Sanguinaria are of the same family, or that Apis is the animal counterpart of Natrum Muriaticum!

It must remembered that where medicine depends upon mechanical aids, whose perfection is fallible in direct ratio to the fallibility of the interpreter of the data, precision is impossible. The best instrument of precision that I have ever encountered is true homoeopathy in skilful and devoted hands. Consider the following examples:

Miss X., fifty-ish, with double pneumonia when first seen, lying rigidly still, rusty sputum, temperature of 40°C, marked herpes on the lips and below the nose, stitching pain in the chest on breathing, hard cough, thirst for great quantities of ice water. Bryonia 10M, one dose followed by placebo. Temperature descended by lysis on the third day, but the patient complained of a lumbosacral backache which bothered her much more than the pneumonia. No characteristic symptoms were forthcoming. Aesculus and later Kali Carb. were tried in succession, with temporary but not lasting relief.

Finally she said how strange it was that the backache was much more severe after urinating (urine negative). On repertorizing in Kent only one remedy had this peculiar symptom: Syphilinum. In looking for corroborative symptoms I noticed corneal scars, and the patient said she had had keratitis and iritis some years before. She had certain characteristics of the syphilitic miasm and the backache was troubling her most from dark to dawn. Syphilinum 1M, one dose, produced a two-hour violent aggravation followed by swift and permanent relief.

Mrs Y., also at the mid-century. A history of mucous colitis and liver trouble; complained of spasmodic abdominal colic or gripes. Worse on the left side, preferred heat to cold, and liked pressure though did not double up. Colocynth was of no avail. Mag. Phos. relieved temporarily but the attacks recurred. No diarrhoea, very few symptoms. Finally she said, 'In these attacks I feel as though my stomach hits my backbone.' I asked her to try stretching during the pain and she found it agreeable. Wassermann and blood count negative. Stools tended to be in little black balls. Plumbum 1M, one dose, produced rapid improvement and the colics, which had been coming every day or two for four months, did not recur within five weeks.

Mrs Z., 78, senile dementia, healthy-looking, rosy cheeks, blonde, terribly restless and loquacious, singing, scolding, alternating with laughing and hilarity, incontinence of urine and faeces, marked destructiveness, would tear up sheets and towels; family said she had been a spoiled beauty all her life. Cuprum 50M, one dose, greatly improved both the mental and excretory phases.

These are simple, everyday instances of the power of precision in homoeopathy, but the results could certainly not be achieved without sedatives in regular medicine. Homoeopathy is arduous, but its rewards can be reaped for both the patient and the prescriber, especially if he or she will remember the sentence by the French aviator Saint-Exupéry: 'Perfection in its finality is not when nothing can be added, but when nothing can be taken away.'

Precision Prescribing
in Acute Cases

Man of 72 with history of empyema and rib resection five years ago has a bronchial cold with fine moist râles in the left lower posterior chest. No fever. Slight cough. Shallow breathing. Boring pain in left side of the chest. Stitch catches him on breathing in.

Boring pain in side of chest (Kent, page 852): Bismuth, Bromium, Ferrum, Muriatic Acid, Senega. Left side (Kent, page 852): Mercurius Iod. Flavus, Senega. Stitching pain on inspiring (Kent, page 864): Muriatic Acid, Senega.

Prescription: Senega 1M, one dose.

Result: Pain and cough gone next day, chest clear of râles.

A lady of 68, depressed in the morning, complained of stinging pain in the ankle and constriction of the right wrist.

Stinging pain in ankle (Kent, page 1096): Agaricus, Berberis, Euphrasia, Kreosotum, Laurocerasus, Mancinella, Natrum Carb., Platinum, Pulsatilla, Sulphur, Zinc.

Constriction of the wrist (Kent, page 965): Cocculus, Mancinella, Silica. Sadness in the morning (Kent, page 75): Mancinella.

Prescription: Mancinella 10M, one dose.

Result: Relief of pain by next day; felt surprisingly cheerful.

A young man of 20 has had neuralgia around the left ear daily for two years, so severe he gets drunk to stop it. Specialists in two major cities were unable to relieve him, even with strong sedation.

Suicidal (Kent, page 85). Thoughts of death (Kent, page 17). Desires company (Kent, page 12). Guilt feeling (Kent, page 6). Sensation of falling or sinking through bed (Kent, pages 99–101). Aggravation dry weather (Kent, page 1357). Pain in left ear (Kent, page 303). Ailments from anticipated pleasure (Kent, page 60). Cold foot sweat (Kent, page 1183). Ingrowing toenails (Kent, page 1019).

Discussion: Only one remedy runs through all twelve symptoms. The runner-up was Sulphur with 8 and the remedy given was Causticum 10M, one dose.

Note that 11 of the 12 symptoms apply to the man and not the ear; however in Hering, under Causticum, we read 'non-suppurative seventh nerve pain in the ears.'

Result: Slight pain for two or three hours after the dose, none whatever for the next three months, at which time slight recurrence. Causticum 10M, one dose. No further pain to date (two months).

Woman of 48 has abdominal distension 'like a drum', cannot pass the gas. Cold knees in bed, tight spasm of the anus, arthritis of the right hand – finger.

Cold knees (Kent, page 961): Apis., Carbo Veg., China, Colchicum, Ignatia, Lachesis, Mercurius, Natrum Mur., Nitric Acid, Phosphorus, Pulsatilla, Selenium, Sepia, Silica, Veratrum Alb. Spasm of the anus (Kent, page 632): Causticum, Colchicum, Serratia, Tabacum Tympanites of the abdomen (Kent, page 545): Carbo Veg., China, Colchicum, Lachesis, Mercurius, Phosphorus, Sepia, Silica. Arthritis of the finger (Kent, page 1060): Colchicum, Nitric Acid, Sepia, Silica.

Prescription: Obviously Colchicum 1M, one dose.

Result: Rapid relief of distension, anal spasm and cold knees. Fingers painless in about a week.

Woman of 30 has intestinal virus. Abdominal cramps better doubling up, worse pressure, Diarrhoea brown, scanty, odour of bad meat, watery. Itching anus after stool. Vertigo worse motion. Nausea from odours. Boils on the buttocks. Temple headache. Hoarse. Exhausted and chilly.

Cramps better bending forward (Kent, page 575): Aconite, Causticum, China, Colchicum, Colocynth, Kali Carb., Lachesis, Mag. Phos., Plumbum, Rhus Tox., Stannum, Phosphorus. Scanty diarrhoea (Kent, page 641): Aconite, China, Colchicum, Colocynth, Kali Carb., Plumbum, Stannum. Itching anus (Kent, page 622): Kali Carb. Vertigo worse motion (Kent, page 101): China, Phosphorus. Nausea from odours: (Kent, page 508): Colchicum. Boils on the buttocks (Kent, page 999): Phosphorus, Plumbum. Temple headache (Kent, page 168): China, Kali Carb., Plumbum, Rhus Tox., Stannum. Diarrhoea, odour of bad meat (Kent, page 640): China, Rhus Tox. Diarrhoea, watery (Kent, page

643): China, Colchicum, Colocynth, Lachesis, Phosphorus. Exhausted from diarrhoea (Kent, page 1416): China, Phosphorus.

Prescription: China Off. 200c, one dose every two hours for three doses.

Result: Diarrhoea stopped before the third dose, and patient recovered brilliantly.

Lady of 74 has had hypertension for many years. Sudden loss of power of the right arm and leg, with thick speech. Face and tongue drawn, blood pressure 230/140. Pupils sluggish, fibrillating heart. History of having a bowel complex. Rectal condylomata. Terror of the night; anguish and anxiety from sunset on; inability to sleep; hot, not chilly.

Discussion: one symptom, the terror of the night, was so overwhelming that combined with the sleeplessness and rectal difficulty, after trying two or three other remedies, without success, the repertory was thrown to the winds. The patient was given Syphilinum CM and peace reigned.

Medical Gynaecology

An allopathic physician who is a friend of mine said, 'What can your homoeopathy do for women's diseases?' Then I began to turn over in my mind cases which showed with any degree of satisfactory incident some of the things that homoeopathy could do for women's diseases. I report just a few of them here.

The first is a case of a fibroid which definitely diminished in size under the influence of the homoeopathic remedy. A woman of 46 with one child, living and well, came to me with the chief complaint of futility. 'There is nothing wrong with me, doctor, I just think that life isn't worth living, and I want you to do something about it.'

I took her case, took her chronic case with great care over a number of interviews, and found that from a diagnostic standpoint she complained of facial acne, menstrual disorders and a feeling of complete exhaustion. Aside from that she was conscious of no symptoms.

Her menstrual symptoms were as follows. She had periods at least every three weeks, sometimes a little oftener, with bright red flow, with actual haemorrhages perhaps twice during the period, and the period was somewhat protracted. She would also have, every three months or so, a period of about ten days between her menses when there would be spotting and bleeding. This irregularity had been going on for three years. She had never been to a doctor about it and never done anything about it. She also had, as one might imagine, a chronic backache and chronic headache, which did not bother her much.

The symptoms that she would give me were few and far between. She was one of those people who say: 'Here I am, I am futile, now kill me', and you cannot get them to tell you things. Finally this one came out, when I started to examine her: 'The odour about me is too disgusting, especially right after my period. I simply cannot live with myself, and the same is true of my perspiration – it is really dreadful.'

I immediately thought of despair, futility, with terrible odour – she was an exceedingly chilly patient; yet I did not give her at first what I ought to have given her, which was of course Psorinum. Because of certain other generals which she had – very much worse in thunderstorm weather, craving salt, being excessively thirsty for ice water, a marked aggravation at twilight time, and this flowing. On examination, there was also a tremendous fibroid in the left side of her pelvis, a fibroid which came two fingers above the umbilicus (she admitted realizing that her abdomen had been getting bigger and heavier). Instead of giving her Psorinum I gave her Phosphorus 1M, just one dose. She did not get much better – she did not please me at all. Then I left the Phosphorus and gave her Psorinum 5c, one dose. She came back after her next period and said it was the first period that she had had in years which was not early and not haemorrhagic.

I let her run on that dose for five months with constant gradual improvement on her part. She noticed no aggravation at all after the dose, but she was a very unobservant person. At the end of three months I examined her again, her fibroid was down to the level of the umbilicus. Presently she began to slip. I let her slip for a couple of weeks, obdurately, although she was cross, and she even had a period at which she had haemorrhage again. Then when I saw she was really worse, I gave her Psorinum 15c, one dose, and let that ride for five months, after which time the tumour in her left pelvis was three fingers below the umbilicus; she had had three periods which were prompt, not early, and non-haemorrhagic. The terrible odour of which she complained was better, and she herself was far from futile and no longer talking of drowning herself. Of course the end is not yet. She still has this fibroid and occasionally has a little spotting from it. I told her what she had, after consulting with her husband. I said that ordinary medicine would advise her to have it out, but that I would not, and that I wanted to see what I could do for her with her remedy. She agreed that no matter who advised having it out she would not do so.

I felt perfectly certain that as she was still having periods and was not yet at the menopause, and as she showed no improvement after the Phosphorus, and did show marked diminution after the Psorinum, that the homoeopathic remedy did something with the fibroid.

Another case, also of fibroid, but this time in a woman of 21, had rather an interesting childhood history. She showed the following:

As a child she would never let anyone wash her, she had always hated water; she also used to crave sweets and be spanked for craving them; also as a child she had chilblains terribly and had a hernia. All those things would make one think of a possible dose of Sulphur, some day. None of those symptoms appeared in her recent condition.

Her recent condition, the thing for which she came to me, was over-frequent menstruation, and too profuse. She would menstruate about every three weeks and spot on for ten days after her nine-day period ended. In her menstrual history I found she began to menstruate at ten and a half, and that she menstruated from that time regularly twice a month for about seven years, was unexamined and it was never stopped.

Recently she had not had quite as frequent menstruation, but there was drenching with it, a steady flow, bright and profuse and some pain, but not violent; slight nausea before her periods and soreness of her scalp and swelling of the glands of her neck – a general aggravation before the time of her period.

This girl had certain marked symptoms of Phosphorus: craved salt, was worse at thunderstorm time, worse in damp weather, complained of continual exhaustion, was losing weight. A rectal examination showed a distinct fibroid about the size of a two and a half months' pregnancy.

I thought that in an unmarried girl like that I had better have corroboration. I sent her to one of the best obstetricians and got a written report from him confirming this fact. This girl was engaged, and he said to her, 'By no means can you get married now. Considering your age I don't advise X-ray therapy or operation. I don't know what to do for you except build up your health. Meanwhile your engagement is indefinite.'

She came back to me with this report, and after that I put her on Phosphorus 1M, one dose, and ran her up through a series of Phosphorus, at long intervals. Her periods became more regular and she began to put on weight, and her general condition became better. After six months I sent her back to the obstetrician and again he said, 'There is an amazing thing – this fibroid has gone down.' She said, 'Has it gone down more than you would expect?' Because she had a secret delight in being able to tell him what had done it. He said: 'It has. You are very lucky. If you want to make a date for your wedding you may, but you must not have children yet. What have you been doing?' She told him, and he threw up his hands. Then he added, 'Come back to me again in six months.' And she did, after going slowly up the scale of Phosphorus, and feeling better. Six months afterwards he said if she had come to him then for the first time he would not have known that she had a fibroid condition, and that she could get married and could even start a family if she wanted to. That we have in our records in writing, which is a great joy to us.

She then developed another interesting variant. She began having terrific pain in her left pelvis after menstruation. The pain would go to the back and down the front of the thighs. Nothing helped it. At this time she also had a white, sort of albuminous leucorrhoea which she told me she used to have long, long ago.

Then she said, 'I have a passion for onions; I have always liked them, and I want onions every day in the week.' I thought, this is interesting; with the discharge, the fibroid, craving onions, and this left ovarian pain which Thuja has, I gave her a dose of Thuja 10M, since when she has been much better. She then went back to her Phosphorus (she seemed to call for that again after three or four months).

Certain other gynaecological conditions are much less interesting, because there is no possibility of checking up what good you do.

One patient who came to me in the 1920s had a history of terrific menorrhagia and metrorrhagia. As a girl her doctors had done a dilatation and curettage on her; after that she almost bled to death and had to be transfused. She was not homoeopathic at that time. Although she was then 23 years of age, she was given X-ray treatments, which entirely stopped the bleeding. She began to get hot flashes, had no more periods, fell in love, got engaged, and got married. The doctor who had given her the X-ray treatment said, 'It will come back', but it did not come back, and after two years from that time the same doctor said, 'I guess I was mistaken, you will have to adopt a baby.'

She said, 'I am desperate. My husband is the last of his family, we must have a child, and I have had no periods since the time of the X-ray. Can homoeopathy do anything?' I did her chronic case and she too was Phosphorus, and I think that if she had had Phosphorus it would probably have checked her haemorrhages.

I put her on Phosphorus, one dose, repeated it four months afterward, and five and a half months after she began treatment with me, which was four years after she had had her X-ray treatment, she had a period. She telegraphed me in great excitement, and thereafter continued to have periods, although slightly irregular.

Another case was one with a local thick, yellow, stringy elastic discharge in a very beautiful and very calm young woman. I accent that because the remedy I gave her stands in the book for beautiful and calm people – Kali Bichromicum. She did not have a symptom in the world that I could find except this discharge. She had been under the care of a regular obstetrician who was going to do a repair and various local treatments, which she objected to. She had two doses of Kali Bich. 1M at two-month intervals, and her discharge practically disappeared. Whether it would have stopped anyway is always open to question, but it was so typically a Kali Bich. discharge that I feel it might be added to our list.

Then there was a case which really is mental, and yet comes in under the sphere of the sex organs. It was a case of onanism, in a girl of twenty-seven who had done it from the time she was a child, whom I had had as a patient for terrible aphthae of the mouth. I put her on Kali Mur., which helped her very much. She confessed the onanism one day and apparently it was very serious. She was life's greatest snob, which she had no reason to be, and was also a great one for washing, washing, washing, which goes psychiatrically with that state of affairs. She certainly had a superiority complex, and practically no symptoms, but just on the mental haughtiness and insistence on cleanliness, and onanism, I decided on Platinum 200c, one dose.

Before doing that I gave her placebo and told her it would cure her. She was neurotic – I wanted to see what would happen. She called me up a few days afterward and said: 'Your medicine doesn't do any good.' I knew it would not. After having tested that on her I sent her the Platinum. In two weeks she came again and said, 'I don't know what you gave me, but for the first two days after your dose I was much worse, and from that day until this I haven't a sign of it.' I think she went four months on that remedy, and then she came around and said, 'It's coming back.' I gave her another dose, 1M, and at that time she was relieved. She then moved away, and I have not heard from her since.

Sterility and Multiple Miscarriage

No one is more popular than a long-awaited stork!

Of a series of couples who had tried every anti-sterility examination and technique without conceiving over a period of one to eight years, all but two had started babies one to six months from the onset of homoeopathic treatment. Of the two not yet successful, the woman in one case has had regular periods for four months for the first time in her life, and the husband in the other case shows a sperm count and motility test that is almost back to normal. Silica was the wife's remedy; a blonde, linear, boyish woman, deaf from childhood, fanatical housekeeper, weepy and timid. Even her hearing is 15% better. Of the other couple, the man, a cheerful redhead, with a too ardent past and a passion for salt, found Phosphorus his need – three doses during fourteen months.

The most frequent remedies for women unable to conceive, in my experience, are Natrum Mur., Sulphur and Calc. Carb., and for men Pulsatilla and Thuja.

Fatigue, over-absorption in business, thyroid deficiency, marital maladjustment, lack of vacations, and improper diet are also factors to be considered. Paramount in importance is the giving of the constitutional remedy to both prospective parents.

Multiple miscarriage is almost synonymous with Syphilinum, especially if it occurs in families with a history of a gravely physically handicapped birth, or Down's syndrome or other forms of mental handicap, or stillbirth. Sepia runs very high. This is not to be confused with single miscarriages, where the range of remedies is far wider. A third remedy to be considered is Secale, especially if there is any history of ergot administration.

Homoeopathy is exceptionally useful in these two distressingly important conditions.

The Way of Homoeopathy
in the Exanthemata

One of the many boons of homoeopathy to the modern parent is its power to free them from the fear of the contagious diseases. It does this by a medley of means. In the first place, it shows the usefulness of these supposed scourges of our young; to wit, that they are a means of ridding the system of some of its inherited taints, of the accumulated miasms of past generations. Children come out stronger, and often with changes for the better in their personalities, afer an exanthem wisely handled by a true homoeopath. To be sure, although the acute course is either brief or mild, out-croppings follow from the deeper layers which call our attention to the need for a chronic remedy. So much the better – the patient might not have noticed the chronic signposts, nor done anything about them, had it not been for the acute trouble. These symptoms from the deep are unlikely to be the conventional sequelae: none such should develop, with proper handling; but rather minor items which the wise doctor interprets into radical help for the child's constitution. Never discharge your acute cases in children till they have had a chronic to follow through. I find the adults who are sickly in a deep chronic way to be those who have *not* had the exanthems in their youth. And many who seem healthy in maturity die sudden deaths, and they also have usually *not* had the children's diseases.

Mothers have a few instincts left, even in these times, and one is a distinct aversion to having their children shot full of this and that preventive serum or vaccine. Blessed and sane instinct! When they realize that the same good end can be accomplished by mild internal protection in high potency, without introducing foreign blood rhythms and with no fear of bad reaction, they are delighted.

If children have been exposed to, say, whooping cough, I ask the parent whether this would be a convenient time to have them get it, in case they need to, by inner necessity. If so, no protection, if they are in a good state to stand it. If not, then a prophylactic remedy; if they get it the case will be mild; if not, no harm is done. For I believe that the potency, instead of suppressing Nature's legitimate urge to measles or whatever, gives Nature an out, releasing forces and rousing the body to combat the incipient evil in itself.

The Way of Homoeopathy in the Exanthemata

May I give you a few cases in illustration?

Case 1: Master B., an interesting but self-willed boy of 13, product of a disharmonious wealthy background – good soil for an eruption! – came down with scarlet fever. Throat abscess had been lanced. Sudden profuse, repeated haemorrhages occurred, eight in an evening. Pronounced not surgical, probably from the stomach. Liver and spleen enlarged and tender. Called in consultation, I found the patient plethoric, blond, capricious, cantankerous, disobedient; blood bright, gushing; constant nausea, clean tongue. Ipecacuanha 200c, 3 doses, one hour apart if needed. No further bleeding after twenty minutes from first dose. Three days after, case study showed Arum Triph. and Ammonium Mur. as the two most similar remedies. Arum was given, 10M., 1 dose, with relief of corrosive saliva, etc. This might have carried the case safely from the start. The follow up was a dose of Natrum Mur. 1M. Swift recovery after the Ipecacuanha. Was the loss of blood therapeutic? Was the Ipecac. more truly related to the child than even I realized in the emergency prescription?

Case 2: Master A., aged 9, small pallid boy of tubercular stock on both sides, came down with whooping cough. Red face with cough, better in the air, worse 2 a.m. to 6 a.m. Drosera 1M., 1 dose. Only slightly better for three days then cough incessant, weak, short, running from one spell into another; postnasal dripping; ulceration of the alae nasi. This latter peculiarity, together with the incredible continuance of the cough, led to Corallium Rub. 200c, 1 dose. Brilliant improvement for exactly one week. Return of cough, though nose clear. Corallium Rub. 1M., 1 dose. Startling amelioration for ten days. Return of cough as before caused me to give Sulphur 200c, 1 dose. Aggravation for several days of general condition rather than cough. Then cough returned in full vigour. Corallium Rub. 10M., 1 dose and a speedy end to the trouble. Follow up: Sepia 1M., 1 dose. Boy gaining weight for the first time in a year and a half, rosy and peppy. Would Corallium Rub. 10M. have settled the whole thing in the beginning? Was the Sulphur an error? Or did it lay some foundation for the Corallium to hold by?

Case 3: Master M., 7, mumps, bilateral, hard swelling, constant need to swallow a lump, sensitive to weather change, oily sweat without profit, intense thirst for cold. This textbook picture responded at once to Merc. Viv. 10M., 1 dose. No symptoms appeared calling for a chronic: as this child comes for a chronic remedy every two months or so anyway, none was given. This is a very psoric child. Did no symptoms develop because the case was so perfectly covered by the Merc.? Or because the chronic remedies clear away enough anyway?

Case 4: Master R., 10, slight measles rash on neck, Koplik spots. Only symptom subjectively was severe photophobia and aching eyes, with slight yellow pus in canthi. Euphrasia 1M., 1 dose. Rash blossomed, eyes cleared, in three days felt well. Two weeks later, earache, flushed face, soft pulse, calm; Ferrum Phos. 1M. Hives followed; Sulphur 1M. brought him round fast.

DISCUSSION

Dr McLaren: About the first case, Dr Hubbard says it is a good thing for children, probably, to have these children's diseases, and I agree with her – so long as they are mild. Any case I have ever attended where Arum Triphyllum was indicated has always been very severely ill. In other words, I don't think you get Arum Triphyllum indicated in a case which is not very ill. Had the Arum Triphyllum been given first, I think she would not have needed the Ipecacuanha. To my way of thinking it is a much deeper-acting remedy than Ipecacuanha.

With regard to the second case, the dose of Sulphur; probably the Sulphur might not have been given just at that time, but I think the result and the good health of the child were probably due to the Sulphur.

Dr Moore: I have just one comment. It was given by Dr Hubbard but it wasn't emphasized. That is, where the Drosera is used, one dose!

Dr Grimmer: I am inclined to think with Dr Hubbard that these acute exanthemata are beneficial in the main, that they do take a great deal of the psoric miasm away, especially if good health evolves under the remedies. No disease will evolve ordinarily, if we watch it. I think that is why a lot of the shots that are given nowadays do harm rather than good. They are suppressive, and these suppressions come out later in changes, in pathological conditions in kidneys and vital organs. I think there can be no doubt but what the acute diseases are, as Hahnemann says, explosions.

Dr McFall: Would you call whooping cough and diphtheria exanthemata?

Dr Hubbard: No, I should not.

Redeveloping Suppressed Discharges and Eruptions

The one sure way to know that the remedy chosen for a case is indeed the simillimum is to observe old symptoms recurring in the reverse order of their appearance. It is gratifying to have your remedy work from within outward, with amelioration of the mental state and the patient's general sense of well-being, but it is not enough. Many more or less similar remedies may induce amelioration in this direction. To have improvement following your dose going from above downward, in addition to from within outward, is more reassuring; but for full satisfaction you must see the distressing symptoms disappearing, the most recent first, and the recurrence of old ailments in the reverse order of their coming.

Even though all three of these laws of Hering's are demonstrated, you can still not claim to have given the perfect simillimum unless one single dose suffices to produce a gradual and steady improvement, approaching nearer and nearer to complete cure, as a line approaches infinity. Some of our best prescribers claim that one dose of the perfect simillimum should, as they put it, unlock the door to permit the vital force to progress to complete recovery without further aid. This is the ideal, and in some instances is feasible. In many cases, however, inherited ill-health and the infringement of spiritual and physical laws throughout the past life of the patient may make this impossible. It may be necessary to repeat the dose after a long interval on a higher potency plane, or even make one or more changes of remedy as the case is unravelled.

Granted that the homoeopath has the skill to find the perfect simillimum, and that such remedy as really fits the case has been proved and is accessible to the practitioner, what are the factors which may prevent the complete cure? Can the vital force be weakened so that it cannot fully respond, even to the perfect opportunity? Or is – as some claim – the dynamic always equally vital and ready to leap to the task of cure as soon as the way is cleared by the remedy? Or is it possible so to sap the vitality by the wrong thinking and hygiene of years, if not of generations, that the channel is clogged? A second factor in the equation of recovery is the pathological one – the degree to which the tissues are maimed, whether by disease, drugging or surgery. Other factors that interfere with true cure are the failure of the patient to regulate his thought and life, and the unwise interference of the homoeopath after the first correct prescription.

For any or all of the above reasons, the cases which follow cannot be claimed to be true cures. They are given to illustrate the return of old suppressed symptoms, or the throwing out by the body of disease products, in the course of the action of the homoeopathic remedy.

Case 1. Mrs F., age 63. Chief complaint: frequent colds. Main symptoms: proud, self-contained, melancholic temperament; abnormally fond of sweets; gouty family, sporadically painful joints without modalities; very irritable recently, especially in the late afternoon; went grey as a girl of twenty; recurrent right-sided quinsy; good appetite but can only eat a little at a time, bilious attacks every few weeks with irritability, her only relief is from hot drinks. Physical examination and laboratory work practically negative. *Prescription:* Lycopodium 200c one dose and four doses of Sac. Lac., one every night and morning.

A fortnight later the patient returned feeling much more vigorous. She showed me a dry scaly eruption on both forearms and on the right palm which had come out on the third day after the dose. She admitted to having had such a right-sided palmar eruption years before, which had been 'cured' with zinc ointment. I warned her against local applications, explained my joy at the eruption returning and gave placebo. The rash cleared in another ten days. Two months later (this was mid-winter), the patient reported no colds for the first time in years at that season, no bilious attacks, joint pains more frequent now in the lower extremities rather than hands. General condition less vigorous for the past week or two. *Prescription:* Lycopodium 1M.

To my great interest a rash similar to that following the first dose, though less severe, reappeared five days after the repetition of the remedy. It cleared in two or three weeks. This was over two years ago, during which time the patient has had Lycopodium 10M, one dose, followed three months later by Lycopodium 50M. Five months later I gave Sulphur 10M, because of the appearance of burning soles and palms at night and faintness at 11 a.m., with entire disappearance of the late afternoon aggravation. Following the Sulphur she has needed no medication for over a year until an acute coryza a month ago. She has had no further eruptions, joint trouble or appreciable symptoms of any kind.

Case 2. Miss B., age 54. Chief complaint: eruption on neck, face and scalp of right side, burning not itching, shooting pains, screams if touched. This eruption, vesicular at first, was a week old with slightly enlarged right cervical glands. Diagnosis: cervical herpes zoster. *Prescription:* Ranunculus Bulb. 1M and placebo, one every two hours. One week later the patient reported relief within about three hours. I then took her chronic case. She was a pallid, repressed, sentimental little woman with dark hair and eyes, mildly chilly, brooding temperament, very averse to consolation, with a lifelong history of severe headaches over the right eye extending to the occiput and nape, which would come on in the late forenoon. She was worse before menses, which had been early and scanty; liked to be alone; right-sided complaints always; always headachy before thunderstorms; timid about robbers; disliked salt strongly, history of spots of eczema on the right hand years ago with cracks in the skin of the knuckles; consciousness of beating of the heart, worse lying down, with sensation as though the heart turned over; frequent panicky sensations in the pit of stomach, light-headed in the morning. Physical examination showed poor nutrition above the waist, good below, occasional extrasystoles, blood pressure 168/90, otherwise negative. *Prescription:* Natrum Mur. 1M and placebo.

Returned one month later feeling much better; only one slight throbbing headache since dose, heart no longer skipping. Marked eczema of right palm which she said had returned a week after the dose, and an eczematous patch below the right clavicle. Placebo. Eczema persisted for four months and then cleared spontaneously; blood pressure on several occasions between 130/80 and 138/80. Severe headache ten months after first dose of Natrum Mur. Right-sided throbbing at 11 a.m. occasioned Natrum Mur. 1M and placebo. This was five months ago, no symptoms since.

Case 3. Mrs Y., age 48. Chief complaint: utter indifference to and disgust with husband and children, increasing during past two years, knows it is groundless but cannot help it. Has been suicidal, depression worse before menses, accompanied with swearing from which she cannot refrain. Says she has lost her sense of humour. Two children living, four miscarriages at third month; terrible headaches as often as twice a week, right frontal, better from motion and pressure, especially from walking in the air; psoriasis of the scalp and face for eight years (has been partially removed with local ointments); red tip of nose, ten years' duration; menses early, scanty, dark, used to be membranous, pain as if everything inside her were being pushed out, relief when flow comes, terrible

205

depression ten days before period, unbearable odour at end of period; attacks of shivering, psychic, uncontrollable; lowest ebb from 4–5 p.m.; warm-blooded; early waking; does not crave sweets; history of kidney pain several years ago, severe backache, worse before thunderstorms; foot-sweat in childhood, which stiffened her stockings, odour bad, 'relieved' by foot powders. Patient of narrow, flat build. Physical examination showed old cervical lacerations, haemorrhoids, slight facial psoriasis, bad teeth. *Prescription:* Sepia 200c and placebo. (Lycopodium, Lachesis and Sulphur also repertorized high).

One week later the patient returned jubilant saying that her family sent me a vote of thanks. Her husband later told me that in that one week family peace was restored, as it had not been in several years. Psoriasis quite red and angry-looking. The patient declared she was feeling much better mentally and more vigorous physically but now had a foul green lumpy leucorrhoea. Questioning brought out that she had had such a discharge at age eighteen which had been stopped by douches, and again two or three years ago after her last miscarriage, when it had been checked by local painting and douching, since which time her mental symptoms had come on. I explained the danger of suppressing it and gave placebo. Six weeks later the patient said she had had only one headache of any severity since beginning treatment, and her period had been much more normal without any desire to swear, although the odour was worse. As the general mental state was again somewhat depressed I gave Sepia 1M and placebo. Some months later the leucorrhoea had changed to a slight yellow, odourless discharge, periods still early but otherwise normal. Since that time I have seen the patient regularly once a fortnight and she has been steadily better. She has had one attack of kidney pain, like the one years ago, and a mild attack of flu, but there has been no further medication of any kind except placebo. Her psoriasis has practically cleared on the face, come out and cleared again on the forearms, and there are now a few patches on the abdomen. The childhood foot-sweat has not returned, but I am waiting for it.

These cases are samples of what the single remedy, even in the hands of a beginner, will do towards ridding the patient of disease, by reproducing suppressed eruptions and discharges.

DISCUSSION

Dr Allen: I want to warn the husbands here not to go home and give their wives Sepia. I learned a few years ago that Sepia was a wonderful remedy for a flat wart. My wife has a large flat wart on her cheek and she had been wanting me to fulgurate it. I avoided that. About a month ago I gave her Sepia, 1M. The wart was somewhat smaller, but she developed a violent psoriasis on her feet. I am in trouble.

Dr Farrington: There are homoeopaths who feel that the matter of suppression and the matter of bringing out an eruption on the skin is bunk; nevertheless, we know it is an absolute fact and that in some cases a cure cannot be established as permanent until the old symptoms return. This is especially true of asthmatic conditions. Long ago I stopped asking patients who appeared in the office complaining of asthma, 'Did you ever have the itch?' I now say, 'When did you have the itch?'

Many years ago I treated a little girl of six who had caught cold and was wheezing and rattling. She sat up in bed like some old woman with asthma. I went through my usual formula: 'When did this child have an eruption?' Her mother said, 'Well, when she was two years old, and strange to say, she has had these attacks since then.' I said, 'She will never be well until that eruption comes back. I will give her a remedy now that will help this, and then you can bring her in later.' I gave her Ipecac., which immediately relieved the acute attack, but I did not see the litle girl until two or three months afterwards when she had another attack. I repeated the Ipecac. In four or five days' time a slight eruption appeared over the face and chest. The child never had another attack.

Dr Boger: When there is an eruption all over the body which the patient cannot endure, then you will find out whether you are a prescriber or whether you are not. If you are homoeopathic enough to resist doing anything until it runs itself out, then you are an artist. That holds not only in regard to eruptions on the body, but also in regard to bad leucorrhoeas that we establish in women. For a woman to wait until the leucorrhoea drains out those tubes and reduces the hypertrophy requires a good deal of patience, sometimes on your part as well as the patient's. I counsel that when you come to that point, possibly a pretty low potency may help you out. I have seen Ignatia 7c or 8c, for instance, do some wonderful work where it had been given high previously without effect.

Dr Royal: I want to illustrate the disappearance of discharge and the evil effects. Ten or fifteen years ago, on a warm day, a girl came into my private office and handed me a paper with a name on it. Following her was a woman with a heavy veil over her face, and behind her a man, her husband. I asked what I could do for her. The husband took up the thread there. He said, 'We came here because we heard that you are a homoeopathic physician and that you didn't believe in local applications. Our physician has always been an old school physician. I am a pharmacist myself, so that I know what has been given.'

So I said, as I usually do, 'What may I do for you?' to the woman. She drew up her veil. Her face was so covered with an elevation that I never saw its like. I could hardly call it an eruption. Her physician had called it lupus, an aggravation of what she had had for some twenty years. She was a sight to see. Then I began to say, 'Tell me all about it.' In the first place, I took her family history and found that this lupus had developed soon after she was born. About nine months before, as I remember, she had been up the lake for her vacation. She enjoyed bathing. She thought she was through menstruating, but she was not. At any rate, she was going to risk it, and she went in bathing. The water was cold. She had not menstruated since. About six weeks afterwards these blotches began to come. She went to her physician and he put on some ointment that would put them away for a while, and then they would return. Finally, his local applications did not do any good and the blotches spread.

The next symptom was what attracted my attention the most and probably led to my remedy. She kept coughing, coughing, coughing. I got my mirror and had her open her mouth, and on the vocal chords there were half a dozen little papillae that you would have called warts if they had been on the hand; but they were in her throat and they kept her coughing and coughing. You know what the remedy was, of course. I gave her one dose of Thuja 1M.

Now for the results. I cannot get these results in a week or two or three, and sometimes not in a month. I do not have the ability, somehow. But about six weeks afterwards, she began to menstruate, the first time she had menstruated in some seven or eight months. Next, these things in the throat disappeared, and then afterwards the face began to clear up. They came up several times. After that, they all disappeared and there was no repetition.

She came up one day and said, 'Now, doctor, these are all gone. Here is my old scar that is left, but my husband says it is not as large as it was.' I said, 'All right, here is some medicine', and gave her placebo. I told her I thought it would pass away. In about four or five months she came up again and said, 'I have no trouble with my cough and my menses are regular, but I wish I could get rid of that scar.' I gave her the second dose of Thuja and I guess it took six months, but it nearly all disappeared.

Laurocerasus – A Case Study

Laurocerasus, the common or cherry laurel, is seldom used, although it appears at length in Hering and Allen. Because of an almost miraculous alleviation in a desperate case, I want to bring it to your attention.

I was called in consultation by an ardent young homoeopath. I found the patient sitting in a big chair gasping for breath, with blue lips, hectic malar flush, staring frightened eyes, coughing in short racking spasmodic hacks, skin cold yet craving air, though not desiring fanning, with clubbed fingers and markedly oedematous feet which were icy up to the knees.

Physical examination showed a mitral and an aortic heart murmur, double pleural effusion, huge liver, tender and pulsating, fluid in the abdomen, probable hypostatic pneumonia, irregularity and at times flutter of the heart, pulse soft and weak. Practically no urine was being passed.

The chief complaint was cough: starting at 9 p.m. to 10 p.m. and constant through the night. Sputum scanty, jelly-like, dotted with bloody specks. Salty taste. Cough better for cold drinks and cool air; loss of urine with cough. Skin was cold and dry, but warmth did not help. Cold drinks craved, gurgled on going down. The patient was worse for emotion and wet weather and better for company. Great fear of death. Smothering and suffocating sensation. Worse for a long time after coition. Youngest child one month old. Duration of heart disease many years, collapse after childbirth. Craves sours; milk disagrees. She had been subject to long-lasting fainting spells.

This patient had been given Phosphorus CM, and two or three days later Sulphur CM, by her doctor. To say that palliation was clearly indicated would have been humorous, had it not been tragic.

Prescription: Laurocerasus 200c, two doses one hour apart. Within twenty minutes relief set in. That night she had two brief coughing spells and her first good rest in many days. Laurocerasus had done its work.

One feature of the case was not according to Hoyle: the cough of Laurocerasus is usually better lying down, which hers was not. (Laurocerasus and Psorinum share that symptom of amelioration from

209

lying.) However, many Laurocerasus symptoms are relieved by sitting up.

Let me bring out a few characteristic points of this remedy. Coldness better for cold (like Camphor, Ammonium Carb., Secale). Cyanosis. Spells of sleepiness and long-lasting faints. Suppression of urine with suffocation, in cardiacs. Gasping dyspnoea. Racking cough worse *or* better for lying. Left-sidedness; chest, nape stiffness, tongue swelling. Fluttering heart with soft pulse.

Also: loss of consciousness, facial distortion, sensation of a cold draft on the face, throat spasms, audible gurgling on drinking, hunger after eating, with emptiness; sensation of a lump falling from above the navel through to the back; diarrhoea with green mucous stools, flatulence, cramps and hiccough with cold skin relieved by cold; menses early, profuse, thin, dark clots, with pain from sacrum to pubis (Sabina from pubis to sacrum), with icy tongue and stinging nipples and dysmenorrhoea.

Laurocerasus is often overlooked in lack of reaction, when the well chosen remedy does not act. Here it vies with Sulphur and Opium.

Stauffer stresses its value in the results of suppressed exanthemata, as well as in chorea, epilepsy, apoplexy, asphyxia neonatorum and terminal tuberculosis.

It should be compared with Ambra, Ammonium Carb., Arsenicum Alb., Belladonna, Camphor, Capsicum, Cuprum, Drosera, Kali Carb., Lachesis, Opium, Phosphorus, Psorinum, Pulsatilla, Sulphur, Tart. Emet., Valerian, Veratrum Alb. and Zinc.

Constitutional Remedies in the Treatment of the Nails and the Hair

Some of our best prescribers stress the importance of objective symptoms which cannot lie. We all know the importance for diagnosis and prognosis of minute observation and sensing through odours, gait, skin texture, etc. – the deep processes of which the patient is often unconscious. There are physicians who claim that by a thorough knowledge of certain small parts of the body they can diagnose the hidden condition of the whole, and even of its parts. There are those who feel the study of the tongue will teach you much, or of the iris of the eye, or of the sensitivity of the nasal mucous membranes. I have a passion for hands, and hence study fingernails to learn what may be read from them.

The nails and hair, and indeed the skin, are supposed, like the bones, to be related to the ego. They often show the outward manifestations of otherwise invisible processes. Let us think what can be observed in the nails. We first eliminate peculiarities of the nails due to cosmetics or occupation, including that of the housewife, or injury, or tobacco. General medicine recognizes clubbing of the nails as a sign of chest trouble, or cyanotic nails in certain types of heart disease, and ridging of the nails longitudinally as possibly related to endocrine deficiency. White spots on the nail suggest myocardial difficulties. Horizontal, wavy depressions in the nails suggest acute illness and wear away without return, but there are also little hollows in the nail which I have observed in a number of cases of combined hyperthyroid and heart disease. In my experience, longitudinal ridging of the nails often goes with emotional overstrain and kidney involvement. Split nails in the mind of the laity mean acidity. Thick crumbling, misshapen ones suggest the tubercular habit. Brittle nails may also be sycotic, or designate a disturbance in the silica content.

The repertories suggest various remedies for these nail conditions. Cracked nails: Antimonium Crud., Natrum Mur., Silica; split nails: Antimonium Crud., Silica, Squilla and Sulphur; crumbling nails: Sepia, Silica or Thuja; brittle nails: Alumina, Ambra, Calc. Carb., Castor Eq., Dioscorea, Fluoric Acid, Graphites, Nitric Acid, Psorinum, Silica, Squilla, Sulphur and Thuja. White spots on the nails first suggest Silica but also Nitric Acid, Sepia or Sulphur, and spotted nails in general include also Alumina, Arsenicum and Tuberculinum. Black nails are an indication for Arsenicum or Graphites. For hangnails we think of Calc. Carb., Lycopodium, Mercury, Natrum Mur. in particular, Rhus Tox., Sabadilla, Sepia, Silica, Stannum, Sulphur and Thuja.

In general, overproliferation of metabolic disturbances of the nails suggest the great sycotic remedies, whereas deformed or misshapen nails suggest the syphilitic miasm.

It has been a pleasant surprise to me how swiftly the indicated remedy, based on the totality of the symptoms, will improve the quality and appearance of the nails.

Case 1. Delicate, flower-like lady of forty-five came for chronic constipation, with receding stools, uterine fibroid, weepy, desires cold food and ice cream, stockings always damp, nervous and poorly before and during thunderstorms, lack of self-confidence, fastidious, frequent colds, boils and wens, tiny warts, succession of styes, nails very delicate and constantly breaking, hair dry and brittle. Silica 1M, one dose. In two weeks the nails looked perfect and had stopped breaking. Other symptoms greatly improved. In the course of the months the fibroid reduced so that it could not be found. Nails became brittle again after two months; on repetition of Silica 1M, one dose, they became normal again and have remained so.

Case 2. Woman of thirty with recent thyroid difficulty, slight exophthalmos, pulse 104, fine tremor, diarrhoeic tendency, salt craving, prostrated in the sun, worse in the morning, nails spotted and with depressions. Natrum Mur. 1M, one dose, repeated after eight months during which time nails cleared, pulse 88, eyes better.

Turning our attention to the hair, we all know its relation to the endocrines and its value as an index of general vitality. For instance, mousy or lustreless hair suggests tuberculosis, as does excessively fine, silky hair. Bushy, wiry, crinkly or unruly hair suggests the sycotic miasm. Loss of hair, unless after an acute disease in young people, especially if in patches, suggests the syphilitic diathesis, as does early or irregular greying of the hair. A single white streak in the hair is often psoric. Mousy hair suggests Medorrhinum, Psorinum or Thuja. Matted hair: Mezereum, Natrum Mur. or Psorinum. Easy tangling: Borax, Fluoric Acid, Graphites, Psorinum, Zincum. Early greying: Lycopodium, if in spots Psorinum. Falling of the hair: Arsenicum Alb., Antimonium

Crud., Aurum, if in spots Fluoric Acid. Baldness: Baryta Carb. and in babies Silica. Great dryness of the hair: Calc. Carb., Kali Carb. as well as Medorrhinum, Psorinum, Sulphur and Thuja. The quality and sheen of hair may be improved with Arsenicum Alb., which is used to make the coats of horses and dogs glossy. Falling whiskers call for Calc. Carb., Graphites, Kali Carb., Natrum Carb., Natrum Mur. or Phosphoric Acid, and falling genital hair for Natrum Mur., Nitric Acid, Selenium or Zincum.

Unruly eyebrows or too wiry hair suggests Medorrhinum. Sudden access of hair on the limbs suggests Medorrhinum or particularly Thuja; if on a child's face, Calc. Carb., Natrum Mur., Oleum Jecorum, Psorinum or Sulphur.

Case 3. Girl of twenty-three, greatly worried over sudden sprouting of thick hair on arms and legs, otherwise very healthy, left ovarian pain at menses, oily skin. Thuja 200c, one dose. Pain has not returned and hair growth has definitely gradually decreased until it is hardly visible.

Case 4. Boy of nine, skinny, pale, mousy hair, tubercular history, moles, osteomyelitis, excessive sensation of heat, craving for air, ravenous appetite, restlessness, difficult disposition and aversion to people. Fluoric acid 1M, one dose. Disposition miraculously changed, parents say. Fever subsided, gaining weight, hair has more life and burnished glints in it, uppermost osteomyelitic opening healed, lower one on ankle open and discharging, restlessness gone. Later received Thuja 1M, one dose.

In each of these incidences the condition of the hair and nails has been but one objective symptom in the totality, yet it has helped to guide to the true remedy; the change in the hair and nails has been gratifying and amazing to the patients.

To the Patient's Surprise

Br-r-r-r went the telephone for the seventeenth time during a busy office hour. 'Doctor', said a radiant voice, which I recognized as that of a depressed and skeptical schoolmarm patient, 'it stopped almost before I got out of your office. And not a drop since, though you recall I'd been flowing three solid weeks profusely. And my hands don't sweat for the first time in years; and I hardly sweat at night now. Do you do it with mirrors?' 'Lady, thank the oyster', quoth I.

My friend the woman business executive rode home with me in my one-horse Chevrolet and anointed its fawn-coloured plush upholstery with everything she had eaten for lunch. As she fled into the air murmuring apologies between retches, I said, 'Come see me some time, you need a dose of Petroleum.'

A week later she came. Recalling my teacher's admonitions, I resolutely put Petroleum behind me, and did her case with care. Carsickness since childhood, from starting and stopping (like the pitch of a boat, not its roll); vesicles on the hands; vulvar itching; chilblains of the toes; cramps of the thighs and feet; eczema under the breast; cracks of the hands in winter; granular lids; diarrhoea; asthma for ten years. Petroleum was given, 1M, one dose. Next week she called me, 'It's a miracle', she said, 'not a sign of car-sickness, had a bit of asthma but felt fine despite it, and some diarrhoea, and two chilblains. But I haven't been like this in years.' The good news lasted two months. Then she came wheezing into the office, still feeling fine, but I must fix the asthma. If I must, I must. Just common-or-garden asthma? But at last one gem: she would cough and then sneeze, which would relieve. Only one remedy has just that in Kent – Osmium, which in the 1M relieved the attack. But not for long. (Oh sin, to follow the lure of the keynote!) Attacks began at 6–7 p.m. with marked abdominal bloating, and came regularly every other day. China has asthma 6–7 p.m., and now she does not – much to her surprise!

Mr Y, having been turned down by life insurance companies as an active TB case, came to me fifteen months ago, spitting blood in lumps, with a chronic cough with sweet green sputum, afternoon fever, skeletally thin, with a terrific mitral heart murmur from childhood. He simply could not afford to stop working or go away. The X-ray was not cheering, either. But Stannum was cheering. Three doses in five months, with no further haemoptysis, fever, sweat or prostration, and a slow but steady gain in weight. He worked hard all that summer with one month's vacation. In August constipation set in, sheep dung variety, and he could not sweat; chronic hoarseness came. Alumen 10M, one dose, set all these to rights. He gained two pounds. In January he told me of his distress at impotence for the last few years. Agnus Castus 200c made him normal in a week, but a month later the Stannum had to be repeated. In March he spat blood again, but only dark thread-like clots; he felt vigorous, but always too hot and restless, and craving air and activity. He ate three times his normal diet and did not gain. Iodum 200c, one dose. No more blood, gained four pounds, heat (which was not fever) and abnormal hunger gone. He has worked nights, moved, and done prodigies meanwhile. The impotence is gone, to the patient's surprise. . .

Taking the Baby's Case

Homoeopathy can do some of its most brilliant work with babies, yet these cases can give no vivid history or picturesque roster of symptoms. The 'language of the patient' is not a spoken one. To be sure, the anxious mother will deluge you with comments. Give her the same silent attention that you would render an important adult chronic in your office. When she has finished, you *may* already have the scaffolding of your case, but what concerns us here are those instances in which her story is of little avail. Often she will merely tell you the textbook symptoms of a disease. If she is not used to homoeopathic treatment you must educate her to watch for modalities. If the case needs a remedy immediately, try out your modalities. Open the window so that a draft blows on the baby. If it coughs, you have learned something. If it stops coughing and breathes easier, you would never give it Rumex. Uncover it, or pile clothing on it to see if it kicks it off; bolster up its head or remove its pillow, and watch the signs of discomfort or relief. Turn a bright light on it or shade it from the glare, and observe. Give it a drink of water, cold then hot, and note its refusal or avidity; its coughing or its relief; its vomiting; its choking, etc. Pick it up, and walk it up and down slowly or fast; touch it and jar its crib; lay it first on one side and then on the other, then on its stomach, and note relief or aggravation. Give it something sour: if, unlike most babies, it drinks it eagerly, think of Hepar Sulph. or Pulsatilla. Slam the door to see whether noise aggravates. Nothing is so important as these modalities.

Next, enquire carefully into the circumstances just prior to the illness of your baby. What was the role of fright, punishment, anger, wetting, chill, wind, food or foreign bodies in the onset? Was the onset sudden or gradual? On your next visit go to see your baby at the time the mother tells you it is most aggravated.

Use your eyes. Has the baby one red cheek and the other pale; one hot foot and the other cold? Is its pillow yellow with sweat or its socks drenched? Does it drool? Are its orifices red? Is it puffy over the eyes or white about the mouth? Does it chew like a ruminant, or burrow its head in the pillow, or arch its back, or clench its fists thumbs in? Look at all its discharges. Listen to it in attacks of coughing, belching, etc. Observe its

216

colic. Note its tongue. Note its attitude toward you and toward the approach of anyone it is usually fond of. Sit and watch it, relaxed, with receptive mind. If you still see no picture of the remedy, give it Sac. Lac. and come again soon.

If it is a chronic case without many symptoms, study the parents, particularly the mother. Question her about her pregnancy and its symptoms and the symptoms of lactation. The baby may need what she needed then. Question the mother particularly about suppressed eruptions, suppressed sweat and previous medication. After all of this, you should be ready to *begin* to prescribe.

Dot and Carry One

In discussion of this case, Dr Grimmer brought out the artistry which is often involved when a master prescriber is at work. He said, 'I could not help but say a few words about the artistry with which our good doctor gets to the simillimum. She had very little to go on, but she could see sadness in that little, dried-up, broken bit of humanity. Only a homoeopath could enter into that sphere to see those things . . . she saw it in a flash.' — Ed.

The office bell rang insistently, the secretary called me and said, 'There is a gentleman here with a baby in his arms and he says that she is dying; can you see her at once?' The current patient was asked to wait and the breathless father followed by a tense mother brought a tiny bundle into the office and unwrapped her. She looked more like a tiny, hairless monkey than a human being, sunken temples, pinched nose, pallor, extreme emaciation, hardly breathing. The father explained that he had just taken her out of one of the finest hospitals in the city where she had been born three weeks previously, a third child, normal labour.

She had been unable to eat and was steadily and rapidly dwindling without any noticeable symptoms, no respiratory disease, no vomiting, physical examination negative. The doctors had tried everything with no result except increasing emaciation and feebleness. I still do not know on what I chose the remedy, except a process of elimination. It was definitely not a Calc. Carb. baby. It looked utterly dehydrated and unspeakably sad and wistful. I really thought it was going to die in the office. It kept protruding its tiny tongue and pursing its lips. I put a powder of Natrum Mur. 10M under its tongue and told the parents to take it home, keep it very warm and feed it warm water and warm raw certified cow's milk with a medicine dropper. Within two hours the mother telephoned to say that the baby looked a little more lively, had a better colour and was breathing strongly, and she then made a steady gain for several days. I was called to see her again because her hands were stiffening and the thumbs turning in and she had a bluish look. Cuprum 10M, one dose. The next day she was relaxed and eager to suck, and made a steady progress into a plump and happy normal baby.

Asthma in a Child of Four

A plump, smiling girl of four; blond hair, brown eyes, very red lips, dry skin, sweaty scalp with stale odour, though clean. Only child. Normal birth, nursed ten months; vaccinated at nine months; diphtheria antitoxin, three shots at one year of age. Soon after this a cough developed with asthma. Attacks every two or three weeks and then more frequently. Attacks always follow anger or excitement. Child hits at people and sends them away during spells. Coughs in paroxysms till she vomits. Cold sweat with attacks. Red then blue in the face, must sit up to breathe, worse by the ocean. Sleeps in the knee-chest position. Dislikes being touched in attacks. Obstinate and contrary. Frequent colds. Loves her bath. Worse in wet weather, yet has asthma also in dry weather. Fearless, full of fun. Fond of sugar and fats. Attacks at 9–10 p.m., wakening her from sleep; she cannot expire; better for cold, ice and ice-cream, worse for hot drinks. Scanty bright right-sided nose-bleeds often (polyp found). Holds her throat when coughing. Coughs on going out into cold air. Loses her urine when angry. Ate newspapers and chalk. History of eczema on face, hands and elbows 'cured' with zinc ointment in babyhood. Sweaty feet. Ipecac. 1M, one dose, and Sac. Lac.

Relief for a month, although attacks recurred in mild form. Slight rash on right arm two days after dose. Worse again, so repeated Ipecac. 1M. More rash out on abdomen. Sweats in first sleep. Marked expiratory grunt. Little if any help from this dose.

Called two weeks later. Child sitting up sneezing and blue in the face; cramps in the legs, spasms with the cough, thumbs in, wants ice-water which gurgles as it goes down. Hysterical and spoiled. Blue nails. Screams. Cuprum 1M, one dose.

Child so well that parents took her abroad, no return of asthma on the sea. One complete month without attack, difficult breathing, a cold or any distress.

Was Cuprum the remedy all along? Or did she need both? Will Medorrhinum follow some day? I think so. And later, perhaps, Calc. Carb. and then Sulphur.

Difficult Cases

The poet's saddest words are 'It might have been', but the homoeopath has a more optimistic experience. As the cases which follow are briefly submitted, think how they might have been and rejoice at the beauty and precision of the system which Hahnemann gave us.

Case 1. Miss A., 11 years old, out of school for over a year five years ago, in hospital for nine months where the diagnosis was rheumatic fever, with pains chiefly in the knees and the left hip; was in a total body cast; had three operations for osteomyelitis of the right thigh and left foot; had five blood transfusions; has been pale, anaemic, stunted and feeble ever since. Patient referred to a homoeopath by the family of a boy of nine who was brought through osteomyelitis by homoeopathy without any operation, and who, after three years, is able to play football and do full athletics. The inner side of left thigh is discharging thick, yellow pus, offensive and sweetish; swelling around the fistulous opening with tenderness. Child had serious ear trouble in infancy, and measles just prior to the onset of the bone trouble. Marked foot sweat, offensive, stiffening the socks; fear of and worse before thunderstorms; sweat of the head, great chilliness and constant weeping. *Prescription:* Silica 200c, one dose and placebo.

One month later she looked brighter, better colour, had gained two pounds. Two splinters of bone were extruded shortly after the remedy; a scab formed over the fistulous opening, which itched. Sac. Lac. Two months later child developed a brown leucorrheal discharge which stiffened the underwear. Thighs completely healed, swelling and pain in the knees, which she cannot straighten. Scar of the left foot (previously operated) oozes on and off, pain in the left ear which had troubled her as an infant; gained two and a half pounds. Six months after the initial visit, repeated Silica 200c, as thighs again painful although knee is now straight. Child has been going regularly to school, at first on crutches and after a couple of months without them. Dives and swims, rides a bicycle and has joined the Girl Scouts; has missed only two days of school this term.

Eleven months after she was first seen had a slightly painful cyst of the left breast and was craving sweets, no longer chilly but unduly hot, especially at night, itching of the eyelids. Sulphur 200c, one dose, and Sac. Lac. The month after this she is better in all ways save that the leucorrhea is very green and profuse. She has an empty 'all-goneness' at eleven in the morning and is craving sours; Sepia 200c, one dose, and Sac. Lac. The cyst is better, foot-sweat better, steady gain in weight, no deformity save the operative scars, and looks and seems a happy, active youngster.

Case 2. Mrs B., 31 years of age, has been in an asylum with a diagnosis of manic-depressive psychosis, and was released in the custody of her mother. Very abrupt, slightly exophthalmic, pale, dark girl with late menses, a tendency to brood, phobia against going away from the house; is a heavy salt eater. Natrum Mur. 10M, one dose, and placebo. Repeated after three months and again after six months. In the seventh month, Natrum Mur. 50M.

Three months later she developed swift impulses, threatened suicide, was abnormally hungry; the exophthalmos, which had been decreasing, returned suddenly, and she complained continually of being too hot. Iodum 1M one dose, and placebo. Steady gain for almost four months, when it was repeated. Seven months later, Iodum 10M. After emotional strain, a sudden recurrence of the manic phase with prayer and singing yielded to Stramonium 10M. Fairly steady mentally and going out more over a period of a year. Suddenly, owing to emotional factors, a violent attack in August of this year with picking at flocks, staring look, great pallor, inclination to take off the clothing, cataleptic rigidity at intervals. Hyoscyamus 200c. Improved slightly. Two days later, Hyoscyamus 50M, within two hours of which no more removing of the clothing or catalepsy, knew her surroundings better. Was finally able to have a talk with her 'boy friend' and found definite nymphomanic symptoms which the family had withheld from me. Patient suddenly began to wash everything and bathe continually, and was extremely egotistical in all her talk and action. Monthly period at about this time, black and stringy and scanty. Platinum 10M one dose, and within six hours the family reported that she was more normal than they had seen her in a couple of years, and for the two months since that time she has remained so. Although the acute phase lasted about three weeks we were able to keep her at home with constant supervision. Certainly without our remedies she would have been, at least for a period, in an asylum again.

Case 3. Miss C., teacher of physical education, 26 years of age, had been troubled for a year with her sacroiliac. Strapping, osteopathic adjustments, long rest in bed, then a cast from the waist down for three months and finally a fusion operation were all of no avail to cope with her pain. She felt certain she would have to change her profession, and in despair was persuaded to try homoeopathy. The symptoms were clear for Lycopodium, although the patient was round-faced, rosy, a jolly blonde. Lycopodium 200c gave almost instant relief of backache and sciatica in right side.

She resumed her teaching and although slightly stiff on bending, continued painless for seven months, when upon return of same symptoms the remedy was repeated. Five months later had Lycopodium 1M for a second recurrence. For two years she felt very well and did her full work at teaching physical education. Then she developed aggravation on foggy days and before storms, relief of her pain on motion, severe pain in heel without swelling or apparent reason. Rhododendron 200c brought swift relief. Two months later she developed a sinusitis, which Silica 200c cleared. She has since had two doses of Rhododendron and three of Lycopodium over the space of a year and a half, and considers herself in excellent health.

Case 4. Mrs N., age 48, with a history of chronic bronchitis and liver disturbances, sent for me one morning in agonizing pain under the right ribs, drowsy, sweating alternating with chills, high fever, 103°F, sensation as though the right side of upper abdomen would burst, with violent pain cutting through under right shoulder blade, tongue yellow, thickly-coated, stool clay colour, loose, scanty. On examination, a mass the size of a grapefruit in the gallbladder region, exquisitely tender and tense. Urine negative, no jaundice. The attack had followed a meal rich in fats combined with sad and shocking news. As you can imagine she received Chelidonium 10M, three doses two hours apart, and placebo. That evening she was reported comfortable although sore and bruised, and the next morning the gallbladder, though still slightly tender, was no larger than an egg. She was subsequently quite weak for several days and then developed what she told me was an old symptom of violent headache, like a nail driven in. Thuja 30c three doses not only relieved the headache but helped her in every way, and on studying her symptoms previous to the acute attack, it was evident that it was one of her deep chronic remedies.

Case 5. Master T., twelve years of age, six feet tall, has been diabetic for several years and on a strict diet. Conventional symptoms of Sulphur and later Silica, each given at two or three monthly intervals, in single dosage over a period of two years, without insulin. He is now able to eat full diet, has gained in weight, no longer has the itching or sweaty feet and remains sugar free, a normal, happy, athletic boy.

Case 6. Little Miss S., whose father had been syphilitic and her mother sycotic, a heavy, squat, unattractive child of four, with Hutchinson's teeth and the stigmata of hereditary syphilis in palate, ears, etc. All her teeth were black and decayed almost before they came in. The child was on a sensible, high vitamin diet, green vegetables, raw fruit and so on. She complained of head and wandering bone pain. Syphilinum 1M.

Through the last seven years I have watched the development of this child into a stocky but pretty and wholesome girl, whose second teeth are perfect. Time forbids a full list of the remedies. Sulphur, Calc. Carb., Mercurius, Magnesia Mur., Graphites, Cina and Capsicum have played their part; recently she has needed a dose of Sepia and subsequently Thuja, both remedies deeply germane to her mother. The study of the interrelation of remedies between parent and child is a deeply interesting one.

One last case. Mr W., 37 years old, four and a half years under my care, preternaturally thin, almost a walking skeleton, complains of tickling sensation in the right chest just below the nipple, and a sensation of tightness there and of spitting up 'gobs of bright, clotted blood'. Weight 118 pounds. History of anaemia as a boy, tonsils out thirteen years previously, acute rheumatic fever which left him with a loud blowing systolic murmur, mitral regurgitation. An X-ray of the chest was ordered. They reported bilateral, upper lobe tuberculosis, possibly active. Examination of the chest revealed fine crepitant râles below the right nipple and definite change of breath and a few fine râles in both apices posteriorly. Probably a small cavity in the right upper lobe at the back. His sputum, which was scanty, was in green fleshy lumps with a sweetish taste. He slumped in a chair. *Prescription:* Stannum 200c, one dose and Sac. Lac.

One month later no cough, gained a pound in weight which, for him, was tremendous. Apices clear to auscultation. No return of blood spitting, but the last few days had recurrence of the tickling, tightness, etc. below the right nipple. Repeated Stannum 200c one dose, which alleviated, but only for a couple of weeks, so he received Stannum 1M one dose.

This patient had a sick child and was doing a one-man job, and simply had to continue at work, as he said, 'if it killed him'. He adhered strictly to the regime of fresh air, extra sleep and high diet, but in the four and half years since has never missed a day at work, although he has taken a month instead of the customary two weeks vacation each year.

Four months after the Stannum he returned complaining of great dryness, inability to sweat, hoarseness, marked constipation in little hard balls, and aversion to starch. His weight was up to 124 pounds. Alumina 10M one dose and Sac. Lac. Three months later a recurrence of blood spitting and green, sweet sputum called for a repetition of Stannum 1M, which he needed again in another three months. Two months later the picture changed. He became unusually hot and hungry and restless and mentally disturbed, and told me what he never had before, of a relative in definite mental difficulties. Iodum 200c, followed in five months by Iodum 1M. No further blood spitting.

Three months later, blood spitting again with old tickling in right lung, weight on the chest, loss of weight, down to 121 pounds. Stannum 10M, three doses and Sac. Lac. Six months later, having been checked and given placebo in the interim, a return of the stools in balls and of the great dryness, one single clot of blood; Alumina 1M.

He had a couple of doses of Bryonia, one of Pulsatilla, one of Rumex and one of Sanguinaria in the course of the next year for beginning colds or coughs which never made any headway. Just a year ago the Alumina 1M was repeated. The beginning of this year, although there has now been no blood spitting for one and a half years, there was a return of the green sputum, and he received another dose of Stannum and is still working hard without night sweats, loss of weight or any apparent disability. It was interesting to see how the three strands, Stannum, Iodum, and Alumina weave in and out in this case.

One could go on indefinitely adding to these cases in which permanent disability, operations, prolonged confinement and prolonged illness have been avoided through the beautiful exposition of our homoeopathic remedies.

Nosodes May Save the Day in Acute Cases

A great many skilful homoeopathic physicians, especially those who use the lower potencies, are not addicted to the employment of the nosodes. Those who specialize in chronic constitutional prescribing find them invaluable. One of our greatest prescribers, when repertorizing any case, made a point of determining not only the four or five most similar remedies, but also which of the miasmatic nosodes had the greatest bearing on the whole history. He even classified the polychrests in their relationship to Hahnemann's three miasms.

The usual practice among experienced homoeopaths is to use a nosode when the case is, as it were, stuck – to put it in order and bring out clearer symptoms for a deep remedy in one of the three kingdoms, mineral, vegetable or animal. Many use occasional doses of the suitable nosode as an intercurrent, to dynamize the vital force or to reach deeper into the inherited weakness.

It is startling even to the veteran prescriber to find how effective a nosode may be in acute cases. Let us begin with some examples of the least used of the four main nosodes: Syphilinum.

A woman of 74, fibrillating heart, blood pressure 230/140, suddenly suffered a cerebrovascular accident with loss of speech, inability to write, complete constipation, deviation of the tongue to the right, inability to focus the eyes and complete inability to sleep, with terror of the night. Dreadful anxiety from sunset until morning. Uncontrollable restlessness at night only. Upon examination the patient was found to have old rectal condylomata. Arsenicum 1M did nothing for her. On sitting watching her the next day I was struck by the retroussé nose, the narrow palate arch, the peculiar small ears and stubby hands which point to the syphilitic miasm; remembering the formidable night aggravation, sleeplessness and rectal difficulties of Syphilinum, one dose of the CM potency was given, following which peaceful nights and steady progress in speech clarity and mobility took place.

A woman of 88, cancer of the colon, pessimistic, restless, talking of guilt and suicide, unable to sleep even under sedation. Violent linear pains, worse at night. Syphilinum 10M, one dose, made her a pleasant, resigned, painless patient.

A cerebral palsy child, aged 7, brought to me for asthma, previously treated with antihistamines, antibiotics and sedatives, without avail. The child grimaced, was constantly restless, speech un-understandable, a look of pent-up anger, severe asthmatic attacks mainly at night. Unable to eat or sleep. History of several gamma-globulins to protect her against measles. The father who brought the child in shared the stigmata with his daughter. Syphilinum 1M, one dose, brilliant relief, eating, sleeping, no wheezing, marked improvement in speech and gait.

A woman of 72, immobilized for a broken hip, suffered excruciating pain at night only with what she called piles. Complete rectal spasm preventing any bowel evacuation. Rectal examination showed condylomata as large as walnuts in a ring around the anus, ulcerated. Patient deeply depressed, has tried all sorts of medication for rectal relief. Syphilinum 200c, three doses, shrank the swelling, relieved the pain, permitted comfortable evacuations and a cheery patient who could sleep without sedation.

A woman of 47, history of severe asthma for many years, very thin, attacks always at night, active and well by day. No symptoms other than the asthma, except that the attacks were concomitant with linear headaches and often with a linear pain vertically in the front of the chest. Syphilinum 200c, one dose, gave her her best winter in years.

A child aged 9, vomiting headache, found to be connected with the ingestion of milk. Allergy specialists found her violently allergic to milk, which she loved. Family history of tuberculosis. Restless, whining, delicate girl with many stomach aches. Relief of headache in the wind. Tuberculinum Bovinum 10M. After this the daily headaches were completely absent for four months and the child was gradually enabled to drink milk.

A woman of 43, eczema of the palms of the hands since six years of age, violently aggravated in the last two months. A concert pianist who must fulfil a longstanding public engagement and could not even practise because of the swelling, stiffness and dripping oozing of her hands. The patient had an alabaster complexion, heart-shaped face, sloping shoulders, always wanting to travel, have something new and change things around. Her husband said she had always had an extreme terror of dogs. Tuberculinum Bovinum 200c. Patient reported that after two or three days of aggravation her hands became almost normal and usable. She was able to play her concert. After several months there was a slight recurrence and she wrote for another dose.

A man of 52, suddenly discovered blood in his urine. Fever of 101°F, great weakness and restlessness. On examination there was some tenderness over the left kidney. He was excessively thin, although he ate well, and had a scar of an empyema rib resection of twenty years before. A jolly, cheery man, refusing to believe that he was ill or should stay in bed. Strict bland diet, two quarts of pure spring water a day and one dose of Tuberculinum Bovinum 1M. As a result, his urine became free of blood and pus within two days, and after three days there was no more fever or kidney tenderness. He was gaining weight and back at work.

A plump, apparently healthy baby of nine months who had very severe colics. Bowels normal, abdomen distended with gas during the colic. History of gonorrhoea in the father. During pain the infant turns onto his stomach and draws up his knees in the knee-chest position. The usual physician had not been able to affect this colic. After one dose of Medorrhinum 10M there was peace in the household.

A woman of 35, opera singer, a Brunhilde type with bushy vital hair, stricken with acute arthritis, particularly in the fingers, ankles and toes. Unable to rehearse or perform, fever of 102°F. History of a leucorrhoea recently stopped by local treatment. Joints and pain worse by day, comfortable nights. Relief in wet weather. Medorrhinum 10M brought back the leucorrhoea and relieved the joints within three days.

A woman of 37, actress. Recently overweight although she diets. Cysts of both ovaries following a trichomonas infection suppressed four years before. Told she must have a hysterectomy. Craves salt and sweets. Craves ice. Hot drinks have nauseated her for ten years. Fear of the ocean, even though a champion fresh water swimmer. Has lain in the knee-chest position to sleep all her life. Medorrhinum 10M. Two months later the gynaecologist could not find the ovarian cysts. She has subsequently had a baby.

A boy of 11, asthma and hay fever for years. Characteristic relief of asthma from lying flat. Chilly, sleeps with the windows shut and a towel over his head. Psorinum 10M brought back a forgotten rash from years before and he is now a runner without asthma or hay fever.

A child of 4, chronic running ears for the last two years. Foetid odour like a chicken house. Child never looks clean though loves its bath. Father had asthma in his youth. Child is sensitive to thunderstorms. Psorinum 10M cleared the ears permanently within a week.

Hahnemann's names for the miasms may be unfortunate, but his observation of the profound dyscrasias were salient and invaluable. Read the small philosophic volume of Hahnemann's *Chronic Diseases* and J. H. Allen's two precious volumes of *Psora* and *Sycosis*, then study H. C. Allen's *Materia Medica of the Nosodes*, and become nosode-conscious in acute as well as in chronic prescribing.

The Run of the Mill

A young couple stepped tentatively into my office. The wife looked like a 13th century Madonna, thin and worn, holding in her arms a little, pallid, slant-eyed boy of about a year and a half. The father wept quietly as he told me that several clinics and specialists had pronounced their little boy a Down's syndrome baby and had said that nothing could be offered but custodial care in some institution. They had heard of homoeopathy and asked me if I thought anything at all could be done for him.

The child was thin and pasty-looking, his mouth open, drooling slightly, with a sort of snorting snuffle every few breaths; his head shape was within the limits of normal and his ears were normal. He had no teeth. He could neither stand nor sit without support, nor creep, and his head would wobble if he got off balance. The fingers of his hands were spread widely apart and back, and had spatulate tips. He was totally unable to grasp anything. The mother said he could neither drink from a cup nor suck at a bottle; she fed him with a spoon. When I picked him up the musculature of his back and limbs was pitifully flabby, like a rag doll. He seemed perfectly formed except for the typical mongoloid eye-casings. He did not smile or reach for bright jewelry; he frequently put his head back and rolled his eyes toward the ceiling and then flopped his head down on his chest. The parents begged me not to give them a ray of hope if there was none. A more inexpressive and hopeless trio I have rarely seen. The child had had no colds or childhood disease, no eruption, convulsion, fright or accident.

What to do? All I could see was triple grief. I asked the mother to tell me about her pregnancy and labour. She had experienced a deep grief in the early months of her pregnancy, no nausea, easy labour, no instruments needed. This was the second child, the elder one being, they said, well and normal. No history of syphilis, convulsions or insanity in the family. Laboratory work under the previous doctors was all negative, including Wassermann, blood count, etc. The boy received one dose of Natrum Mur. 10M on the tongue, which he made no effort either to swallow or spit. I explained to the parents what homoeopathic remedies can often do in mental handicap and asked them to give me a try for at least three months, seeing the child every fortnight. I told them it might take several years to get much of anywhere.

Two weeks later the child looked almost rosy and had a gleam of intelligence. The muscles of the back had better tone, he rolled his head and eyes less. He had begun to have a thick catarrh and almost a wheeze. The mother volunteered that he could now roll in bed and that he had taken to doing the queerest thing, sleeping with his little behind, as she called his buttocks, up in the air. The father was not present this time and I asked the mother if she had at any time had a sudden, creamy, profuse discharge from the womb. She said, 'Why, yes, the year before this boy was born; but it was soon cleared up at the clinic.' Medorrhinum 1M, one dose.

Two weeks later when I picked the baby up he grasped my hair. The snuffles and snorting were entirely gone, he had cut two teeth without trouble, could sit alone and was trying to pull himself up in his pen. He had a curious symptom of protruding the tongue between the lips and there was a gurgling sound when he drank. The mother told me he had been exposed to chickenpox and I found a few small spots on the abdomen. He had a short, concussive cough. I explained to her that it would do him good to have the chickenpox and have it thoroughly, but that he would need a remedy to help the vitality bring it well out, and gave him Cuprum 1M, one dose. He skipped the next visit because he blossomed out with a strong chickenpox rash. He himself seemed bright and better than he had ever been during the illness. When he returned at the end of a month he had gained three pounds, no longer stuck out his tongue, grasped my finger so tightly I could hardly extricate it and clutched the paper weight and pencils on my desk, and was beginning to make sounds such as 'Dada' (he was by this time two years old). He felt far heavier than before, now had occipital head sweat with sour odour and was starting to cut two more teeth. Calc. Carb. 10M was given, on which he is still riding and gradually improving.

I have had occasion to do the mother's chronic case. Her remedy was Sulphur. I should judge the father's to be Natrum Mur. How far along toward normality will homoeopathy be able to bring this child?

Little Miss P., aged three, walked stiff-legged into my office, holding to the nurse with both hands. She had never spoken. She had her quota of teeth but was very under-nourished. She would sit all day on the floor in the corner, not playing with any of her toys. I was unable to see either the father or the mother. Apparently she had been a normal infant until her daddy, to whom she was devoted, was called into the army, and she did not improve when he returned a few months ago. First class clinics had pronounced her as 'one of those spastics', although her neurological examination was negative. No history of injury or polio. Natrum Mur. 10M, one dose. The nurse called back two days later and said she could not understand it, that Miss P. had started to use three or four words, like 'mama' and 'spoon', and was walking less stiffly and even alone for two or three steps. When she returned in a month she walked about the office picking up things, and played with the handles of the desk. Three months have elapsed, she is gaining weight and making steady progress. No further remedy as yet.

Summoned in the middle of the night to a hotel, I found a boy of four with tense thigh muscles. He was unable to turn in bed, and screamed if you touched the thighs, though otherwise lethargic and drowsy. He had a fever of 103°F and some rigidity of the neck. He had recently returned from the West and had been, apparently, perfectly well when he went to bed that night. Throat, chest and abdomen were negative; no twitchings or convulsions; no particular perspiration; stool and urine had been normal the day before. No history of wetting or unusual emotion. The arms could be moved freely and were not tender. The joints were normal. Gelsemium 1M was given, hot packs to the thighs ordered continuously through the night, and a homoeopathic paediatrician, who is especially interested in poliomyelitis, summoned. He confirmed the diagnosis of acute polio. By the time he arrived there were fibrillary muscle twitchings and the child had urging to stool and urine, but could not pass either. Nux Vomica 30c, three doses, two hours apart. After about four hours the twitchings and strainings ceased, the muscle tenderness and spasm relaxed, and three days later the child was taken in a taxi to a paediatrician's office for a checkup. He has been active and in excellent health the six months since then and has neither wasting nor any other sequel.

An emergency call to a suburb revealed a boy of fourteen with a temperature of 105°F, lying half on his right side, with a pillow under his left ankle and knee. On entering the room the sour odour, typical of the sweat of rheumatic fever, was strongly perceptible. The left ankle and knee were swollen but not red, exquisitely tender, and the parents said that since calling me, Master B. had complained of pain in the left hip. The bed was a mess, though all the rest of the house most immaculate. The mother apologized, saying the boy kept moving and wriggling as he could not endure the pain lying still, yet the change of position brought only momentary relief. He was frightened and crying. His pulse was 130, heart racing but no murmurs. The inner throat appeared normal and the family denied any recent sore throat or cold. However the boy said, 'I didn't tell you, Mummy, but three weeks ago I had a sore throat and the glands hurt here on the left on my neck.' An electric heating pad was around the boy's knee and a hot water bottle propped against his ankle. No time needed to repertorize this case. I asked one question, 'What time of day are you worst?' 'In the evening', responded his father and mother together, 'after midnight he seems to quiet down.' You know the remedy: Rhus Tox. 10M. Next day the fever was 102°F at its highest, no more pain in the joints. Temperature normal the next day, pulse in the 90's. The boy was kept in bed as a precautionary measure for three weeks, during which time there was no more fever or sweat, no heart murmur and no discomfort. He has looked and felt better since this illness than ever before.

These few cases are routine to any homoeopath, yet they show how beautifully even 'run of the mill' prescribing can help the children fortunate enough to have homoeopathic treatment.

The Direction of Cure –
'Inside Out'

From embryology we remember that the skin and the nervous system develop from the same layer, and my cases here are those of the skin. I also describe one more case at the end, which is not skin, but, to put it mildly, a tumour. I personally think it was a sarcoma, but as it was not operated upon, nobody can be sure. In this case the 'inside out' still applies, because the mental symptoms disappeared first and the physical later.

To start with the first of the skin cases, that bane of the regular physician, eczema:

Case 1: Mrs O., age 34, never heard of homoeopathy. She had such terrible eczema of the hands that she was incapacitated from earning her living as a pianist. It is interesting how fate brings forward the one aspect that you need and use. She was impeccably dressed and quite exquisite – platinum-silver hair, grey eyes, alabaster skin, immaculate – rather frightened, coming to a strange kind of doctor. A cosmopolitan lady who had toured Europe to play. She was singularly symptomless except for these poor hands, which were bound up. I unrolled the gauze and looked at them. They were a mess – cracked and bleeding – just horrible hands.

The one interesting thing in her history was that twenty years ago, when she was a girl, she had had violent eczema of the hands and had been hospitalized. They had given her every known salve. Nothing happened. Nature was too strong for them. Finally they gave her X-ray treatments. She smiled – 'and that cured me.' She subsequently trained as a pianist and had no trouble with her hands until two years before I saw her. Then the whole thing came back again, worse than ever. She had gone from one doctor to the next but still could not play, and was practically in a decline, as a real artist is when thwarted.

There was no family history that would help, no history of tuberculosis, very few symptoms. I looked at her. Her hair was mousy under the dye, her skin was too lovely, her temperament was too excessive under restraint, and I thought for once I was going to follow instinct, so I gave her Tuberculinum 10M, one dose. I have seen her only twice since then, but every two weeks she writes from wherever she is, or calls up if she is near enough, and says, 'I don't need to come in. My hands are wonderful. I am playing. I am so grateful, but you had better send me some more of those little pills because I don't have enough. Last night I only took three, instead of four, and I didn't do quite as well.'

Case 2: Something apparently quite trivial – a girl of fourteen whose father brought her in. She was a fat little girl, shy and flippant when papa corrected her, as he did. She was weepy when we talked about her symptoms. She had eczema of the face, poor child, bleeding and cracked – what a mess! She had lovely blonde hair, and a pretty frock, but her face was just a battlefield.

She had a history of first menses a year ago, pinkish, three days, no symptoms and none since. Thyroid profile was normal. What to do? Cracks, fatness, flippancy, weeping! She was moderately constipated in spite of a sensible diet – Graphites 10M, one dose.

Two weeks later a very pretty girl walked into my office, without papa, with a smiling face all clear except a couple of tiny places on the cheeks, and her first remark was, 'I had a period two days after I saw you.'

Case 3: Master G., aged 7. The poor child has had all the conventional allergy tests, some eighty of them. The only thing they found him allergic to was wheat. If he passes by a bakery he begins to scratch; so mama cut out all the wheat. Try to feed a nice, healthy exuberant seven-year old and let him go play in other people's houses without wheat. If he had wheat he busted out all over, like June, face, elbows, knees, back, everywhere but his stomach.

He was a cute youngster, blond, intelligent, happy, cheery; chilly, however. I said to the mother, 'Doesn't he have anything but this allergy to wheat?'

'Oh,' she said, 'of course, he has always had a sniffle.'

I asked what she meant by 'sniffle'.

She said, 'He never gets up without using up two or three handker-chiefs. He doesn't sneeze a great deal, but he does sniffle and he blows his nose, and it runs.'

I said, 'Oh, he has hayfever.'

'Oh no. They say it is not hayfever because he does it twelve months of the year.'

'Does he cough?'

'No.'

'Does he have headaches?'

'No.'

Sniffle, eczema, wheat – nothing else. I thought, what do we do with this one? So I gave him my favourite potency in the entire materia medica, Psorinum 15c. Why I hang my hat on 15c, I do not know, but it does so much better for me than anything else. Psorinum – I love that bottle!

His mother called me up. She is very ignorant of homoeopathy. She is quite a social lady and cannot tell you a symptom. I do not know how the child has grown up. She said, 'You know, it is a funny thing. David still has his eczema, but he doesn't sniffle.' I replied, 'That's something. Why don't you feed him some wheat?'

She said, 'Feed him wheat?' 'Yes, feed him a little wheat and see what happens.' 'If you say so.'

I said, 'Call me up after the weekend', so she did and said that David had had a couple of pieces of bread each day and nothing happened. The eczema had become no worse and he did not sniffle.

So we let him ride, and in the course of two or three months the eczema was gone, and David was no longer sniffling. He was eating all the crackers and all the bread and biscuits he wanted. I forbade her to give him chocolate, to which he was not allergic, because in my experience chocolate and eczema just absolutely do not gibe. If you have eczema, you cannot have chocolate.

Case 4: An older person called me up and said, 'I have been to three doctors, all of whom you know personally – none of them are homoeopaths – and I think I had better leave them.'

'Well', I said, 'they are nice, honest doctors. What ails you, madam?' 'Eczema.' I grinned into the telephone and said, 'All right, come along.'

She was a lonely and frustrated woman of fifty-six, long, lean and efficient, somebody's first-class secretary. She had her eczema in only one place, on the vulva on the right labium majus, which was swollen. There was a great patch like red shoe leather, and it itched so much that she nearly lost her mind. When I first looked at it I thought, 'My heavens, this is a skin cancer!'

I said, 'What have they been doing to you for this?' She went into everything, starting with lotions and ending with X-ray. When I heard about the X-ray, I knew why it looked that way.

'Do me one favour', I said 'Put nothing on it unless it be lanoline, calendula cream, or fuller's earth – ever heard of it? It feels cool and comfortable and absorbs any sweat. Now let me hear the story of your life.'

235

The chief *motif* of her life was resentment. She supported her mother, who had lived with her all her life and was now dying of cancer. She began by saying how wonderful her mother was and, before she left the office, she said, 'I wish she would die. I wish I could kill her.'

Then she said, 'Oh, I never have said that in my life. I don't mean it.' I said, 'Oh, yes you do, dear. Oh, yes, you do, and your cure has begun.'

Afraid of being alone – she had thought of parking her mother somewhere but could not bear to live alone. Wants somebody always there. Quite exhausted – the other doctors had told her she was so exhausted she ought to take a vacation for six months, but she cannot. She has to have the money. No reason for the exhaustion – negative chest X-ray, negative urine, negative blood. They all said the exhaustion was psychogenic. She was very chilly; she walked the floor while she interviewed me, up and down, up and down, like an animal at the zoo.

She amused me enormously by bringing a bag to the second interview, a big bag entirely full of other people's medicines, which she put out in rows on the desk. I asked why she had brought them and said, I am going to give you one little dose.'

One of my complaints (and I do not have too many) about Kent's *Repertory* is that when you look up 'Resentment', what does it tell you? 'See Malicious.' That is not right. Resentment is not malicious, but that is where you have to look for it. So I took that as Symptom 1. I finally got out of her that her itching was worse at two in the morning, woke her up at that time every night. I also happen to know her socially, and the one thing I have ever observed about her – and which you could not miss – is that she owns more expensive and fantastic hats than anyone else I ever knew. If you saw her every week she would have a different hat on, and I know there is not one of them that is reasonably inexpensive, yet she lives way uptown in a small apartment and saves money madly. You would almost say she is miserly except for the hats.

There are two mentals, avaricious and vain. Take resentment, avarice, vanity, exhaustion, prostration out of all degree, restlessness, waking at 2 a.m. and eczema and what have you? Arsenicum 200c (because she is fairly old), one dose.

She likes us. She is going to stay with us. She is telling the other doctors that we have helped her.

Case 5: Oh, the bane of my life, an eight-month-old baby from a horribly psoric family. Papa is a minister. I do not know why, but ministers' children (and I am one) have tough lives. The baby was born excellently, everything under homoeopathic care, everything very fine, and suddenly

Miss R.B. bloomed out with an eczema. She is a fat baby, weighs a ton when you pick her up – these little Calcarea babies! Her mother tells me that even at three or four months, if any paper was nearby, her fist was at it and she put it in her mouth, or she would chew the sheet – she would eat anything she should not.

Her face was just a blood-stained mask, even though they kept her nails cut and filed. When they brought her in to me I said I had never seen anything so pathetic as this poor child. She was a great milk guzzler, a bottle baby. We stopped the milk and tried goat's milk, and skimmed milk, and canned milk, and dried milk, and none of it made any difference. It was not the milk.

I gave her, almost desperately, a dose of Calc. Carb. 10M. It did something, but not much. After two or three weeks the mother said, 'This isn't doing it.' She knew about homoeopathy. I said, 'Tell me more.'

She replied, 'Her diapers are frightful. It is as though I had spilled ammonia on them.' 'Does she take lots of water?' 'Oh, she is an elegant guzzler. She drinks water; she drinks milk.'

'What else?' 'Well, she seems to like everything fatty, that is one thing. And her poor little tail!' 'Has she eczema around it?' 'No, but it is all little cracks and hurts so awfully when I try to dry her.'

I said to myself, 'Cracks on the tail, cracks on the face, ammonia urine, a baby eight months old. Come up, Nitric Acid bottle.'

So I gave her a dose of Nitric Acid. You would think that was a remedy for more mature people, but I had a child of five in my own family with frightful whooping cough and haemorrhages, and Nitric Acid cured him in twenty-four hours, so you never know. I gave Nitric Acid, and the mother called up in the next ten days and said, 'It was wonderful! She is fine.'

I thought, 'Aha, for a while', so the next week she called up and said, 'I must bring the baby in.' It was a Sunday. 'She has glands as big as a house.'

She brought her in, and at first I thought she had the mumps. Her poor little parotids and cervicals were swollen and stony hard, not tender, not red, no sore throat. She could take lemon juice, which people with mumps cannot take. The glands in the groin were as big as a pullet's egg and so were the glands under the arm; blood count normal, no fever. Where do we go from here? I went to the Kent *Repertory* and sweated blood, and finally found that I just had to give the child a dose of Conium 10M, one dose. The glands went steadily down. The child felt steadily better and the eczema cleared up. I do not know why.

The end is not yet. That child is deeply psoric and will need to be monitored, as I told the mother, for at least another three or four years. But it is interesting – I learned from that that you must give the indicated remedy even if it does not have one of the chief complaints.

Case 6: Here is one brief case which is neither 'outside' nor 'inside'. A child was brought to us who had had a sore throat, temperature of 104°F. He was seven years old, I guessed, and his father had had rheumatic fever. I did not like it. He had symptoms, vaguely. His right leg, behind the knee, bothered him a little, so I gave him a dose of Rhus Tox. 200c. We did his blood count and it did not show much – it failed to show what it ought to have shown.

His urine was all right, and I said, 'Bring him back in two or three days.'

His mother brought him back and said, 'This child has a lump which I discovered when I bathed him. It is behind his knee, a little on the outside.' I felt a lump and thought, 'Oh-oh!' It was as big as a pullet's egg and hard as a stone. It had a ridge in it like serrated rock. If I ever felt a really cancerous growth, that was it. He had a couple of little almond glands in the groin, none elsewhere, and had seen a surgeon who told the mother he should go instantly into hospital to have the lump out; that it was a sarcoma of the bone. I thought it might be that, too.

The mother was very homoeopathic and said, 'I want you to try with the remedy.' I said, 'If you promise me I will see your child regularly and often, if the family is willing, I will take a chance, but I warn you, I don't know.'

She said, 'He has the following mentals: he is the devil temperamentally, he is cross and obstinate and thrashes around. I can't do anything with him. He weeps. He has a big, square, Calcarea-looking brow.'

I looked in the *Repertory* for lumps in that position, stony hardness – Calcarea Fluorica. Sort of pathologically I gave him Calc. Fluor. 10M, one dose. He had no further doses. His mentals cleared first and the lump stopped growing, but did not decrease. We saw him every two weeks thereafter and the lump went steadily and slowly down. Six months later I could find it only if I knew I was looking for it, and the following month it was gone. I wish someone could tell me whether it was a sarcoma.

Nervous Moments

You will not accuse me of needing Gelsemium or Argentum Nit., or even Lycopodium or Silica, when I assert that even the best homoeopath has his or her 'nervous moments'.

At these crucial times not only the life of the patient is at stake, and the doctor's reputation, but the furtherance of faith in homoeopathy in some small but devoted purlieu.

Case 1: Woman, age 46, complains of swelling and stiffness of the joints, markedly worse in wet weather, bathing, or even drinking water; bitter taste, bright yellow coat on rear of tongue; right-sided flatulence, worse on waking, cannot bear tight clothing, loose a.m. stools; violent impulse to harm her children; suicidal, has to restrain herself; red naevi. Natrum Sulph. 10M, one dose.

Marked improvement for two months, when return of symptoms called for repetition.

Case 2: Woman, age 84, diabetic; 4 plus sugar in urine cleared and blood sugar of 203 lowered a year ago by diet and Phosphorus 1M., one dose, followed in a few days by Digitalis 10M because of slow intermittent pulse, nausea and frequent urination. She then went south for the winter and felt so well she omitted medication. On returning she had sudden terrific diarrhoea, scanty stools, collapse, no sweat, dry mouth, blueness, icy fingers and toes, cold yet insisted on uncovering; acetone 4 plus, sugar 2 plus; apparently dying though not comatose. Camphora 10M, one dose.

Acetone cleared, sugar reduced to least trace; sat up in chair in twenty-four hours.

Case 3: Woman, age 40; one child; hysterectomy many years ago; has sudden profuse thick yellow burning leucorrhoea, two days' duration, with bearing-down sensation. Craving for sours since onset; all-gone sensation, nausea. Violent, burning urination and frequency; pain up the rectum on urinating. Smear 4 plus for gonorrhoea. Sepia 10M, one dose.

Second smear on third day, 1 plus. Distress almost gone. Smears at one-week intervals all negative thereafter. Monthly checks since negative. General health better than in years.

Case 4: Man, age 42, scalp eczema for many years, spreading. Patches circinate, red rims, dry, scaly, itchy mostly in the late afternoons; right lumbar backache, urine negative. Desires sweets lately. Irritable, marked inferiority complex; blood pressure low. Lycopodium 10M, one dose.

Two weeks later red rims to eruptions gone, less itch, looking and feeling better.

Case 5: Boy, age 3, treated by sulfanilamide by suburban doctor for streptococcal sore throat. Local condition and fever controlled, but child dwindling, low persistent fever, very low white count. Cannot bear top button of shirt closed, wakes from sleep cross and miserable. Left tonsil swollen and purplish, pain on empty swallowing, desires cold drinks, choking on eating. Pulse 120; yellowish facies; mitral systolic murmur (recent). Grandparents persuaded mother to try homoeopathy. Lachesis 1M, one dose.

No fever after second day. Normal rosy cheeks returned. Pulse 108; throat better and choking gone. In one week murmur gone, pulse 90, child active and gaining; thriving steadily ever since.

Case 6: Man, age 38, with oozing, itching, cracking eczema of scrotum and groins, which had resisted salve and X-ray for months. Stout and gaining weight. Marked aversion to sweets of late. Worried, constipated, with knotty stool covered with mucus. Chilly. In three weeks, better, but relapsed in last two days. Graphites 10M, one dose.

Not heard from for eight months. Not long ago his wife told us, 'It was like a miracle. No more eruptions or trouble since.'

Case 7: Man, age 53, life-long 'migraines', start with eye symptoms; sour burning from mouth to stomach; sour vomiting after which he can eat again; must move with headache. They come on after he gets home from mental strain or on days of rest. Iris Versicolor 50M, one dose, controlled each one but did not stop tendency.

Chronic case study came to Graphites. After a 1M dose, no vomiting or migraine for months.

240

Case 8: Man, age 48, diagnosed as multiple sclerosis by full tests including spinal tap; recommended to try homoeopathy. Case repertorized to Alumina, Phosphorus and Silica. Alumina 1M, one dose. Relief moderate for five weeks. Repeated. Progressing slowly but favourably three months later. Aluminium Silicate may follow.

Case 9: Sea captain, age 64, walked into my office with a pulse of 180, BP 188/70, complaining of choking spells at night, on waking, with loss of breath. Cannot wear stiff collars. Craves air. Burning feet. Lachesis 10M, one dose. Pulse 90 but irregular, fibrillation. No more chokes. BP 140/70. No decompensation. Caught cold in chest muscles; intercostal neuralgia. Bellis 1M relieved. After this, Lachesis repeated and the cold did not take hold. Times of fibrillation, weak pulse, worse at night; restless. Aurum 200c, one dose. Little result.

Crataegus Oxyacanthus 30c four times daily for a week, gave slow steady improvement.

I do wonder whether Crataegus 10M, one dose, would have helped more. It is one of the remedies I have not succeeded with in high potency.

Case 10: Man, age 42, very thin, dark. Spitting of bright blood by thimblefuls. Occasional cough with green thick sweet sputum. Weak feeling in chest. X-ray shows active bilateral tuberculosis, one healed cavity. Fever each night 99°–100°F. Sputum positive. Marked double mitral murmur since a child. For financial and family reasons this man must work. Extra feeding, air and rest advised. Stannum 200c, one dose.

No more blood spitting after second day for three months. Gain of over two pounds. Cough and sputum stopped. No longer feels tired. Carried for over three years on Stannum and Alumen at two to three months intervals (with one dose of Iodum for a cold), never stopping work except for two weeks' vacation yearly. No blood spitting in over a year. Holds his increased weight. Chest negative for acute findings. No fever or sputum.

A lifetime of strict homoeopathy has taught me, in nervous moments, to study the cases and the materia medica more; to go into training to keep oneself fit and intuitive, and then homoeopathy will not fail you.

Oddities

The ability to ask is the leading requirement of man in the modern age. Next comes the capability of really *listening*. Third in importance to the homoeopath is what one of our writers calls not 20/20 vision but 20/20 *observation*. To listen, to ask, to observe. To recognize the position of man in the cosmos and his individual dignity; that man is the physical expression of spiritual causes. To understand that illness has purpose and value; that functional illness is a boon; that healing is one of the laws which occurs in *sleep*. Tell me your illness and I will tell you what you are!

The homoeopath must know which are the constructive illnesses (childhood diseases, colds, fevers), and how the patient can profit by them; and which are the destructive ones, where nature needs help to cope. As the Austrian philosopher Rudolph Steiner said – himself a patient and pupil of the famous Paracelsus student and homoeopath, Dr Emil Schlegel – 'The first physician was the angel with the flaming sword.'

These thoughts may seem odd, but oddity is related to genius and intuition. There is a polarity, a correspondence between the upper and lower organic spheres in man. If there is distress above the diaphragm, seek its causes *below* (migraine from liver, intestines or ovary); and vice versa (if abdominal complaints, look for emotional and rhythmic trouble *above*, as in heart disease, disguised as indigestion). Some cases follow, in which such odd thoughts connived with the repertory to find the helpful remedy.

Case 1: Pale, slender woman of 30 with a tubercular history, complains of a small dry cough which hurts the skin on her right side. The skin is also sensitive to clothes, rubbing and even a draft of air. She is nauseated only when standing. Her chest is sore to light touch, but hard pressure helps. Fever but not sweaty. Looks alarmingly exhausted. No appetite. Chest clear. Had a dose of Tuberculinum two months before.

One thought first of China, but there were no gassy symptoms, no loss of fluid, no vertigo and no difficult disposition. The most distinctive of the three symptoms was the excessive *sensitivity of the skin*. Kent's

Repertory, 5th edition, page 1331, in high degree: Apis, Belladonna, China, Hepar Sulph., Lachesis, Lyssin, Mercurius, Petroleum, Phosphoric Acid, Plumbum, Silica, Sulphur. *Light touch bothers but hard pressure helps*, page 1407: Belladonna, China, Lachesis, Mercurius, Phosphoric Acid. And third, *nausea only on standing*, page 510: eight remedies, of which only one appears with both the others – Phosphoric Acid. I found that she had been grieving and working far beyond her strength. Had the remedy been Phosphorus, with her tubercular history, I would hardly have dared to give it. Intuition backed up the repertory. Phosphoric Acid 200c, 3 doses four hours apart. She called me in three days sounding like a different woman, not only relieved of her curious cold but deeply fortified.

Case 2: Handsome blonde of 44, looks Scandinavian but of Germanic origin. Bilateral chronic cystic mastitis. Almond-sized gland in left axilla. Lumps chiefly in the outer quadrant; not hard, not attached, no skin dimpling. Fearful of cancer, several of her family having died of it. Exquisitely neat person, business executive. Told me she feared the responsibility of a higher job which had been offered her. Said she had always been desperately shy and feared losing face. Toenails deformed and brittle. Chilly but likes cool air. Kent, page 838 in high degree: Carbo An., Conium, Phytolacca, Silica. The patient wept as she told me of her shyness. Key symptom: lack of self-confidence despite extreme competence. *Prescription:* Silica 10M one dose. Two weeks later both breasts completely clear, gland entirely gone from the left axilla. Patient said she had not felt so well in years and added that her ankles, which had been swollen for many months (and which she had not even mentioned) were thin again.

Case 3: Widow of 65, plump, a worrier. Chief complaint: left arm numb, especially while sitting. Heart normal, teeth and sinuses normal. Sensation of heat in the left leg below the knee. Frequent sore throat on the left side. Kent's *Repertory*, page 1036, *numbness of left arm*: Aconite, Baryta Carb., Cactus, Graphites, Lachesis, Medorrhinum, Phosphorus. *Sensation of heat of left leg*: Aconite, Graphites, *Prescription:* Graphites 200c, one dose, with complete relief.

Case 4: Divorcee, age 30, animated blonde, woke from sleep with a sensation of being paralyzed, felt as if she were going to die, heart pounding. Same thing two weeks later. Sensation as if electric shock in her head on falling asleep. Three weeks later suddenly fell to the floor with vertigo, and thereafter four or five times fell to the left. History of goitre, right side. Vertigo on looking downward. Examined for brain tumour, negative. Terrified at suggestion of brain tumour. Eye grounds normal, ear and sinus examinations negative. Tentative diagnosis, Menière's disease. *As if electric shock*, Kent, page 230: Alumina, Cicuta, Phosphorus. *Vertigo on looking down*, Kent, page 100: Phosphorus in high degree. *Complaints from fright*, page 49: Aconite, Ignatia, Lycopodium, Natrum Mur., Opium, Phosphoric Acid, Phosphorus, Pulsatilla., Silica. *Goitre right-sided*, Kent, page 147: Phosphorus. Kent, page 99, *Falling to the left* does *not* have Phosphorus, despite which, because she is a chilly, volatile, scary, trembly type, I gave Phosphorus 1M, one dose. No trouble since.

The Unique Scope of
Homoeopathy in Chronic Disease

Homoeopathy is a system of therapeutics and preventive medicine, based on a philosophy of disease, a natural law, and empiric results. It is a therapeutic specialty, and yet of universal application. Its forte is in the functional stage, when there is little pathology, even when no diagnosis is possible; and in prevention and chronic disease. Acute disease is self-limited – one either recovers or dies; homoeopathic results are brilliant here, even with lower potencies. Chronic disease does not of itself tend toward cure, and most non-homoeopathic chronic medication is only palliative. For real results with chronic disease we need the high potencies, the single remedy, and the single or divided-single dose. We must know the philosophy of aggravation, repetition, and the use of nosodes. We must know how to unravel a tangled case, bring to light the hidden hindrances, and then aid the vitality to cure. We must peel our onion, layer by layer. We must apprehend the deep-seated condition (Hahnemann's miasms), and know the relationships of our remedies. We must have in our blood and bones and spirit the portraits of the remedies, so that we can recognize them in their protean forms.

Apropos of the remedy pictures, the homoeopath will recall Kent's description of Ignatia – the over-cultivated, spoiled girl who has returned from art training in Paris on the verge of a nervous breakdown, who thinks she has fallen in love with a chauffeur; or the Sulphur portrait – the ragged philosopher, the unsuccessful inventor, the great unwashed, with frayed collar and dirty cuffs, nibbling candy and discussing who made God.

In chronic work we must also have a new concept of pathology – as an end product, as a beneficent localisation, not to be lightly removed; and realize that our remedies can work on the cause and shrink the fibroid, slough out the polyp, or decrease the cyst. We must have a new viewpoint on bacteriology – that germs are concomitant rather than causative, and so must turn our attention to the correction of the terrain. Bacteria inhabit everyone, but only those with a low threshold of resistance develop disease from them. Our remedies influence the constitution so that lice and worms depart.

We must also have a new respect for disease, and not nip the outward and visible to the detriment of the inward and not yet visible.

Many prescribers doubtless use homoeopathic remedies skilfully, and often as adjuvants in acute disease. But how many have gone to the trouble of learning the technique of constitutional prescribing? It is a speciality, yet a general one – one that can help you signally whether you be specialist, surgeon, internist or old-fashioned general practitioner. Doctors do not cavil at post-graduate study to become experts in their chosen field – they would not attempt cranial surgery or diabetology without long and complicated training. Yet they think themselves homoeopathic on a smattering of superficial knowledge of one of the most delicate, rewarding and – yes – dangerous specialties. Many who do not know the beautiful precision of the science of homoeopathy, and the exacting art of its practice, feel that because general medicine is less crude than it used to be, homoeopathy has lost its point and will fade into harmless disuse.

Let me enumerate some of the advantages of homoeopathy: it gives to the doctor a real confidence, which the patient feels. It appeals profoundly to commonsense and to human nature in its desire to be understood, to be valued as a complete being, to be listened to. It appeals also to the Scotch blood in us all, being an enormous saver of time and money; and gives patients a sense of wellbeing of the whole man which so contributes to efficiency. Even those patients whose symptoms are purely functional know that you are interested in curing them. It is not the disease that is important but the person who has it, and the road to cure is marked by the symptoms.

Homoeopathy is a kind of cosmic optics, each patient a prism refracting the vital ray according to his structure, and by these brilliant patterns the true homoeopath can help them. Homoeopathy does not engraft drug diseases, nor clog the cure, nor cloud the picture. Whoever saw a case in ordinary medicine recapitulate its symptoms? Yet after the constitutional remedy, if we are on the right track, Hering's three laws of cure obtain: from above downward, from within outward, and in the reverse order of the appearance of the symptoms. When the symptoms follow this course, real cure is being effected.

Homoeopathy avoids suppressions, including operations, and the premature and external closing of vents, such as the stopping of catarrh with strong local applications, foot sweat with drying powders, and skin eruptions with repressive salves. It regards certain acute diseases, such as measles, as vents for inherited or innate taints. Homoeopathy helps in prognosis through the type of aggravation brought on by our remedies, and its helps in diagnosis through the remedies called for by the symptoms and the organ relationships of these. It is a superb palliative in incurable conditions, and the best social security from the health standpoint. The greatest of all its gifts is the reinforcement of the patient's own vital force. Acute disease reveals chronic weaknesses, though it may hold them in abeyance during its course. After every acute illness, even a cold, there should be a follow-up remedy, so that the new aspect of chronic illness may be removed. The homoeopathic simillimum in acute disease will minimize chronic sequelae. Patients under steady homoeopathic treatment should never develop mastoiditis or sinusitis. When patients have true homoeopathy for several continuous generations the results are impressive.

It is not too much to say that every human being needs a constitutional remedy. Which person does not have certain minor deviations from that complete unconsciousness of our body which constitutes health? A wart here, a pile there, an itch, a discharge, a craving for salt, an aggravation before storm, menstrual pain or sweaty feet, brittle nails or canker sores. The Chinese pay their doctors to keep them well – a part of the immense passive wisdom of that subtle race. Modern medicine advises check-ups every six months or so. A splendid idea, but crude and fragmentary. We are frequently revising our business, our characters and our investments, trying to better ourselves and climb ahead; in chronic constitutional homoeopathy we have a definite means of increasing our vitality and efficiency, warding off the tedious and limiting annoyances of insidious chronic diseases.

The use of homoeopathy in chronic disease is complicated. A special method of case-taking is essential to good results, establishing the modalities of the symptoms, evaluating them into a totality of symptoms which is the language of nature asking for a remedy. Once this is procured, it remains to find the most similar remedy. It is much the same in prescribing as in diagnosis: long experience and minute observation, made almost subsconsciously, contribute to a hunch as to what is wrong with the patient or what remedy he needs. But even as thorough procedures are essential to diagnosis, so is the technique of repertorizing and materia medica checking vital to the selection of the simillimum in complicated cases. Even acute cases need this if they are not immediately clear.

Chronic case remedies are often more visible than the acute ones. Consider a violent acute lumbago which I repertorized. The three remedies which came highest were Sepia, Alumina and Magnesia Mur., none of which one usually connects with lumbago. Sepia 10M, three hours apart, gave brilliant results. On the other hand, a schoolgirl of fifteen came for chronic headache almost daily for seven years, never free of them for a week. Simple pain-killers had been of no avail. Pain hammering, 10–11 a.m.; late and irregular menses; craving for salt; oily pimply skin; history of long grief; did not want sympathy. No need to repertorize here – Natrum Mur. 10M, one dose, which was followed by one more headache and none since.

In some cases which present for acute conditions, the chronic remedy will cope with these from the start. If the chronic remedy that you see is the complementary of the acute remedy, then this is almost sure to be effective. If there is a history of repeated similar acute attacks, an immediate chronic is especially indicated. Sometimes the converse is true, and a chronic case must be opened with an acute remedy; for instance, hay fever is a constitutional condition, but in the beginning of an attack an acute remedy gives relief and clears the way for the more searching constitutional remedy.

I discuss the chronic remedy of the patient rather than remedies in chronic disease, because the homoeopathic mind works that way. *It is the patient who matters and not the disease.* Yet I must also give two cases to illustrate the power of the remedy in chronic disease.

Case 1: Tuberculosis. Tall, skeleton-thin man of 35 came for blood-spitting, sensation of weight under the sternum, dragging pain to the right of the sternum, green salty sputum, terrible weakness, exhausted at mid-day, better by dusk. Physical examination showed severe mitral murmur, slight fever, altered voice and a few moist râles over the painful area. X-ray of the chest showed bilateral tuberculosis. Patient could not afford to stop work. *Prescription:* Stannum 200c, one dose, rest when not working and a sensible lifestyle, high calorie diet, cod-liver oil. One week later heavy feeling gone, no more haemoptysis, gained half a pound, felt fresh and strong. Repeated Stannum 200c, one dose, after two months. At the end of three months, while working hard, the patient had gained three pounds and felt better than in years.

Case 2: Diabetes. Elderly lady, acutely dizzy for weeks, staggers, extreme weakness, 'Oh God!' feeling at pit of stomach at 11 a.m., crazy for salt, fidgety and sleepless, eats little and often, violent thirst for ice water. Physical examination: blood pressure, heart and eye grounds normal, 4% sugar in the urine. *Prescription:* Phosphorus 200c, one dose, and a moderate diabetic diet. Able to go out after the third day, sugar down to 1% in two weeks, much stronger and not dizzy.

The Simillimum as Psychiatrist

The following brief cases would be classified in ordinary medicine as psychiatric.

Case 1: A woman of 50 whose opening gambit in consultation is that family life is grim. She is continually angry at her husband (a charming and able man, but impervious) and like a good wife she never shows it. She has itching without eruptions all over, headache as a band around the head, clenches her teeth, and has toothache in sound teeth. At her job she feels constantly humiliated by people who know less than she does. *Prescription:* Staphysagria 10M, one dose. Two weeks later she reports that she has not felt as well in many months. No itching, no headaches, job and home going well.

Case 2: Young man of 20, cerebral palsy, unable to speak intelligibly although he is mentally clear and bright. Can sing but not articulate. Constant twitching and wringing of the hands, so marked that he cannot get food to his mouth. Had been given strong tranquillizers with little effect. These were stopped and Tarentula Hispanica 10M, one dose, was given. On seeing him again in a month, he shook hands and conversed clearly with me about the farm animals he was tending. He ate his meals more easily. He had lived under the same pleasant conditions for over two years without marked improvement, until the dose. In an effort toward controlled experiment, no other factors or treatment influences were changed.

Case 3: An efficient woman of 60 had nervous prostration following the long strain of nursing a relative. Complete exhaustion. Could not leave her bed. Nausea and vertigo from the least motion. Blood count high to normal; heart and blood pressure normal; urine perfect; no pathology in the genito-urinary tract. Only one key symptom: sensation of emptiness. *Prescription:* Cocculus Indicus 10M, one dose. This patient went to work the next day and continued for two months with her old vigour. At the first sign of recurrence of the emptiness and exhaustion she received Cocculus CM, one dose, and is functioning well.

Cases

Case 4: Beautiful blonde of 27, hospitalized seventy-two times in the last fourteen years following skull fracture (shown by X-ray). Her ignorant stepfather had refused the recommended hospitalization and seizures ensued, more frequent near the menses, eight or ten a day. Incredible and almost constant headaches, not yielding even to strong sedatives for the last two years. *Prescription:* Arnica CM, one dose. Head pain reduced, enabling omission of analgesics. Electro-encephalograph negative; eye grounds negative. Final diagnosis in the most recent of the many hospitals was hysterical epilepsy. Complete amnesia followed on being told this verdict. Based on hysteria she has convulsions, worse before menses, and disproportionate nausea in a beautiful young blonde. I prescribed Cuprum Metallicum 10M, one dose, and placebo, which was followed by one more convulsion and then none for weeks. She has recovered her memory and resumed work. I sent her to a psychiatrist to teach her to deal with the problems behind her recurrent hysteria.

Case 5: Housewife of 50, turned against her husband, children and household work; total indifference. Complains of violent left-sided headache, constant until her attention is distracted. Marked nausea. Varies from abnormal quietude to darting movements. Immense relief from violent motion. *Prescription:* Sepia 10M. Has subsequently sent the rest of the family to homoeopathy.

Case 6: Young man of 21, diagnosed as mentally retarded from birth, has been hospitalized most of his life and on large doses of tranquillizers recently. When spoken to he stares into space, repeats the question or remark, and after a long interval answers logically. Constant fidgeting of the foot, although otherwise abnormally still. All drugs were stopped. *Prescription:* Zincum 10M, one dose, which gave noticeable improvement for three months. Upon relapse, Zincum 50M, one dose, was given, followed by an even longer amelioration. Now carries on normal conversation, works in a shop successfully, though still under supervision. Care has been taken not to alter other factors of environment in these cases.

Let no one say that the high potencies cannot aid mental conditions in a spectacular manner.

First published in the *British Homoeopathic Journal*, Jan. 1966, and included by permission.

A Provocative Prescribing Puzzle

A 57-year-old diplomat, who had been under homoeopathic care for some dozen years, was referred to me in consultation. A full chart of his case had been sent in advance of his visit. I prefer to interview the patient first and read the chart afterward, so as to be unprejudiced and, as it were, receive the language of nature on a *tabula rasa*. This charming gentleman displayed considerable anxiety about his condition, although to my practised eye he looked rather well. His chief complaint was that six months previously he had had a sudden pain starting in a small point in the middle anterior chest, going to the heart 'like a fire' and extending diagonally through and down the back like a small pin. He felt that this original pain had followed on one of two things: fast eating of Swiss cheese on black bread or a dive from a diving board into his pool.

There has been no sharp pain now for two months until this past weekend, when he planted peach trees and the pain returned. He had noticed that he tends to get the pain when he becomes annoyed at his secretary or excited by television. Emotional causes bring on an increase of the pain, which changes in character. Recently he trembles with the pain. His wife does not see his shaking, so probably it is internal. The pain is better in a warm place. Cold weather really distresses him. It is worse in a damp warm place or muggy humid weather; even the bathroom during a hot shower bothers him. There is no shortness of breath or nausea.

He describes himself as a 'misanthrope'. He says, 'People leave us a sorriness – if you help, it is worse.' He is afraid to speak in public. He fears leaving his daughter alone if he or his wife should die, or his wife by herself, or lest she die before him. He keeps trouble to himself. He is a cautious man, yet his self-confidence is good. He keeps anger in. His best time of the day is 4 to 6 p.m. and in the evening. Although perfect on waking in the morning, he feels poorly after getting up, and says that he starts life at 10.30 a.m. each day.

All his life he has easily swallowed the wrong way. He likes to eat much and rapidly, but feels better when he eats little and not often, or even when he fasts. He likes salt and smoky things. He enjoys beer,

251

which aggravates, and has pain in the liver from cognac, but can take Scotch. He has small internal piles and says there is a connection between his piles and what he calls his heart pain. His heart, he says, feels better when he does not eat.

He was born in the mountains but prefers and feels better at the ocean.

He sometimes has a sensation of fullness in the chest on laughing. Four years ago he had a spell of vertigo with a sensation of turning from left to right. Recently his feet sweat, with odour.

He is afraid of sex, which he enjoys and needs, for fear it will bring on his heart pain, which however it has not done to date. His wife fears it for him, hence ensues what he calls 'heroic estrangement'. He is very musical. He likes the past and all its ways. On being asked about his friends he said, 'I had one friend and he died.'

Conclusion: Natrum Mur. 10M.

On re-reading the file sent to me, for my amusement I repertorized the case on the basis of the symptoms it described, without regard to my personal impressions. The symptoms from the past came out to Phosphorus first, Pulsatilla second, Calc. Carb., Sepia and Lycopodium. Why such a different picture? The doctor who referred him to me had not had him very long, and in her accompanying note she said, 'He has Weltschmerz and is taciturn. I like him especially.'

What made me choose Natrum Mur.? – the man himself, the key statement being 'One friend who died'. Better not eating, mid-morning aggravation, fear of the sex he needs. This is a singularly interesting case from the point of view of the evaluation for symptoms and the intuitive perception of the personality of the patient.

When and When Not to Operate

A homoeopathic surgeon is 'precious beyond rubies'. By that I mean an able operator, a wise case manager and an encouraging and definite personality, who adds to these criteria of all good surgeons at least an appreciation, if not a working knowledge, of the aid that is possible for the surgical patient through homoeopathy.

To be sure, those following homoeopathy properly need less frequent operations than other patients. Why is this? Because, aside from mechanical conditions, the states that require surgery are end-pathology conditions, the result of defective physiology rather than the primary processes of the body; in other words, surgery copes with end products rather than with functional beginnings. The most brilliant sphere of homoeopathy is in the functional stage, when there are many symptoms and few irreversible organic changes.

Let me illustrate the case of a woman who had fibroids, not very big, not bleeding, not giving any trouble appreciable to her, which were found on a routine check-up, with subsequent hysterectomy. A few months after this she developed symptoms referable to her gallbladder and took them to her gynaecologist, who decided to remove the gallbladder. As she did not wish to undergo another operation so soon, she consulted me. The symptoms pointed clearly to Nux Vomica, which she received with relief to her acute difficulties, followed later by Sepia, her constitutional remedy. Her diet was altered, her weight reduced, and she was saved the necessity of this operation.

On the other hand, a patient was referred to me who for five years had had a lump in the breast, involving the nipple and adherent to the skin. She had been under excellent homoeopathic treatment during the preceding five years and was herself in good condition, although involvement of the glands of the axilla was starting to progress. I advised immediate operation without radiation therapy; in my opinion and that of the surgeon we used, the operation should have been performed long before. Had this woman been under constitutional prescribing many years earlier she would, I believe, have been far less likely to develop cancer.

Another example. Kidney colic with actual stones can be coped with by a homoeopathic remedy, and in a large number of cases, particularly with early treatment, the constitution can be so regulated that subsequent gravel and stones do not occur. Many breast lumps which are not cancerous can be made to go away and kept from recurring with a remedy, and many duodenal ulcers can be healed with a remedy even without too prolonged or trying limitations to the diet. But it is wrong to say that surgeons are not needed even in patients under competent homoeopathic care. The question of judgement, as to when and when not to operate, is the most delicate part of the surgeon's business and no less essential to the family doctor and the homoeopath as well.

Certainly one operation leads to another. A patient who has had many operations is dreaded by the homoeopath; on the other hand, the patient who refuses operation even when the pathology requires it is a danger to himself and his physician. Try to educate your devoted homoeopathic patients to the fact that careful prescribing under frequent supervision should be done, preferably in consultation with a surgeon who understands homoeopathy, both at the beginning and at intervals during the treatment. For instance, if I wish to try reducing small fibroids with a remedy, I would want my gynaecological surgeon to check them at the beginning and then frequently during the course of treatment. Often they can be cleared, but sometimes not.

A homoeopath should know when critical conditions like volvulus or intussusception can be resolved by a remedy such as Plumbum or Cuprum, or when it is necessary to life to have an emergency operation. Such things as varicose veins, haemorrhoids and ulcers, a good homoeopath rarely has to have operated. The criteria to remember are: will the operation constitute a suppression or an obstacle to complete cure, if cure seems possible; or will the operation be the removal of the end product of a disorder to be resolved by the remedy, acting in effect as a foreign body; or is it, as in the case of a large tumour, actually dangerous? He who knows what the remedy can do, and what it cannot do, is the best and most constructive physician.

Operations Obviated by Homoeopathy

All patients, like Gaul, are divided into three parts, at least as regards surgery: those who have an irresistible desire for it, at any price; those who will never submit to it, no matter what; and those who can be swayed by sense or consequence. For the first, I commend them to Irvin Cobb and his *Speaking of Operations*. May they continue to 'enjoy poor health', and vie with their neighbours! As to the second, I embrace them in spirit, for one can do one's homoeopathic best with them. It is to the third group that I would speak, as follows: Operations can be obviated by good homoeopathy in a large percentage of cases, and particularly so in the chronic homoeopathic patient. One of the advantages of our work is that we can raise the threshold of disease susceptibility and prevent illness – or rather, nature's need of illness – particularly in adults.

To diverge for a moment into the philosophy of sickness. Acute disease in the adult is an outcropping of chronic trouble, whether brought on by unhygienic (that is, unnatural) thinking or living, or by the occasional need of a vent, or by a suppression, or by any lowering of the vitality which permits a sickness to develop, often with its concomitant bacteria getting unruly, instead of remaining harmless guests of the healthy economy. Acute disease in the child is necessary and admirable in the form of the so-called 'diseases of childhood' – the exanthemata, for instance. Hence our objection to the suppressive prevention of these valuable illnesses by the conventional methods of sera and vaccines – in addition to the resulting introduction of foreign growth rhythms from animals, and the introduction by injection methods which violate Nature's protection. It is to be hoped that the child will not need to have certain other kinds of disease, such as rheumatic fever or malaria. But if it does, proper homoeopathic remedies should bring the young patient through fortified, and not weakened.

The best preventive for chronically recurrent attacks in the adult or child is the constitutional homoeopathic remedy, chosen by individualization based on the totality of the symptoms, since this represents Nature's own request and guide. The same can be said for frequent attacks of so-called surgical troubles – tonsillitis, appendicitis, sinusitis, haemorrhoids, duodenal ulcers, bleeding fibroids and many others.

An acute remedy must be picked if the case is first seen in an acute stage, and it must be the simillimum. If the disease is a tricky and dangerous one like appendicitis, follow your blood counts, your pulse and temperature ratios, the look of your patient, and have a good surgeon in consultation who also knows what wonders your remedy can do – to protect your reputation and reassure the family. Watch like a hawk – and be *sure* you have the right remedy: nine out of ten cases will clear without surgical intervention. Then insist on treating chronically to prevent recurrence. Returning attacks in children can be well controlled. In my hands Sulphur often does yeoman service here; Phosphorus too, where the abdomen is full and exquisitely tender, and when you might think of Belladonna save for the nausea from hot drinks and the false appearance of well-being in a child whom you know to be critically ill.

Once I was badly fooled by a boy: lower right quadrant tenderness with rebound pain, temperature 104°F and W.B.C. 20,000 with 80% polys, pulse slow (72). The family wanted operation, so I weakened and sent him in to hospital, but not before giving him Pyrogen 10M, one dose. The surgeon agreed on appendicitis – on operating, behold right mesenteric glands and nothing else. Appendix perfect.

Let me cite another case as a counterpoint. Woman, age 69, no history of 'indigestion attacks' or appendix upsets; under homoeopathy for years, sudden attack of right lower quadrant pain with vomiting, rebound tenderness, W.B.C.10,000, polys 78%, fever 100°F, pulse rapid but good; held her side and flexed knee; thirsty, wanted to be left alone. Bryonia 1M, one dose and placebo. Averse to operation. Blood count rose to 14,000, polys 92%, fever 102°F. Rectal examination showed tender mass in right fornix. Became restless, worse at early night; Rhus Tox. 1M. Next morning the fever was lower, pulse 120 – nervous moments! The surgeon said, 'Pray, but not operate.' Pyrogen 200c, three doses, once an hour. After the second dose the patient had a chill and turned blue (perforation), followed by diarrhoea for several hours of masses of foul pus. During this she felt better and went on to a quick recovery. No symptoms of ileocaecal or ovarian pain or adhesions. Bowels perfect. Health excellent thereafter. 'Pretty lucky', said the surgeon. 'Three cheers for my subsequent health and homoeopathy', said the patient. Do not misunderstand me – some-times we must all recommend operation for fulminating cases, first seen too late, or unwisely purged. In my experience the ones cured medically do far better.

Patients and doctors both need to remember that surgery is not merely mechanical, but tends to be suppressive and close a vent before the cause is cured. The law of cure in chronic disease – that the symptoms disappear in the reverse order of their coming – is blocked by an operative scar as a stream is blocked by a dam. Let Nature find her vent under the guidance of the remedy.

Surgery may be needed for the removal of a mechanical obstruction, but cure the *process* first before you cut out the end product (pathology), or else disease will follow in more vital regions where it cannot be cut out.

In cases of chronic tonsillitis where there are foci leading to fast hearts, dyspnoea, exhaustion, neuritis etc., such remedies as Lachesis, Sulphur, Tuberculinum, Silica, Graphites, Sepia and Argentum Nit. do wonders. The following case is an example of this.

Man, aged 26, right rib resection at age 4 for empyema; Tbc in both parents' families; gaining weight fast (200 lb). Chief complaint: exhaustion on least effort; chronic hoarseness for two years; nausea on rising in the morning. Burning in epigastrium, better by cold. Wants only cold food and room and air. Craves sweets. Thinks he has gastric ulcer. Deep-sounding cough without modalities. Lungs negative, also lung X-ray and gastric series. Heart found to be 120–140 at rest, regular, no murmurs. Electrocardiogram normal. 'Never a sore throat' – but tonsils, though small, are unhealthy-looking. Slight tic – twitch of head. Diarrhoea from anticipation. A worrier. Argentum Nit. 10M, one dose.

Two weeks later stomach brilliantly relieved, no morning nausea since second day after dose. Cough almost gone, less hoarse. Tonsils look 50% better. Heart 98. Ran four blocks without thinking. After two months, slight relapse: Argentum Nit. 10M. Pulse 78, less tired, throat looks almost normal. Urinating much, losing false fluid weight.

Cases of breast lumps, fibroids, fistulae, mastoid, proven duodenal ulcer, gallstone colics, kidney colics, thyroids, piles, bony exostoses of the foot, varicose veins pronounced clearly surgical, and spinal pain where fusion operations failed to help, have yielded to the remedy without recourse to surgery.

The Avoidance of Surgery

The homoeopathic attitude towards operations is based on its philosophy of non-suppression and pathology. Such pathology as fibroids, tumours, cysts, even warts and wens, are considered as end products, the result of a diseased process in the constitution. In homoeopathic case-taking one uses polyps as an objective symptom, say, in the sense of a tendency of the constitution to form polyps. Together with such an objective symptom one uses the haemorrhage or nasal obstruction, with their modalities; and also – and chiefly – the mental and general symptoms of the patient. By means of this totality, of which the surgical pathology is but one item, the simillimum is chosen.

Such constitutional treatment tends to clear up the cause of the pathology, and to shrink the actual tumour. If there is still a mechanically annoying mass left when the patient in himself is cured, and the symptoms subsequent to pathology are obliterated, this may be considered residual and be removed surgically without detriment to the patient. If, however, it had been removed before the tendency to its formation had been cleared up, a recurrence in that or other spots would be expected. Or, even graver, some affection of a more vital organ would be sure to follow.

These connections between operative suppression and subsequent development of dire chronic trouble are usually not traced except by the homoeopath. Analogous to this process is the development of asthma following upon the suppression of eczema. Moreover, if a barrier is erected by surgery before the chronic case is cured, Hering's third law of cure – the return of the symptoms in the reverse order of their appearance – is unable to operate; the cure is either held up, or else a method of avoiding the obstacle caused by the surgical interference must be found. Whether such a method exists is a question in my mind and in the discussion I would like your experience in this matter. My own view is that the vital force, in the course of its reverse operation, may be able to find a vent or channel through some other point of least resistance. For example, if fibroid bleeding cannot be brought back, or if suppressed leucorrhoea redevelops because of surgical removal of the womb, then a substitutional diarrhoea or coryza or haemorrhoidal bleeding or eruption may take place. I have seen these results follow, although whether as an alternative course because the original line was blocked, or whether merely as a second method of outlet, I do not know. Even where there has been no apparent suppression I have seen, under the constitutional remedy, the healing of one vent and the breaking out of a discharge of a different nature in another orifice. But this has been in the correct order, from above downward, and may simply mean the passage of the disease down and out.

Let us for the moment consider the most frequent types of operation, beginning in the order of the repertory, from above downwards: eye, ear, nose and throat operations, empyema, gastrointestinal including rectal, genito-urinary, bone, glands and skin, including varicose veins and ulcers. Homoeopathy has power over strabismus, with deep remedies like Tuberculinum or Psorinum, as well as smaller remedies like Cyclamen; over cataract with Calc. Carb., Silica and Cineraria; over chalazion with Staphysagria, over pannus with Hepar Sulph.; over glaucoma with the indicated chronic remedy, often Phosphorus. In lieu of ear operations we have a host of remedies for acute otitis media, not forgetting Dulcamara, Nitric Acid, Hepar Sulph. and the Mercuries; for chronic otitis there are Silica, Fluoric Acid, Graphites, Psorinum and others; in mastoid, Capsicum, Aurum, and indeed the indicated remedy. My last mastoid case cleared up under Rhus Tox. given on modalities of the patient as a whole.

In the nasal tract, polyps will yield to Calc. Carb., Sanguinaria, Phosphorus or Teucrium, and severe recurrent epistaxis to the indicated remedy rather than to cauterization. Sinuses can be made to drain with any of the host of chronic remedies, notably the Kalis, Silica, Lycopodium, Mercury, Sticta, and so on. Tonsils and adenoids in their chronic state respond to Tuberculinum, Baryta Carb., Calc. Carb., Natrum Mur., Silica and others; glands of the neck to Rhus Tox., Lycopodium, Calc. Carb., Phytolacca and the Barytas. Empyemas and lung abscesses will often clear with such remedies as Kali Mur.

Gastric and duodenal ulcer will yield to Anacardium, Arsenicum Alb., Argentum Nit., Calc. Phos., Conium, Kali Bich., Graphites, Lycopodium, Phosphorus, and other similar remedies. Even in strangulated hernia, Nux Vomica will sometimes relax and reduce the hernia while the operating room is being prepared. Lycopodium or Sepia prevent hernia development better than trusses. Plumbum has its place in intussusception, and a great number of acute remedies apply in appendicitis, notably Belladonna, Rhus Tox. and Phosphorus. In the rectal sphere Ignatia or Ruta may be useful in prolapse; Nux Vomica, Aesculus, Aloes, Sulphur,

Collinsonia and Ratanhia, or indeed the indicated constitutional remedy, will obviate pile operations. Fissures and ischiorectal abscess should never be operated – Silica, Sulphur, Nitric Acid, etc., will cope with them better. Gallbladder surgery can be indefinitely postponed very often with Calc. Carb., Bryonia, Chelidonium, Podophyllum, Magnesia Mur. or even Colocynth; and nephrotomy with Lycopodium, Berb. Vul. or Ocimum; and bladder stones controlled with Sarsaparilla, Terebinth, etc.

Prostate operations can be staved off with Staphysagria, Cannabis Sat., Sarsaparilla, Causticum or Cantharis. Fibroids yield to Calc. Carb., Phosphorus and a host of others; ovarian cysts to Apis, Colocynth, Lycopodium, Lachesis, Podophyllum or Thuja. Many prolapse operations can be averted by Sepia, Murex or Lilium Tig.; abortions, leucorrhoeas and metrorrhagias are managed best by the indicated remedy, both acute and chronic. Urethral caruncle has responded for me to Clematis, Cannabis Sat. or Cantharis.

Many a sacroiliac fusion for persistent secondary sciatica can be avoided by Rhus Tox., Tellurium, Gnaphalium or whatever the indicated remedy may be. A spinal tumour, two years ago, disappeared under Calc. Phos., and spinal fusions need not be done if judicious use of our great anti-psorics were made. Varicose veins and ulcers respond to constitutional treatment. Some of the worst I have ever seen have healed under Pulsatilla, Calc. Carb., Graphites and Anthracinum.

Osteomyelitis gets a quicker and better result under such remedies as Phosphorus, Mercurius, Silica, Fluoric Acid or Thuja than by repeated operation.

This does not mean that we are not grateful to the surgeons. In mechanical conditions such as cleft palate or club foot, and in emergencies too far advanced for the remedy, or in accidents, they are invaluable. But the plea of the true homoeopath is ever for the chronic remedy first.

DISCUSSION

Dr Bond: In a toxic thyroid, would the thyroid crisis of the heart be considered as an end product of the disease, and too far advanced to cope with by the true homoeopathic remedy before real damage was done to the heart, or death ensued, or would the homoeopathic remedy handle that just the same as any other condition?

Dr McLaren: Some acute cases are so violent in character that you will lose them, no matter what you do. That applies to toxic thyroid as well as to angina pectoris or any other disease.

Dr Hubbard: In the mild cases where there is no urgency, I think it is correct for the doctor to try his remedies. If there is no improvement, under whatever system he employs, he will have to call in the surgeon. He should not wait too long because of the damage which will accrue to the heart. A number of these cases will clear up very nicely if you get the right remedy, but it is not always easy to get the right one.

Dr Bond is facing the same situation that all of us have to face, and that is the ability to pick out the right remedy for these drastic cases; therefore, I will ask you to bear further with me.

Belladonna will often pull you out of the hole. Barium Met. has all the flushing of the face and the fast pulse of these cases. Natrum Mur. has the fast pulse, the flushing, the fear, the nervous symptoms, the trembling. It will help you a great deal.

Lycopus corresponds very well to the heart-pulse symptoms. I nearly always give these cases what I consider to be the indicated constitutional remedy and put them to bed, whenever possible, and have them rest. I do not think that any of them will clear up in less than six months to a year. They will be improving all the time, but it will take that long for them to be able to get back to work again, ordinarily, if they are at all severe.

A BRIEF STUDY COURSE
IN HOMOEOPATHY

Review of 'A Brief Study Course in Homoeopathy'

By Lucy Swanton Clark, M.D.

This is the briefest of courses. Each of the chapters is full of gems not to be skipped. They bring to the reader those rare qualities of human understanding, which along with a gift in the use of words, were characteristic of Dr Hubbard. Once having met and heard her lecture, or watched her interview and prescribe for a patient, one became aware of an artist and a perfectionist in her work. She never can be replaced. This small work preserves her essence.

The first chapter gives full credit to orthodox medicine and its accomplishments. However, she points out that it lacks both a law for the use of drugs and a law of cure, so that it has developed mainly a palliative approach to illness, with overtones of suppression, e.g. the removal of eczema by salves and ointments which may give rise to asthma.

Homoeopaths need the basic scientific training and procedures of diagnosis and the use of laboratory data, as well as a sound grounding in physiology, pathology and pharmacology. Their special skills begin when starting therapy, for they bring to this crisis of cure a broader concept of illness, a special knowlege of what the remedies will do, and a special approach to each individual patient and his symptoms.

It is interesting to review the main points of difference between orthodox medicine and homoeopathy. These are:
1) In homoeopathy there is a natural law of cure – 'like cures like' – a medical principle dating back to Hippocrates but first investigated by Hahnemann.
2) The basis of homoeopathic therapy is a *vital* rather than a physiological (palliative, isopathic or suppressive) process, stimulating the patient's own vital forces toward a cure.
3) The single remedy is used. This is the basis of provings and of the materia medica, with a few exceptions in which two may be proved in combination, e.g. Merc. Iod. cum Kali Iod. The use of polypharmacy

does not allow one to know what each component remedy can do, either in a proving or in therapy under homoeopathic laws.
4) The minimum dose is used, based on the Arndt-Schultz law:
  – small amounts of a drug stimulate,
  – moderate amounts will paralyze,
  – large amounts of a drug may kill.
  In other words, the action of small and large doses of a drug on living matter is *opposite*.
5) The homoeopathic materia medica consists of provings – the results of remedy experimentation with small doses of drugs, specially prepared, on relatively healthy humans.
6) Diseases are named for classification purposes, to denote the symptom complex picture which appears when departures from normality occur.
7) Individualization is essential in homoeopathy, to get the symptom picture on which one is to prescribe.
8) Suppression is one of the greatest dangers in homoeopathic medicine in terms of true cure.
9) Chronic disease is a constitutional matter, and has a relationship of inestimable importance to homoeopathic prescribing. Homoeopathy has its own concept of disease classification, according to underlying miasms.

Homoeopathy is thus a therapeutic specialty in the use of remedies specially prepared and prescribed according to an orderly concept of disease and health. This concept includes: (1) the Law of Similars, (2) the Arndt-Schultz Law of Remedy Action, (3) Hering's Laws on the Direction of Cure, and (4) chronic disease patterns.

Health to the homoeopath is a state of harmony among the parts of the body, and also between the person as a whole and his total environment, including weather, work, recreation and food. In real health, the life force in each individual is vigorous. Changes in this life force, or vital force, produce symptoms. These symptoms help point the way to the similar remedy, which can stimulate the vital force and thus bring about a return to the state of health – that is, a 'cure'.

Disease to the homoeopath is a state of disharmony involving at least three different factors: some morbific influence, the susceptibility of the person affected, and the rôle of the patient's individuality in modifying the form that the disease takes, thus leading to a symptom picture which is highly individualistic. Symptoms are the language of the body expressing its disharmony and calling for the similar remedy.

To say 'A case well taken is a case half cured' is a truism for all medicine, but especially so with homoeopathy. Taking the case from the homoeopathic viewpoint is thus an art, following a definite procedure, pattern and grading of symptoms. Several sections are devoted to this procedure, and several more on how to study the remedies with suggested texts. How to select, give and follow the results of a prescription, how to make a prognosis on the basis of these results, and the importance of Hering's Laws, are all discussed.

Dr Hubbard includes her famous observations and warnings, some of which she learned from the master prescribers who were her teachers. The following is the one on 'Repetition or Changing of a Remedy':
1) Never repeat when the patient is improving and feels better.
2) Never change when the symptoms are following Hering's Laws.
3) Never change when a discharge or eruption follows the dose.

The last chapter is on 'The Value and Relation of Diet in Homoeopathic Prescribing'. Nutrition is one of those large and vital subjects about which little is taught in medical school, and about which there still exists much ignorance and superstition. Other such subjects are care for the dying and bereaved (what a blessing Ignatia has been here), the effects on health of pollution and the environment, and the contributions and limitations of other healing disciplines, including acupuncture.

Dr Hubbard points out that special diets and good hygiene for some conditions are important in homoeopathic prescribing:
1) To help detoxify the system.
2) To help obtain a true totality-symptom picture, and thus to find a true simillimum.
3) To allow the simillimum to work uncontaminated and in a prepared ground, while watching for Hering's laws to develop.
4) To help eliminate the need for medicine wherever possible, through good hygiene, environment and diet.

One can see that homoeotherapeutics, when well done, can be a great preventive and curative force within the whole field of medicine. Orthodox medicine needs homoeopathy, and homoeopathy needs orthodox medicine, in a symbiotic relationship, for the good of mankind.

On First Attempting to Prescribe Homoeopathically

Before discussing the problems of actual homoeopathic practice, let me describe some of the difficulties in the ordinary practice of medicine which led me to an interest in homoeopathy. When I was a student at Columbia Medical School, I was much disappointed at the paucity of therapeutic information. There was pathology and bacteriology galore, and fascinating drill in diagnosis, but being a woman, and therefore a practical soul, I hankered after the means of cure. Most of what we were taught in therapeutics was hygiene, nursing procedures, diet, hydrotherapy, etc. A large proportion of my class, who had intended to go into general medicine, took up surgery or other specialties because in those fields there was something definite to do for the patients. From medical school I went to Bellevue Hospital for two years' rotating internship, and there again I met the prevailing therapeutic nihilism. Our chief of service was a wizard at diagnosis, but I always felt that an autopsy was fully as acceptable as a cure, and much more frequent.

One class of patients in the hospital particularly distressed me – those who had abundant subjective symptoms and on whom the diagnostic and laboratory pronouncement was, 'There is nothing wrong with you.' I remember one patient saying, 'Well, doctor, I may be perfectly well, but *I* know I am sick.' And then there were the chronics, not only those with marked pathology, but lifelong sufferers from 'indigestion' or migraine who had been passed around from doctor to doctor with nothing but temporary relief.

Two other problems puzzled me particularly, besides the apparently functional cases and the chronics. One of these was the patient with a classically recognizable disease who did not respond to the usual 'specific' treatment for that disease. For instance, a young sailor with a severe malaria which no amount of quinine influenced in the least, to the consternation of all. The other matter which set me thinking was the wide variety of types of a single disease. I used to wonder why the pneumonia in one bed, who was such a strapping specimen and who had come down suddenly at midnight on the date of admission, was in such mortal terror of dying by noon the next day (which I may add, he did, to the surprise of all of us); and why the besotted-looking fellow in the next bed lay on the affected side with his hand under his chest, motionless, gulping two or three glasses of water at long intervals, complaining of the light and snapping your head off when spoken to; and why the pneumonia on the other side of the ward thrashed about so incessantly, especially in the evening, calling for cold milk. Now I know that although these three had the same disease, and received the same treatment, each would have responded to a different remedy – one to Aconite, one to Bryonia and the last to Rhus Tox. My puzzles, then, were the apparently functional cases, the chronics, the patients who did not respond to the classical treatment of a clearly-marked disease, and the varied types classified and treated according to one diagnosis.

My initiation into homoeopathy began in Vienna. After working at the Allgemeine Krankenhaus in the usual way, I was apprenticed for nine months to a homoeopathic physician in Geneva where I studied, literally, from twelve to sixteen hours a day. Before he was willing to take me as a pupil he gave me a stiff examination in ordinary medicine, including anatomy, fractures, surgical diagnosis, pathology, bacteriology and chemistry, and gave me slides to diagnose under the microscope. He then asked certain questions as to what I thought life was about, why I went into the practice of medicine, what were the chief duties of a physician and so on. These questions perplexed me, as I did not then understand their bearing on the philosophy of homoeopathy. He then asked a leading question to see if I already had any background of homoeopathy: 'What do homoeopaths give for rheumatism?' Having read somewhat in homoeopathic literature I answered that homoeopaths do not give a remedy for rheumatism or for any disease name or diagnosis, although, of course, that certain remedies were more frequently indicated in rheumatic conditions. I said that they give a remedy on the symptoms of the patient who has the disease, in other words on the reaction of the individual in question to any given disease entity. This indeed defines one of the fundamental differences between the homoeopathic approach and that of conventional medicine.

Until the physician's mind has encompassed the differences between the viewpoints of ordinary medical training and homoeopathy, he cannot even begin to prescribe homoeopathically. Let me enumerate for clarity wherein these differences lie. First, he must grasp the principle of *individualization*. Modern medicine lays a good foundation for this through its interest in endocrinology and psychiatry, but except for obvious glandular imbalances, it offers as yet no therapy commensurate with the refinements of differentiation. What does individualization mean to the homoeopath and how does he arrive at it? It involves a subsidiary and new method of case-taking.

After you have the classical medical history, elicited largely by asking questions, you can often make a diagnosis but rarely can you make a homoeopathic prescription. For the latter you need to know the mental state of your patient, and what the homoeopaths call his 'generals'. These are the things which apply to the patient as a whole – his reaction to heat and cold, wet and dry weather and storms, motion, position, food, etc. You need to know how these same factors affect the specific complaints of your patient, in other words the 'modalities' of his particular disease symptoms – whether his headache is better from hot or cold applications, from motion or rest, from lying or walking, from pressure, or food, and at what time of day it is worse. 'Modalities', in other words, mean aggravations or ameliorations of specific symptoms, just as 'generals' mean aggravations and ameliorations of the patient as a whole.

There is a fourth type of thing you must know about your patient in order to prescribe homoeopathically, and that is his rare, peculiar or characteristic *particular* symptoms. These often appear trivial idiosyncrasies to the patient, things that he has always had, or that no doctor to whom he has told them has ever been interested in. These often serve as keynotes to guide you to a remedy. But of what use is all this additional information about your patient? How does this picture of his personality aid you? You have individualized, but of what use is such differentiation, if you have only a standard treatment for the condition that you have diagnosed?

This leads to the second great difference between homoeopathy and conventional medicine. The law on which homoeopathy is based, or if you prefer, the hypothesis, is to be found in the statement of Hippocrates, *'similia similibus curentur'*, which Hahnemann revived and amplified. Hahnemann came to apply this law and made the first so-called 'proving' of quinine. A 'proving', in the homoeopathic sense, is experimenting with a drug in minute doses on a relatively healthy human being. The record of symptoms so produced, on a large number of provers of different ages and sexes, constitutes the basis of our homoeopathic materia medica. The object of proving a remedy is to delineate the remedy personality.

Each of our remedies is to us a living individual, like a friend whom one recognizes whenever seen, not only by his grand characteristics but also by his mannerisms and tricks. We now have on the one hand the remedy personalities, and on the other hand the picture of our patient in his present state. It follows, if like cures like, that we must match pictures and fit the personality of a remedy to our patient, administer it, and watch the results. After one has grasped this ingenious theory and learned to put it into practice, it remains only to see it work. Being a natural sceptic, I was slow to believe the evidence of my senses. Could the astonishing improvements and cures have been coincidence, or suggestion, or faulty diagnosis?

There are certain controls which one can use. Put the patient on the proper regimen, including diet, etc., and see what that alone does for his condition. Then give placebo, with your best manner. In my experience, in nine cases out of ten, the patient will report no progress. When they are discouraged by this unsuccessful first prescription, give them the remedy you have chosen, the simillimum. If you feel reasonably certain that the remedy picture fits your patient, and you have the simillimum, in most cases you will see a swift and beautiful result.

But these are not the only possible methods of control. There are laws of remedy action which are contrary to anything you could expect in an untreated case. When you see these, you know that your remedy is taking hold. They were formulated by Constantine Hering, one of the pioneers of homoeopathy in the United States, and are as follows: The curative remedy acts *from within outward, from above downward*, and *in the reverse order of the appearance of the symptoms*. Take as an illustration a case of rheumatic fever in which, after the customary salicylate dosing, the joints appear to have cleared up but a heart condition develops. Give such a patient the similar remedy and he will complain that his joints are worse again, but *he himself* feels better, and you find that his heart is clearing up. You explain to him that the remedy is working *from within outward*; the more vital organ, the heart, is getting well first, and the peripheral organs, the joints, are again involved. Give him nothing but placebo. Shortly he will tell you that his shoulders and wrists are clearing up but that the pain is now in his knees or ankles. Again you see the law of cure in action, *from above downward*, and you wait. You observe that his symptoms are dis-apppearing *in the reverse order of their appearance*, the heart condition, which came last, going first. If you trust your remedy under these conditions, your patient will make a real recovery without the annoying recurrences. If, on the contrary, you found that the joints in the upper extremities became involved, you would know you were on the wrong track and had not found the simillimum.

One of the knottiest problems for the beginner is the different concept of pathology and bacteriology. Homoeopaths accept the facts of these branches of medicine. The difference lies in the interpretation. Pathology is an end result of some morbid process. The homoeopath is not nearly as interested in the diseased tonsil, the haemorrhoid, the ovarian cyst, the cancer, the tapeworm or the psoriasis, as he is in the constitutional dyscrasia behind these. He is not eager to remove the ultimates of disease at once, but rather to cure the underlying cause. In the course of this cure the ultimate will often disappear, as in the case of diseased cervical glands or fibroids. If not, it can be removed when it has become merely a foreign body, and when the constitution is so changed that it will not ultimate itself in further pathology in a more deep-seated organ.

Similarly, one is taught to consider that bacteria cause disease. The homoeopath is more interested in the individual's susceptibility than in the bacteria themselves. Instead of poisoning the invading organism, the homoeopath prefers to stimulate the body to make itself uninhabitable for that organism, and he does this by means of the similar remedy. To give another instance, instead of killing off head lice with delphinium and leaving the patient susceptible to further invasions, the homoeopath gives a chronic constitutional remedy which removes the susceptibility, and the lice seek better pasturage.

A fourth stumbling-block for the medical mind is the question of suppression. Discharges and eruptions are ordinarily classed with pathology as something to be eliminated by local measures, using chemical applications to stop any discharge from nose, cervix or bowel, or any skin eruption. The homoeopath holds that this is suppression, and not cure, that these outward manifestations are not primarily local but an expression of deep disease, in other words that the body is trying to throw off impurities. They have watched the incidence of more deep-seated troubles following such 'suppression'. The chronic constitutional homoeopathic remedy, given to a case which has been treated in this way, will often bring back the original eruption or discharge; with this there is concomitant relief of recent grave symptoms and an ultimate clearing up from *within* of the original discharge or eruption.

Let me illustrate with a case from my practice. A woman of forty-five came to me for suicidal depression, for which she could give no emotional cause. She dated her mental symptoms definitely from the time when she had had a foul, lumpy, green leucorrhoea 'cured' by local vaginal applications, a few months before. I gave her a dose of Sepia, a remedy made from cuttlefish ink, on her mental symptoms. A week later she returned exuberant, all the depression for which she had been doctored being gone, and said, 'By the way, doctor, I have that awful discharge back again just as it was before.' I was delighted, warned her against suppressing it a second time, and gave placebo. The discharge then lessened and improved in character and she continued, as her husband said, a changed woman. So much for the fundamental differences.

Another problem which confronted me was whether the homoeopathic remedy could influence definite chronic pathology. A girl of nineteen came to me for severe intermenstrual bleeding. On examination I found a nodular fibroid bigger than my fist. A well-known New York specialist had diagnosed it and advised merely general health measures, as he did not want to X-ray so young a girl. Her chronic case worked out on mental and general symptoms to Phosphorus, which happens to be one of the main remedies useful in fibroids. Three months after I gave her this, I sent her to be checked up by the same specialist. He was amazed at the decrease in size of the fibroid and asked her what she had been doing. Six months later he pronounced her normal and sanctioned her marrying.

A further difficulty I experienced was in believing the current statement that homoeopathic remedies can do no harm. *They can!*

Another problem one meets frequently in general practice is that of prophylaxis. Strict homoeopaths believe that vaccines and inoculations are harmful. It took considerable experience for me to be convinced that the chronic constitutional remedy is the best prophylactic.

The Meaning of Homoeopathy

The four fundamentals of homoeopathy, as stated by its founder Hahnemann in his *Organon*, may be briefly put as follows:
1) The proving on healthy persons of substances to be used as medicines.
2) The selection and administration of remedies thus proved according to the Law of Similars.
3) The single remedy.
4) The minimum dose.

Granting that these are the four fundamental tenets of homoeopathy, the question of its status then arises. Is it a system of medicine? Is it a purely sectarian term? Is it a therapeutic specialty? In order to answer this question of status we must get down to simple facts to see, not only how homoeopathy differs from orthodox medicine, but also what they have in common.

We always like to begin with a common basis. What is the object of all conscientious physicians? We would answer, categorically: to cure the sick, to prevent others from becoming ill, and to raise the standard of health in all people. How does modern medicine try to accomplish this? First, by finding out what normality is, through the study of anatomy, physiology, physiological chemistry and so on. Second, by finding out what the varieties of ill health are. Modern medicine emphasizes the fact that many disturbances of health are due to psychic or sociological causative factors. Aside from these it searches for anatomical or physiological changes in the sick person and classifies these changes, when found, under some disease nomenclature. This search is called diagnosis, and modern medicine feels that the possibility of cure depends, in large measure, on the certainty of diagnosis. It defines as pathology the organic structural changes due to ill health which it finds before or after death. It finds that many 'diseases' are accompanied by some variety of bacteria which it considers to be one of the causative factors. In short, modern medicine feels that it must find out all the 'facts' that fit in with its own concept of disease.

To all of this the homoeopath subscribes, but he feels that it is only the beginning of what he must learn about his patient. The spontaneous, characteristic things that each patient longs to tell, be they very general or minutely particular, are of special interest to the homoeopath, for they individualize the case, bringing out that particular patient's reaction to the 'disease' he suffers from. The busy modern doctor feels he does not need to know these salient points, as to him they are not signposts but merely clutter.

At this point modern medicine is ready to try to cure the disease it has diagnosed. What laws of cure does it follow? First, the commonsense principle of rectifying anything mechanically wrong and instituting appropriate hygiene, diet and so on. When it comes to the prescription of actual drugs, those that are given are not uniformly governed by any one law. The intent is to give them on a physiological basis, which means that they are experimented with in laboratories in crude dosage, and mainly on animals. It is more or less expected, by analogy, that what slows the heart in the frog, rabbit or dog will do so in the human.

In addition to laboratory data on animals, many drugs are tried out empirically on patients and pass into general usage in accordance with their success. A few forms of therapy are aimed at the individual as a whole, taken as a type – for instance, endocrine therapy, but the majority of modern drugs are given for a definite physiological effect on one organ or function of the body. They are thus given with no regard to the varying individualities of the patient who may have that organ or function disordered, as for example in the use of cholagogues, digitalis, diuretics and so on. A large part of modern therapy is not even aimed at physiological alteration (the drugs being given according to the law of contraries), nor at chemical antidoting (such as alkalis for acid stomach), but is frankly and only palliative, as in the various analgesics for headaches or neuralgias. Most modern drugging, in short, is aimed at specific symptoms and makes no attempt to get back to the constitutional cause of the disease. The success of this type of therapy is necessarily uneven. Furthermore, much of it is actually suppressive. It is an interesting fact that many cases of apparent cure prove to be those in which the drug given on a physiological or symptomatic basis was, unknown to the prescriber, a similar, in the homoeopathic sense, to the case in hand.

It should be clearly stated that homoeopaths need the accepted scientific training and the procedures of diagnosis and laboratory data. Their special technique begins at the moment of starting therapy, although they bring to this crisis of cure a broader philosophy of illness and a special knowledge of each individual patient.

The Meaning of Homoeopathy

Homoeopathic therapy is based on the hypothesis, ancient as Hippocrates, that like cures like (*similia similibus curentur*). The persistent and enlightened practice of homoeopathy can prove that this principle is a basic law of nature. It must also be demonstrable by laboratory technique, but the systematic working out of this has not as yet been done, mainly because homoeopaths are so beguiled by the practical application of it that they have not given suitable attention to the laboratory end. (Only in recent years has there been a significant effort by homoeopaths to carry out controlled studies using homoeopathic methods. — Ed.)

We have sketched modern medicine's approach and attitude and have shown up to what point homoeopathy concurs. It is also appropriate to give briefly here the main points of difference between the two. These are developed more fully in the rest of the course.

1) That there is a natural law of cure – like cures like.
2) That the basis of therapy is a *vital* rather than a *physiological* one. That is, the vital force must be stimulated to cure the patient and only so can he be really cured, and that any other drug therapy is palliative or suppressive.
3) That the single remedy at a time is all that is needed. This follows from statement (1), because there cannot be two things most similar to another. The single remedy has the further advantage that when one thing is given one can evaluate its action, whereas, if four are given you cannot know which helped, or in what proportion.
4) That a minimum dose is essential. This is based on the Arndt-Schultz law that small doses stimulate, medium doses paralyze and large doses kill. In other words, that the action of small and very large doses of the same substance on living matter is opposite. Under this heading comes the whole potency question; this is considered by many to be the greatest snag in homoeopathy but is, together with the Law of Similars, the key to the whole matter.
5) That the materia medica must, because of the Law of Similars, be composed of the results of remedy experimentation with small doses on relatively healthy humans, that is to say, 'provings'.
6) That disease is not an actual entity, but a name given for classification purposes to manifestations of departures from normality in individuals.
7) That individualization is essential, i.e. that no two people are exactly alike in sickness or in health, and that while even homoeopaths must classify, they draw vastly finer distinctions. For example, to ordinary medicine there is but one disease pneumonia, though with several

sub-types – broncho-, lobar, viral and others; to homoeopathy there are as many types as there are remedy symptom pictures. Any remedy in the homoeopathic materia medica may be called for in pneumonia, although only rarely will one outside of the thirty or forty in frequent use be needed. Theoretically there should be as many types of pneumonia as there are people who have it, but owing to the small number of proved remedies compared to the substances that might be proved, there can only be as many pneumonia types to date as we have remedies for. Homoeopaths, in other words, classify pneumonias as Aconite, Bryonia, Gelsemium, Phosphorus, Tartar Emetic pneumonias, to name but a few.

8) That suppression is one of the greatest dangers in medicine.
9) That chronic disease is a constitutional matter, and that this has a philosophical bearing of inestimable importance on prescribing. One cannot practise true homoeopathy without a concept of chronic disease.

Having given the main points of contact and difference between homoeopathy and regular medicine, we can now return to our earlier question concerning the status of homoeopathy. It is not a sectarian term, although even a slight study of its history will often show how it has been necessary for it to be considered one, both by its opponents and its adherents. It is a therapeutic specialty and, as such, is more easily grasped by the modern student, but *it is much more than that*. 'System of medicine' is a term which conveys little to my mind; it sounds like somebody's textbook or treatise on one of the minor 'opathies'.

Homoeopathy is not an 'opathy'; it is the first part of the term, the 'homoeo', the similarity, which we must bear in mind. It is a method of cure according to law, based, as all great things are, on a far-reaching philosophy. *It is the central core of medicine*, whether recognized or not, and is thoroughly compatible with the best of modern science.

Bibliography
The Law of Cure, Ridpath.
The Patient's Dilemma, T. M. Dishington.
The Principles of Practice of Homoeopathy, C. E. Wheeler.
'A Symposium on Homoeopathy', *The Homoeopathic Recorder*, Vol. XLIV, May 1929, p. 293.
The Organon of the Art of Healing, Samuel Hahnemann.

The Epitome of Homoeopathic Philosophy

Homoeopathic philosophy may be divided into three sections: the theoretical, dealing with how and why remedies act, which is so abstruse that it is best be dealt with by the more advanced student; the didactic, meaning the rules and tenets; and the practical, which comprises the art of applying the results and following through the subsequent prescriptions to cure.

Let us first take a bird's eye view of the didactic aspect. Health, to the homoeopath, is a state of harmony between the parts of the body, as well as between the person as a whole and the cosmos. In real health the as yet unexplained life force in each person is vigorous. It is usually spoken of as the vital force, which in disease is the true curative power. The object of giving the similar remedy is to stimulate the vital force. The object of hygiene and mechanical intervention is to clear the path of obstructions. No remedy can cure disease – it can only at best enable the vital force to function properly again.

Disease, to the homoeopath, is a state of disharmony involving at least three different factors: some morbific influence; the susceptibility of the person affected; and the individuality of the patient modifying the form that the disease takes. Homoeopaths do not try to cure the morbific influence – they try to cure the patient himself. In order to cure the patient the most similar remedy must be given.

Symptoms, to the homoeopath, are the language of the body expressing its disharmony and calling for the similar remedy. For prescribing one must take into consideration the totality of the symptoms. These include: the mental symptoms; the 'generals', predicated of the patient as a whole, which include his reaction to meteorological conditions, time, bodily functions, food, etc.; the particulars, predicated of any part of the patient, and the 'modalities' of these (that is, what aggravates or ameliorates them), and especially such particulars as are 'rare, strange or peculiar'; the causative factors, such as ailments from grief, wetting, riding in a cold wind, suppression of menses, etc.; and the pathological symptoms, indicating the elective affinity of the remedy for certain tissues or organs.

Homoeopathy regards acute disease as an eliminative explosion, which, if handled in the proper homoeopathic manner, leaves the body in a healthier condition. This does not mean that the acute disease should be allowed to run its course: if the symptoms are met at its inception by the simillimum, the disease will be aborted and still the economy will be purified. No acute case under homoeopathic treatment from the beginning should die prematurely, and there should be no permanent sequelae. Acute epidemic diseases often call for one or two epidemic remedies which vary as the disease shifts geographically. In this connection the epidemic remedy is an admirable prophylactic, although the chronic constitutional remedy is always the best preventive. Sequelae following acute diseases are not strictly speaking part of the acute trouble, but are flare-ups of chronic disease aroused by the acute condition.

Chronic disease is not self-limited and shows no tendency to ultimate recovery if untreated. This is the unique sphere of homoeopathy. Practically every person has some symptoms of latent chronic disease, and to the homoeopath chronic diseases form the basis of susceptibility. By taking the totality of the symptoms from birth onwards, a deep-acting, chronic constitutional remedy can be chosen which will aid in fending off future acute disease, and also remove many inherited and acquired encum-brances to the vital force.

Hahnemann divided chronic diseases into three main categories or 'miasms' – psora, syphilis and sycosis. These may appear singly or in combination with each other, as well as with drug disease engrafted by improper treatment. This matter of the miasms is the most difficult and moot question in homoeopathy, but the fundamental thesis of the importance of chronic disease in general is essential.

Having prescribed for chronic disease, if you have given the true simillimum, the symptoms are cured in accordance with Hering's three laws of direction: (1) from within outward, (2) from above downward, and (3) in the reverse order of their appearance. This is never the case in chronic disease untreated by homoeopathy; therefore when it is observed one can be sure that it is the remedy which is curing and that the correct remedy has been found.

Hering's laws are so important that we will give an example. A rheumatic fever case, where the joint symptoms have disappeared and the heart is affected, receives the simillimum. The heart improves, pains return in the shoulders and elbows, these disappear and the knees and ankles are involved, these in turn pass off and the patient entirely recovers. The symptoms went from within outward (heart to joints), from above downward (shoulders to knees), and in the reverse order of their appearance (heart to limbs, instead of limbs to heart). If the symptoms do not go in this order, the remedy is wrong. When a patient on a chronic remedy develops a different symptom, search back in your record or question him rigorously to determine whether this is the recurrence of an old symptom – a good sign, in which case no further remedy should be given. If it is not an old symptom, search the pathogenesis of the remedy given. If the symptom appears in the proving, give nothing; if it does not, the choice of the remedy must be revised.

These laws of cure may or may not apply in acute disease, although usually they do not. If the picture of a chronic disease includes a suppression, especially if the suppression is due to crude drugging, the chronic remedy will sometimes restore the original discharge or eruption, in accordance with the third law of cure. The percentage of cases in which this return from the original channel occurs is relatively low. With good prescribing, however, some exteriorization takes place, even though this may only be a diarrhoea or a coryza. One of the times when the practitioner most needs a thorough knowledge of homoeopathic philosophy is when, after chronic prescribing, he is faced with such a discharge having more or less acute symptoms. He must then decide whether this is a return of an old trouble in its original form, or a compensatory vent, or a new acute disturbance, or an aggravation. If it is the first he should wait and give placebo, explaining the process to sustain the patient's morale. If it is the second he should attempt to do the same. If, on the other hand, it is the third, or if the second is too annoying to the patient, or even dangerous, one should prescribe an acute remedy in low potency (the thirtieth or even the twelfth, and surely not above the two hundredth). After this episode the action of the chronic remedy may not even have been disturbed. Often the acute remedy required will be found among the acute complements of the chronic remedy. If, in the fourth case, the disturbance is merely an increase in one of the patient's complaints, or is found under the pathogenesis of the indicated chronic remedy, it can be classed as an aggravation and should receive no medicine other than placebo, unless dangerous as above. If it is so serious as to threaten life, owing to the chronic remedy having been given in too high a potency, an antidote may be in order. The great point is not to mix up your case and spoil it by giving unnecessary remedies.

In addition to acute and chronic diseases there are, of course, diseases due to drugging or to bad hygiene. There are also diseases which have finally resulted in pathology calling for surgery, as well as troubles that are primarily surgical, such as foreign bodies, fractures, extra-uterine pregnancy, etc.

A word should be said here about pathology and surgery. From the homoeopathic standpoint much of pathology is protective – abscesses, ulcers and tumours are an effort on the part of the vital force at localization and extrusion. Such pathology should not be removed by surgery until *after* the sick constitution which produced such pathology has been cured. Often in the course of cure the pathology will shrink or be absorbed. If not, it remains as a foreign body and is a subject for surgery. Its removal before the cure of the constitution simply means that, balked at that outlet, the vital force will seek another one, either by recurrence in the same form or by more deep-seated trouble. As to surgery, some orthodox homoeopaths hold that any surgery which is not merely a mechanical adjustment (such as ventral suspension of the uterus) is a definite bar to cure; the idea being that in the unraveling of the disease it gets back to where the knot was cut by surgery and can go no further. It requires the keenest judgement to decide when a case has gone too far to be relieved by remedies, and hence that emergency surgery is indicated in a crisis. The homoeopathic remedy should always be resumed after the surgery.

In any of these classes of disease where the patient has been wrongly treated, one should include the symptoms before the incorrect treatment – in other words the original symptoms – in the totality.

Having glimpsed the didactic aspect, we must run over practical philosophy. The unique law which is the basis of all homoeopathy, as already stated, is *similia similibus curentur*. How we arrive at this equation, the actual studying of remedies and patients, is covered in subsequent chapters. The actual handling of a case after the first remedy has been selected is the more difficult part of homoeopathy. First is the necessity of giving the single remedy. This precludes the use of compound tablets, alternation of remedies, or unhomoeopathic adjuvants such as cathartics and analgesics. In a case where the miasms are mixed it may not be possible to cover the totality of the symptoms with one remedy. In such a case, observe which miasm is, so to speak, on top, and prescribe for the totality of symptoms of *that* miasm; when these symptoms have been cleared away, the layer beneath – representing, perhaps, another miasm – may be prescribed for, again by a single remedy. Sometimes the remedy indicated may be one which has power over all the miasms, as for instance, Nitric Acid. The term 'single remedy' does not imply that only one remedy should be used throughout a case, although that is the desideratum, but rather that only one remedy should be used at a time. It cannot be too often stated that one must not give a remedy lightly nor change it frequently. In acute diseases the concept of one single remedy at a time still holds good, although the remedy may have to be changed as the case develops. In this case some of our master prescribers state that the original remedy may be indicated again at the close of the cycle to complete the case. Further details on the single remedy are covered in the chapter on prescribing.

Next in importance to the selection of the single similar remedy is the question of dosage. The classic rule is that of 'the minimum dose'. We prefer the term 'the optimum potency', meaning the potency on a plane most similar to that of the patient at the moment of question. Hahnemann's original choice of the word 'minimum' served two purposes – first, to discourage the enormous crude drugging of his time, and secondly, to point out that the high potencies have a different action from crude drugs. The potency issue is discussed later in the book.

The question of repeating the dose is the next in importance. As a simple rule for beginners, high potencies should be given in one dose with placebo; the low potencies, 30c and under, may need repetition. After giving the single dose of the single similar remedy the student *must watch and wait*. The duration of action of remedies and the factors influencing this are also discussed later. The general rule is to give nothing more than placebo while improvement continues, in other words as long as the patient himself feels increasingly better, regardless of the accentuation of certain symptoms. The beginner must learn not to try to make a good thing better by repetition, as this defeats itself. According to the case, the potency and the remedy, the need for repetition may occur within a few hours in acute disease (or a few minutes in desperate cases) to weeks, months and even a year or more in chronic cases, although waiting is perhaps the most difficult lesson for the eager homoeopath. He must wait with knowledge, or valuable time will be wasted. How is he to know whether the remedy is the right one or is still acting? In acute cases the general wellbeing of the patient should be apparent from within a few moments to two or three days. In chronic cases it can vary from a few hours to sometimes several weeks, and indeed may only be apparent after the second dose. In chronic cases Hering's laws of cure, already mentioned, will show you whether you are on the right track. It is at this point, while watching the action of your remedy, that you must understand the subject of homoeopathic aggravation.

An aggravation is not necessary to improvement, but often occurs even with master prescribers. The usual cause of severe aggravation is an error in the potency, or the presence of marked pathology. Aggravations are of two kinds, disease aggravations and remedy aggravations. The first of these is merely the natural progress of the disease and does not concern us here. The remedy aggravation is a sort of house-cleaning, and is indicative of the prognosis of the case. It has about twelve recognizable forms, which are discussed later. Due allowance for aggravation must be made before considering repetition of the dose. A general rule is that even during aggravation the patient, as a whole, in himself, feels better.

The subject of the second and subsequent prescriptions, one of the most important in the whole of homoeopathic philosophy, will be better understood in connection with prescribing, also discussed later.

Another vital point in homoeopathic philosophy is that of suppression. The causes of suppressions are dependent on so many factors; the results of suppression untreated are dire and frequently unrecognized, and the results of those treated are so brilliant, that a complete chapter is devoted to this subject.

To present homoeopathic philosophy lucidly and logically to a novice is well nigh impossible. The student is urged to read and re-read the appended list of books.

Bibliography
The Principles and Practice of Homoeopathy, Herbert A. Roberts
The Principles and Practice of Homoeopathy, C. E. Wheeler
Textbook of Homoeopathy, Otto Leeser
The Simile in Medicine, Linn J. Boyd
Grundlagen der Heilkunde, Otto Leeser
Lectures on Homoeopathic Philosophy, James Tyler Kent
The Genius of Homoeopathy, Stuart Close
The Organon, Samuel Hahnemann
Homoeopathy: the Science of Therapeutics, Carroll Dunham
Manual of Pharmacodynamics, Richard Hughes

Know the Patient

A great deal of information which is not needed in ordinary medicine is essential for a good homoeopathic prescription. The homoeopath must know his patient, spiritually, emotionally, mentally, physically and sociologically. He must give as much time as he needs to acquiring this knowledge. In a chronic case he must prescribe nothing but placebo until he has it. In an acute case he must know these same factors in so far as they affect the acute condition.

Let us suppose that a new patient arrives to consult a homoeopath. What is the procedure?

1) The physician must be receptive, like a photographic plate ready to receive the image of the patient. He must clear his mind of other pre-occupations and of previous opinions about the patient. He must be tranquil and cordial, and after the first greeting and question, 'What brings you to see me?', or 'Tell me what it is that troubles you', he must be silent.

2) The physician must allow the patient to tell his own story in his own way. Questions or interruptions of any sort derail the patient at this stage, and may cause the doctor to lose essential information.

3) The physician must observe from the moment the patient enters. The office should be so arranged that the light falls on the patient. The main points to be noted are:
   (i) The personality of the patient.
   (ii) His apparent state of mind, both in himself and in relation to the doctor (whether depressed, shy, suspicious, secretive, afraid, ashamed, or whatever).
   (iii) His apparent physical status (signs of disease in gait, complexion, difficulty in breathing).
   (iv) Traits of character as shown in dress, cleanliness, neatness, pride, etc.

4) The physician must record every item which seems important to him, in the words of the patient, both in what the patient says and in what he himself observes. He should do this in a column at the left of his paper, leaving at least an inch blank between the items to be subsequently filled in as the patient reverts to that subject or, later,

when the physician raises questions about it. He may prefer to put facts pertaining to history on one sheet or in one column, those pertaining to actual physical symptoms in another, and mentals in a third, but this requires experience and adeptness. It is safer for the beginner to list them all as they come, and sort them later in the working out of the case.

5) When the patient has come to a full stop the physician may say, 'What else?', and by waiting may often elicit much additional and valuable information. If the patient is reticent or gives only brief and objective data, and the physician is unable to persuade him to give more, this passive method may have to be abandoned in favour of active questioning. The object is to drain the patient dry of what he knows of himself. If the patient is loquacious, time may necessitate the prevention of irrelevancies, and here the utmost tact is needed to keep him on the main track and yet not lose important sidelights.

6) A few remarks by the physician may be in order when the patient is through with his story, relating to the aid that can be given through our remedies and the necessity for special knowledge of the patient as a whole and the many details ordinarily overlooked. This reassures the patient and enlists his co-operation in answering the often rather intimate questions which must follow.

7) The data needed for an ordinary medical history may hardly have been touched on up to this point, and should not be inquired into even yet. If by this time the consultation period is over, provided that the patient is not in acute pain or distress, or has not come from a long distance, a subsequent appointment should be made for the next day if possible. The patient should be definitely told that the physician must do a complete physical examination and the necessary routine laboratory tests at the next visit. Instructions for bringing a 24-hour urine specimen should then be given. This makes the patient realize that in addition to the interest in all details of the case, the physician is also going to be thoroughly scientific.

8) The physician should now take up each item that he has noted on paper and get the patient to tell him more about it. When the patient has exhausted all that he can tell about each item the physician should bring out the 'modalities'. If, for instance, the item is pain in the stomach and the patient volunteers that it is burning, and has no relation to meals and no radiation, the physician must find what aggravates or ameliorates it, what time it occurs, its concomitants and its relation to mental states, if any. When each item has been modified in this way and noted down, the physician must run through

the list and see which of the possible mentals, generals, particulars and modalities have not been mentioned, and question the patient about each of these.

9) All questions that the physician asks must be put so that the patient cannot reply with a simple 'Yes' or 'No', but must think before answering. The physician must be careful never to suggest an answer by the form of his question, and must guard against questioning for the symptoms of a particular remedy which may have come to his mind. If he has seen a fairly definite remedy picture in the patient's story and wishes to clinch it, he must take special care not to lead the patient into the answer he desires, and may even suggest the opposite, and watch the reaction.

10) When the physician has covered the fields outlined above in detail, according to a systematic outline, which the novice should have before him during the interview and which the master will know by heart (a suggested one is given below), he must make sure that he has questioned the patient on every system and function. If not, some important detail, which might prove to be a keynote suggesting the study of one or more remedies, may well be missed.

11) The mental symptoms and characteristics of the patient (which are the most important, if strongly marked) should usually be elicited last, when the patient's confidence has been more fully gained. Especial tact and insight on the part of the physician are needed to evaluate the emotional causes of disease. For instance, few patients would know that ailments from mortification might be the most important symptom in their case, or that suppression of their sex needs or anger might rank as a leading cause in their illness.

12) At the close of the interview the patient must be made to feel that the physician is deeply interested in his case, and that he will spend the hours needed to thoroughly study (or 'repertorize') the case. Also, that the special method of homoeopathy can bring not only relief but a fundamental improvement in the whole constitution, which will tend to ward off subsequent illness and increase the powers and wellbeing of the patient. A thorough physical examination plus routine laboratory work, or any extra tests suggested by the history, must be done on every new patient and at least once a year on established patients. Patients must be instructed as to why they should not use other drugs during homoeopathic treatment, what the dangers of suppression are, when they should report back, and what they may expect as the immediate results of the treatment. One other point which may be valuable is to get the version of the

immediate family or close friends. This is sometimes dangerous, as nervous patients hate to know that they are being talked over. However, the wise physician can take much contradictory evidence and arrive at a more just and sympathetic evaluation of the case.

By this time the physician should have a remarkably accurate picture of the patient in all his phases, subjective, objective and pathological. From this totality of symptoms he can, by correctly evaluating the symptoms as we will show, derive a true image of the patient and the appropriate remedy.

Outline for Taking the Case

A. The patient's story

B. Modalities as applied to each of the patient's symptoms, in the following order
1) *Causes.*
2) *Prodrome, onset, pace, sequence, duration.*
3) *Character, location, laterality, extension and radiation of pain or sensations.*
4) *Concomitants and alternations.*
5) *Aggravation or amelioration.*
   a) Time (hour, day, night, before or after midnight): periodicity; seasons; moon phases.
   b) Temperature and weather: chilly or warm-blooded usually, chilly or warm-blooded in present illness; wet, dry, cold or hot weather; weather changes; storm or thunderstorm (before, during or after); hot sun, wind, fog, snow, open air, warm room, changes from one to other, stuffy or crowded places, drafts, warmth of bed, heat of radiators, uncovering.
   c) Bathing: hot, cold or sea; local applications: hot, cold, wet or dry.
   d) Rest or motion: slow or rapid, ascending or descending, turning in bed, exertion, walking, on first motion, after moving awhile, while moving, after moving; car and seasickness.
   e) Position: standing, sitting, (knees crossed, rising from sitting), stooping (rising from stooping), lying (on painful side, back, right or left side, abdomen, head high or low, rising from lying), leaning head backward, forward, sideways, closing or opening eyes; any unusual position such as knee/chest.
   f) External stimuli: touch, hard or light, pressure, rubbing, constriction, as of clothing, jar, riding, stepping, light, noise, music, conversation, odours.
   g) Eating: in general (before, during, after, hot or cold food or drink), swallowing (solids, liquids, empty), acids, fats, salt, salty food, starches, sugar and sweets, green vegetables, milk, eggs,

meat, fish, oysters, onions, beer, liquor, wine, coffee, tea, tobacco, drugs, etc.
h) Thirst: quantity, frequency, hot, cold or iced, sours, bitters, etc.
i) Sleep: in general (before, during, on falling asleep, in first sleep, after, on waking).
j) Menses: before, during, after, or suppressed.
k) Sweat: hot or cold, foot-sweat, partial or suppressed.
l) Other discharges: bleeding, coryza, diarrhoea, vomitus, urine, emissions, leucorrhoea; suppression of same.
m) Coition: continence, masturbation.
n) Emotions: anger, grief, mortification, fear, shock, consolation, apprehension of crowds, anticipation; suppression of same.
6) *Strange, rare and peculiar symptoms.*

C. The patient as a whole: Physical Generals

7) The *constitutional type* of the patient (endocrinologico-homoeopathic correspondences, lack or excess of vital heat, lack of reaction, sensitiveness).
8) Ailments from *emotions* (see also Mental Generals, below): *suppressions* (emotions; discharges such as menses, sweat, leucorrhoea, catarrh, diarrhoea, etc.; eruptions; diseases such as malaria, rheumatic fever, exanthems, syphilis, gonorrhoea, etc.; pathology, such as haemorrhoids, fistulae, ulcers, tonsils, tumours, other surgical conditions, etc.); from *exposure* to cold, wet, hot sun, etc.; from *mechanical conditions*, such as overeating, injury, etc.
9) *Menses.* Date of establishment, regularity (early or late), duration, colour, consistency, odour, amount, clots, membrane, pain (modalities of), concomitants, aggravation or amelioration before, during or after, both physically and mentally); menopause (symptoms of).
10) *Other discharges* (see also Modalities, 5k above). Cause, colour, consistency, odour, acrid or bland, symptoms from suppression of, symptoms alternating with, hot or cold, partial discharges as of sweat, laterality, better or worse from discharges (before, during or after).
11) *Sleep.* Better or worse from, position in, aggravation after; difficulty in getting to sleep, waking frequently or early, at what hour; somnambulism, talking in sleep; dreams (see also Mental Generals, below), restless during.
12) *Restlessness, prostration, weakness, trembling, chill, fever, etc.*

13) *Aggravations* and *ameliorations* applying to the patient as a whole (see 5a-5n, above).

14) *Objective symptoms* such as redness of orifices or superfluous hair, applying to the patient as a whole.

15) *Pathology* which applies to the patient as a whole, such as tendency to tumours, wens, cysts, polyps, warts, moles; individual and family tendency to certain diseases, or weakness of specific organs or tissues (also related to (7) above and to physical examination), frequency of catching cold.

D. The patient as a whole: Mental Generals

16) *Will.* Loves, hates and emotions (suicidal, loathing of life; lasciviousness, revulsion to sex, sexual perversions; fears; greed, eating, money, emotionality, smoking, drinking, drugs; dreams; homicidal tendencies, desire or aversion to company, contrariness, depression, loquacity, weeping, laughing, impatience, conscientiousness).

17) *Understanding.* Delusions, delirium, hallucinations, mental confusion, loss of time sense.

18) *Intellect.* Memory, concentration, mistakes in writing and speaking.

E. Quick review of the condition of every system and organ, beginning with the head and following the order of Kent's *Repertory*

F. Past history of the patient in seven-year periods

G. Family history

H. Physical examination and laboratory tests

Reading List
Case-taking, G. B. Stearns.
How to Take the Case, E. B. Nash.

Know the Remedies

Theoretically any substance or force may become a homoeopathic remedy. In a large number of instances, varying degrees of potentization are necessary to bring out the remedial powers of substances which are physiologically inert in the crude state. At present no complete list of all homoeopathic remedies exists. At a rough guess, some two to three thousand remedies are in use and new ones are continually being developed. Only a relatively small number of these are thoroughly proved according to the Hahnemannian standard.

The remedies in accepted use are divided for convenience into certain groups as follows:

1) Mineral remedies, including elements, metals, compounds, salts, etc.
2) Vegetable remedies.
3) Animal remedies.
4) The nosodes, which are remedies derived from morbid tissues and secretions.
5) Sarcodes, which are remedies prepared from healthy animal tissues or organs, and include remedies derived from altered tissues and secretions, such as Uric Acid and Thyroidine. This also includes endocrine remedies.
6) Imponderabilia, which include positive and negative magnetic forces, electricity, and sun force.

The information about these remedies is obtained from the following sources: from provings, which means experimentation on the relatively healthy human; from toxicology, which contributes the extreme symptoms, and in part the pathology; from experimentation on animals, organs and tissues in the laboratory; from clinical verification of symptoms by cure; from the clinical appearance of remedy symptoms during medication; and from human pathology which has been cured. The main classical source of the knowledge of remedies is, of course, the proving. The subject of the making of correct provings and their standardization is an important one, but it does not belong within this course.

We then come to actual methods for acquiring and retaining the general picture and detailed knowledge of this multitude of remedies. This is no simple task, as anyone reading the proving of a polychrest such as Calcarea Carbonica will realize. No mind can retain such a mass of symptoms, often seemingly unrelated and contradictory. *One must learn how to study a remedy.*

The most important task in the study of a remedy is to get the feel of it. Since the essence of homoeopathy is individualization, and since each well-proved remedy has a definite personality, the student must get acquainted with the different remedies in the materia medica as if they were friends. He must be able to recognize them from partial expressions, even when he cannot see the whole picture, as he would recognize a well-known person in a group across the room. Experts in prescribing are so saturated with the remedies that they can often choose them intuitively, and although this is dangerous to the beginner it should be the goal of all.

We suggest the following plan for systematic remedy study:

For those who do not contact humans in this way, and indeed for all at first, the study of a remedy must begin with a knowledge of its mentals. The innermost element of man is the most important, and the psychic characteristics and peculiarities of each remedy must be thoroughly mastered. You would not conceive of giving Sulphur as a chronic remedy to a woman in whose linen closet the towels and napery were tied neatly with rose-coloured ribbon. You would not give Phosphorus to one who was abnormally modest, or Arsenicum Album to a sloven. Unfortunately, many of our remedies do not have a fully-developed proving of mental symptoms, but where these exist they are of prime importance.

Many more remedies have clearly marked modalities – in other words, aggravation from or amelioration by meteorological conditions and such things as motion, heat, jar, touch, position, classes of foods or special substances. The marked desires, aversions, aggravations and ameliorations should become etched upon the mind of the student, both those which affect the personality as a whole and those, often agreeing but sometimes contradictory, which modify the affected part.

Of particular importance in the knowledge of materia medica, and often difficult to find in books, are the causations of disease that are typical of the different remedies. These may be mental or general. The student should pay particular attention to the symptoms of ailments from emotion, such as: mortification in Staphysagria; anger in Chamomilla, Colocynth or Nux Vomica; grief in Ignatia; fright in Aconite; as well as to ailments from injury, as in Arnica or Natrum Sulph. Ailments from suppressed discharges are of paramount importance, whether they be from mucous membranes, such as leucorrhoea, diarrhoea, etc., or from the skin, as in the case of perspiration or eruptions, or from operations which close nature's vents, as on fistulae or haemorrhoids. The fourth important variety of causation is the one due to chilling of various kinds, non-mechanical dietary indiscretions, and so on, these being applicable more frequently in acute diseases.

When the student has mastered these various points about a remedy, he should then study the localities of the body to which the remedy especially applies, making a chart of a figure with the vulnerable points of the remedy suitably drawn in. In this connection he would do well to make a diagram of the tongue – its condition is often characteristic and gives valuable hints for prescribing. He may also make drawings of different parts of the body, such as the eyes, representing the various conditions in those organs cured by the remedy. These schemata aid memory by visualization. Not only should the organs influenced by a remedy be learned, but also the tissues – for instance that Bryonia is suitable to inflammation of serous membranes, whereas Belladonna is rarely so.

The student should then pick out from among the welter of particular symptoms those which are 'strange, rare and peculiar', the so-called 'keynotes' of the remedy, and have these at his fingertips as signposts to point the way to further study. In this connection he should pick out similes from literature, such as the analogy between the precocious Lycopodium child and Paul Dombey, as well as expressive epithets such as 'mince-pie fiend' (Carbo Veg.), the 'human barometer' (Rhus Tox), 'gloomy Gus' (Natrum Carb.), the 'false, ragged philosopher' (Sulphur), and others.

He should pay especial attention to the pictures of acute disease in chronic remedies, and to the different types of chronic personality in each remedy.

He should get clearly in his mind the important details relating to the bodily functions such as menstruation, pregnancy, digestion, sleep, and excretion, whether by skin, bowels or urinary tract.

He should make a remedy clock – a diagram showing the time of general aggravation and special aggravations of the remedy in quesion.

Picking out the alternating conditions and the concomitant conditions, and keeping them clearly in mind, is a great help, although rarely done. The second edition of Kent's *Repertory* has a separate heading for alternations, which, in the third edition, are sprinkled throughout the book. It will be very helpful to the beginner to make a note of the main contradictions in symptoms in each remedy, and to think through why this should be so.

By this time the student will be in a position to note, without danger of being unduly influenced by pathology, the different 'diseases' in which the remedy under study is especially useful; and after thoroughly mastering the polychrests he should go back and compare their action in each of the diseases. Very little has been written about comparisons between the physiological action of drugs and their homoeopathic action, but in the study of each remedy its pharmacology and uses in conventional medicine should be studied and compared. Useful hints and analogies are often forthcoming.

The student should correlate the homoeopathic remedy picture with endocrinology, metabolic tests and morphology.

Study one polychrest each week, beginning with relatively easy ones such as Aconite, Belladonna or Bryonia; and then, when the habit of assimilating the remedy is acquired, tackle the essential remedies, such as Sulphur, Calcarea Carbonica, Silica and Phosphorus.

Each remedy should be studied in at least ten different books, so as to allow for the refractions of the personalities of the different authors. No human being sees all the aspects of another individual or remedy. A composite picture is necessary for completeness. We recommend the following books for study, in the order mentioned:

1) Kent's *Materia Medica*; though informal in style, it gives a compelling and permeating picture of the remedies.
2) Nash's *Leaders*; a dangerous book if used alone, but stimulating and comprehensive.
3) Allen's *Keynotes*; in a class with the above.
4) Clarke's *Dictionary of Materia Medica*; not the symptoms of the provings themselves, but the 'characteristics' which give interesting varied information and sparse salient features.
5) Hering's *Guiding Symptoms*, with special attention to the symptoms with heavy and double heavy marks. This is the most solid and practicable of all our materia medicas, although it does not give the picturesque individuality of the remedies as Kent does.
6) Dunham's *Lectures on Materia Medica*; very lucid.
7) Hahnemann's *Materia Medica Pura*; the prime source of the subject, placed late on the list because of the mass of symptoms.
8) Teste's *Materia Medica*, giving suggestive groupings of the remedies; a unique book.

9) Allen's *Encyclopaedia of the Materia Medica*; difficult reading because of the mass of material, but invaluable.
10) Jahr's *Manual*, which has many symptoms not to be found elsewhere.

When the nosodes are studied, H. C. Allen's *Materia Medica of the Nosodes* should be added, and for unusual remedies Kent's *Lesser Writings*, Hale's *New Remedies* and Anshutz's *New, Old and Forgotten Remedies*. For those who read German, Stauffer's *Homoeopathische Arzneimittellehre* is a classic.

The student should also read Farrington's *Clinical Materia Medica*, even though it is confusing, and Hughes' *Manual*, or, better, his *Cyclopaedia of Drug Pathogenesy*, Cowperthwaite's *Materia Medica*, Pierce's *Plain Talks on Materia Medica with Comparisons*, Woodbury's little *Materia Medica for Nurses*, Rabe's *Therapeutics*, and Boger's *Synoptic Key*.

Before finishing his study, the student would do well to outline the emergency uses of each of the remedies and commit them to memory.

As a check to his study he can take the Kent *Repertory* and seek the rubrics in which the remedy he is studying appears in the third (highest) degree.

If the student will follow this outline and get the habit of recognizing remedy types on public transport, at meetings or wherever he may be, his knowledge will be solid and broad, and his time will be saved.

The Evaluation of Symptoms

The evaluation of symptoms is perhaps the most important part of the homoeopathic technique, and to the beginner, one of the most difficult. Certain propositions in relation to it are axiomatic. Owing to the terminology of modern medicine and the training that patients have received from non-homoeopathic physicians, the emphasis which the patient himself places upon symptoms is often entirely misleading. The homoeopath must separate diagnoses and common symptoms (that is, symptoms which are common to any patient suffering from a certain complaint, such as vomiting in a gastro-intestinal case). These *common* symptoms are valueless from the point of view of homoeopathic prescribing, unless qualified by modalities. The homoeopath must discriminate between the relatively worthless common symptom, which may often be the patient's chief complaint, and the precious, minor, subjective symptoms which the patient will inadvertently bring out. The patient may complain of some pain or inconvenience that is relatively irrelevant, and not even be aware of grave and helpful symptoms that are plain to the physician.

On the other hand, just because the homoeopath knows that mental symptoms are most important, he should not hunt in the haystack for a tiny mental with which to open the case. *The symptoms should have the same importance, the same weight or mass, in the patient's case as is assigned to them in the symptom hierarchy.* Take for example a woman who complains of indigestion and admits to overpowering fears – the fear, being a mental, outranks the stomach symptoms; but if this woman had violent pain in the stomach and an unimportant fear, the pain, being a much greater factor in the case, would outrank the fear.

A third axiom is that all rubrics used, or rather symptoms taken to be matched with rubrics, must be really true of the patient, and reliable.

Another is that three or more similar particulars make a general. For instance, if the patient has burning in the head, the stomach, the feet and the skin, the general rubric BURNING is applicable; whereas, if he has burning in the stomach only, it is a particular, or symptom of the part.

If a valuable general cannot be found in the repertory, as stated by the patient, it may be found under the opposite rubric, as, 'cold weather ameliorates'. This is found in the repertory under 'warm air aggravates'. 'Better in summer' is found under 'winter aggravates'. This, again, brings up the nice problem of the interpretation of the patient's words and their translation into terms of the rubrics. Only a knowledge of the exact meaning of words and sufficient psychology to divine what the patient means by what he says, and a thorough acquaintance with every rubric in the repertory, will enable the homoeopath to evaluate the symptoms.

If care and ingenuity are taken it is not only justifiable, but sometimes necessary, to combine rubrics in order to get the exact meaning. There are two ways of combining – by adding all the remedies in the two or more rubrics, especially when the rubrics are small, or by taking only the remedies which appear in all the rubrics taken, which increases the grading of the remedies. An example of rubrics which may be combined by this latter method is: menses acrid, early, bright red and clotted.

Opinions diverge on the proper place of pathology and also on objective symptoms (such as redness of the orifices). In the Kentian method these are placed relatively low, whereas the Boger method, as given in his little *General Analysis*, stresses the pathological generals, as opposed to diagnostic pathology. Stearns favours stressing the objective symptoms, as he feels that these cannot mislead.

There are several kinds of pathology. Disease diagnoses appear here and there in the repertory as, for example, scarlet fever, septicaemia, chorea, apoplexy, etc. Other conditions which are pathological, and yet are symptoms or signs rather than diseases, are found, such as convulsions, dropsy, cyanosis, haemorrhage, etc. There is a third class of pathology, the importance of which consists in the bodily tendency to produce such changes, such as warts, polypi, fibroid tumours, etc. These are the most important of the pathological rubrics, as they indicate the tendency of the whole constitution. A rubric such as empyema, which is found under chest, is a pathological particular and therefore less important, although it may be of great interest in that case to see what remedies have had the power to cause and to cure this condition.

The schema of the importance of symptoms, according to Kent, is:

Mentals: will, understanding, intellect.
Physical generals: time, temperature, weather, position, motion, external stimuli, eating, drinking, sleep, clothing and bathing.
Particulars: strange, rare and peculiar, and the modalities of the particulars. For details see 'Know the Patient' (page 281).

In the Kent method, after taking the complete case, the physician selects any outstanding mentals, grading them in the order given above. He will of course add such mentals as he himself perceives in the patient or as a cause of the ailment. There may be from one (or indeed none) to six or seven marked mentals. The physician then takes the chief generals in the case, ranking them in the order given above. The mentals plus the generals will give him a working basis for the selection of a chronic remedy. When he has repertorized these symptoms down to about five remedies he should then rank the particulars and see how the five remedies cover these. Then he must take these five remedies and study them in the materia medica, in order to select the one most similar to the case. It is obvious that this method proceeds from generals to particulars, and that no special attention is paid to pathology.

In the Boger method, fewer symptoms are used and special stress is put on pathological generals. For instance, if the case presents several excoriating discharges the rubric ACRIDITY, in Boger's *General Analysis*, would be taken; if the patient complains of marked dryness of mouth, rectum, skin, etc., the general, DRYNESS, would be used. In this method the mentals are prominent and take first place, as in the Kent method.

Stearns takes not more than five or six symptoms, of which one is mental, one pathological, one objective and two are physical generals.

Boericke divides symptoms into basic and determinative classes, the basic being the common – diagnostic and pathologic, and the determinative the subjective – modalities and generals. Boericke, like Margaret Tyler, advocates the use of certain large general rubrics, such as lack of vital heat, as eliminative symptoms. Some Kentians consider this dangerous.

It is hoped that the student will not be confused by this variance of method among the masters, and it is strongly recommended that each beginner should master the Kentian technique first, the other variants being short cuts to suit different types of minds.

As soon as the case is taken and the physician sits down to study it, he will find it useful to run down the list of symptoms and mark with 'M' opposite the mentals, 'G' opposite the generals, 'PATH' opposite the pathology, 'P' opposite the particulars, and 'O' for objectives. This should be done in the left-hand margin and should be in coloured ink. For further clarity he may underline any peculiar symptoms in red. The symptoms to be actually used for repertorizing should be written down on a new sheet in the order of their importance. If the Kent method is being used, the symptoms may then be transcribed onto special blank repertory sheets, which greatly simplify repertorizing.

After the beginner has listed his symptoms according to their importance he should reconsider them, checking mentally his symptom list with his impression of the patient, to see if any elements of the case are placed too high or too low; for on the correct evaluation of the symptoms depends the possibility of finding the most similar remedy, which will lead to cure.

The Crux of Homoeopathy –
The Mental Symptoms

One of the prime tenets of homoeopathy is the importance of spiritual factors: 'From within outward, from above downward'. In accordance with this principle the mental symptoms are of the greatest import. This does not mean that some non-prominent peculiarity of the mind should outrank a flagrant general symptom. If the mental symptoms do not speak unmistakably for themselves, the true homoeopath should realize that in this individual the trouble is centred on a more outward and physical plane, at least for the moment. On the other hand, many marked aberrations may not at first strike the mind of a physician who is being consulted for a definite pain in some locality, and these may be of such a nature that the patient himself is unconscious of them. Every expert homoeopath must also be a good psychologist. He must read the character of the patient and scent out the failings and warped attitudes which may be at the root of many bona fide bodily ailments.

Granted that the patient presents symptoms in the sphere of the mind, and that the doctor places a high value on them, how is he to use them in repertorizing his case? Let us take up first the problem of the usefulness of these features in acute conditions. We are all awake to the importance of the intense fear of the Aconite patient, of the irritability and fault-finding of the accountant who needs Nux Vomica, of the irascibility of the Chamomilla baby, of the pitiful gentleness and craving for sympathy of those who need Pulsatilla, even though their normal state is critical and dry-eyed. What is more difficult to perceive is the guidance given to us in acute conditions by what we are accustomed to think of as the chronic mental symptoms of a remedy. Who has not heard the loquacity of a Lachesis angina? or been startled by the abruptness of a girl needing Natrum Mur. after an unfortunate love affair? For the best success in prescribing, acute mentals should never be disregarded. They will often be the deciding factor between two remedies, both of whose modalities fit reasonably well.

In chronic cases, the realm of psychological traits is far richer and more suggestive. The physician knows the temperaments of his remedies, and in clear cases can fit them on mentals alone with beautiful precision to the patients before him, although the majority of mankind are more complicated than this. From some remark that they let fall, from some comment of the family, from some ill-concealed uneasiness or characteristic reaction to a skilful question, from something which crops up during the physical examination, the discriminating homoeopath can select his remedy almost with certainty. However, many states of mind require interpretation – is the patient before you silent and uncommunicative because he is a brooding introvert, or because he is timid, or has he a laugh up his sleeve? Such a decision may make the difference between studying Natrum Mur., Pulsatilla or Lachesis. Or is this same individual reserved because of some hidden mortification which may call for Staphysagria, or through a haughty pride of the Platinum variety, or is he one of the 'stiff-necked' people needing a limbering dose of Lycopodium? If, on the other hand, your patient is excessively communicative, is it the loquacity of Lachesis or Calcarea Phosphorica, is it the lack of mental modesty of Phosphorus, is it the hypochondriasis of Ignatia, or the egoistical philosophical garrulity of Sulphur?

If the mental symptom you see does not appear in the repertory, even under any of its synonyms, what then? You must be very sure that your choice of so important a rubric is correct. Often your patients will not confide in you, do what you will, and yet you may know that their lack of reaction or other symptoms is due to psychic causes. These are the ones you must feel out and sense and often give the remedy for, without making them aware either that they have such psychic causes or that you know it. Do not forget the unspoken influence of sex difficulties: your Conium, your Origanum, your Lycopodium or your Apis. In handling any case where the patient has a marked character defect, be it jealousy, vengeance, temper, obstinacy or what not, use that as a symptom and your chronic remedy will often change the life of the whole family. Above all, remember the grading of the mentals: first, those having to do with the love of life; next, such as affect the creative instinct and love of other human beings; thirdly, those which pertain to traits of character, to desires and aversions; and fourthly, those concerning emotions which are thwarted or suppressed.

Do not let your patients mislead you. Have infinite patience, tact and intuition, and study over and over again the section on Mind in Kent's *Repertory*. Then your patients, homoeopathy and you yourself will be rewarded.

Strange, Rare and Peculiar Symptoms

One important stumbling block in homoeopathy is the 'strange, rare, and peculiar' symptom. What is such a symptom, may it be both a general and a particular, does it affect the evaluation, and is it equivalent to a keynote?

A 'strange, rare and peculiar' symptom may be of two kinds. It may be a symptom which is weird, fantastic, unheard-of, rarely found – such as 'Sensation in a non-pregnant woman of something alive, jumping about in the abdomen', or 'Sensation of the whole body being brittle'. The second class is that of symptoms which though not fantastic in themselves are unusual, unexpected and even contrary to what you could rationally predicate in a given condition. For instance, 'Laughs and sings when in pain'; 'Thirst for cold during chilly stage only, with no thirst during fever'. This latter type, as is evident from these two examples, is peculiar because of the juxtapositions; it is the concomitance that is queer – 'laughter with pain', 'thirst with chill'.

Such a symptom can be a mental, a general or a particular; in the nature of things it cannot be a common symptom. As an example of such a mental, take 'Sensation as if she were double in bed', or 'Constantly washing the hands'. As a typical strange general, take the well-known Camphor symptom, 'Desires heat during the hot stages and cold during the cold stages', or 'Thirsty with aversion to water'; as a rare particular take 'Empty sensation inside the head', or 'Blueness of the nails during chill', or 'Temporary blindness which passes off as the headache develops' or 'Epistaxis brought on by washing the face in cold water'.

A 'strange, rare and peculiar' general, such as 'Chilly but aggravated from heat', outranks other ordinary generals of the same class, unless there is a general which runs through so many particulars that it is the leading feature of the case. For instance, the case has 'Suicidal on waking'; 'Restless when he wakes in the morning'. Here it is the aggravation on waking in the morning which is the most marked symptom, and for repertorizing purposes it outranks even the mentals – suicidal impulses – because these are modifiers of the patient's state on waking rather than his constant condition. Among particular symptoms, also, you give preference to the 'strange, rare and peculiar' ones.

299

Angina pectoris with pain extending up into the occiput would take preference over heart pain extending down the arm, because the former is more strange and unusual. The strange mental symptoms may often be of less value than the peculiar generals or particulars. This is especially true in neurasthenic cases, which often invent and embroider symptoms. In the realm of mentals, especially, we must be sure that a symptom is authentic. Some homoeopaths claim that in mental cases it is safer to repertorize by strange and prominent generals and particulars, and to consider the myriad mental symptoms only as part of the general picture, when choosing from among the few remedies that come out highest from the repertory study. As a rule, then, select the generals and the particulars which are most peculiar, provided always that they are prominent features of the case.

'Strange, rare and peculiar' symptoms often become keynotes, although not all keynotes are strange symptoms. For instance, 'Hunger at 11 a.m.' is a keynote of Sulphur but it is not a 'Strange, rare and peculiar' symptom; the same with the 4–8 p.m. aggravation of Lycopodium. But a keynote which is also a peculiar symptom is the well-known aggravation from downward motion of Borax, or 'The more you belch the more you have to belch' of Ignatia, or the peculiar symptom which is also a keynote of Calc. Carb., Aluminium and Nitric Acid – 'Craves indigestible things like chalk, earth, and slate pencils'.

The individualization which is so essential a part of homoeopathy is greatly helped by the understanding and use of 'strange, rare and peculiar' symptoms. Hahnemann himself especially stressed this point. It is needless to say that if strange symptoms found under only a couple of remedies are permitted to predominate, they may mislead the student. For instance, we had a patient who kept telling us that his twitching was worse during eating and when he sat down at the dining table. This symptom is to be found in the Kent *Repertory* under only one remedy, Plumbum, which was not at all the remedy for the whole of this case.

These strange symptoms are often difficult to elicit, as patients feel ashamed of telling anything so peculiar, so inconsequential or absurd; and yet they will crop up, especially in simple people. Above all where they are generals they prove of enormous value as *parts* of the totality of the symptoms.

Repertorizing

As no one person can carry all the symptoms of all the remedies in his mind, a concordance or index is needed. We term such a symptom index a repertory. There are about half a hundred of these, general or special, based on different systems of studying the case. The most vital ones to know are the basic ones of the two main methods – Kent's *Repertory* and Boenninghausen's *Therapeutic Pocket Book*.

THE KENT REPERTORY: ITS CONSTRUCTION

The Kent *Repertory* is a compilation of materia medica, some earlier repertories (such as Lippe's), and clinical symptoms that have been verified. In order to search successfully in the Kent *Repertory* for the symptoms of your case, as evaluated in accordance with the preceding chapter, you must be thoroughly familiar with the plan of the book, its rationale, and also its inconsistencies.

The plan of the book is to work from generals to particulars, a general rubric first in most instances. The book is based on anatomical divisions, with certain exceptions such as the first section, on MIND; the last one, GENERALITIES; discharges, such as STOOL, SWEAT, URINE, and EXPECTORATION, which appear as separate sections next to the anatomical region producing them; and certain general conditions, such as VERTIGO, COUGH, SLEEP, CHILL, and FEVER, which are also separate. Under each anatomical section the rubrics run in alphabetical order regardless of whether they are pathology, sensations, modalities or objective symptoms (such as 'bores head in pillow'). Each main heading is followed by modifiers (if these exist), in the following order: time, circumstances in alphabetical order, extensions (the point *from* which a symptom extends is the one under which it will be found, not the point *to* which it extends), location with *its* time, circumstance and extension modifiers, and lastly, sensation with its modifiers. For instance, the main section HEAD is anatomical, but under that you will *not* find an anatomical section for occiput – you must look under the sensation in the occiput, as for instance, Coldness or Pain, occiput, in.

Note that certain anatomical regions have no corresponding section in this repertory; for instance, neck, which is found under THROAT, EXTERNAL THROAT, and BACK. EXTERNAL THROAT contains the rubrics pertaining to the anterior neck, such as goitre, glands, torticollis, etc., and BACK contains nape and posterior cervical region. Furthermore, lungs, heart, aorta, axillary glands, breast and milk appear under CHEST; posterior chest appears under BACK; pulse under GENERALITIES; head sinuses are divided between NOSE and FACE; salivary glands are found under FACE instead of under THROAT; lips under FACE instead of under MOUTH; oesophagus is found under STOMACH; and liver under ABDOMEN. There is no section for the circulatory, glandular or nervous systems, as this book is not based on systems (which Boericke's *Repertory* is, in part), but the parts of these systems are found scattered throughout the book under allied anatomical headings. Many symptoms which one would expect to find under the nervous system appear under GENERALITIES, as they indicate a tendency of the whole organism, such as ANALGESIA, CHOREA, CONVULSIONS, PARALYSIS, TREMBLING. Twitching of the parts appears under the anatomical part, such as FACE, EXTREMITIES. Nervous symptoms having to do with the spine appear under BACK, such as OPISTHOTONOS. Meningitis appears in two places, under HEAD, INFLAMMATION, meninges of, and BACK, INFLAMMATION, cord, membranes of.

Similar or allied rubrics often appear in two or more different places, as for instance: Dysmenorrhoea under GENITALIA, FEMALE, Menses, painful; ABDOMEN, PAIN, cramping bearing down, cutting, menses, during; ABDOMEN, PAIN, hypogastrium, in, menses, during; and ABDOMEN, PAIN, menses, during.

It must be noted that many rubrics which appear as particulars under the proper anatomical sections or main headings also appear in the last section, GENERALITIES, in their relation to the body as a whole. For instance, under GENERALITIES, MENSES, comes aggravation or amelioration of the whole person before, during or after menses, while under GENITALIA, FEMALE appears the type and circumstances of the menses, or, so to speak, the particulars. Similarly under GENERALITIES, PERSPIRATION, appears amelioration or aggravation of the body as a whole from sweat, whereas under the section PERSPIRATION are given the quality, occurrence and modalities of the discharge itself. Sweat of any special part is found under the anatomical section in which the part is located, such as ABDOMEN, PERSPIRATION on. Perspiration of the scalp is not under HEAD, scalp, perspiration of, but under HEAD, PEPSPIRA-TION, scalp of. General amelioration by, or distress from, the act of eating appears under GENERALITIES, EATING; and under GENERALITIES, FOOD, are the aggravations and ameliorations from the different articles of food, but under the section STOMACH, aversions and desires for special articles of food appear.

Pathological diagnoses are found frequently in GENERALITIES and occasionally as headings under other sections, but more often as subheadings under the condition involved. For instance, pleurisy is found under CHEST, INFLAMMATION, pleura of, and appendicitis under ABDOMEN, INFLAMMATION, appendicitis. On the other hand, empyema is found under CHEST, EMPYEMA, directly, and goitre under EXTERNAL THROAT, GOITRE. Certain pathological states which are symptoms rather than diseases, such as chorea, convulsions, cyanosis, dropsy, etc., appear under GENERALITIES. Objective symptoms are scattered all through the book and are often small unclassified rubrics, such as brittle nails or gestures under MIND, biting under MIND, and red lips under FACE, DISCOLORATION, red lips.

THE KENT REPERTORY: ITS USE

This repertory is built to work the cases from general symptoms to particular symptoms. We have already mentioned the evaluation of symptoms in Kent's method of grading, MENTALS being the most important, and GENERALS next. Most chronic cases and many acute ones can be worked out by the *Repertory* on the MENTALS and GENERALS alone to within three to five remedies. The beginner should take at least eight of these symptoms, although experts often solve the case on three to five. The beginner must be very sure that these MENTALS and GENERALS are really true of the patient, and that he has not warped the symptom in translating the patient's colloquial expressions into the language of the rubrics. Moreover, a symptom must have the same mass or importance in the patient's case as is assigned to it in the symptom hierarchy. If an important symptom cannot be found in the *Repertory* it can often be found under a synonymous rubric. It is to be understood that the headings under GENERALITIES which are not pathological and not marked 'ameliorated by', or otherwise explained, and which are not sensations or conditions, mean 'aggravation from'. For example, EATING, before, means worse before eating, COITION, after, means aggravated after coition. Many of the ameliorations are omitted and you must look for them under aggravation of their opposites. For instance, there is no 'better in summer'; this is considered equivalent to 'worse in winter'. Sometimes two or more rubrics must be combined in order to be equivalent to a given symptom. If the rubrics are very small, it may be wise to add all the remedies. If at least one of the rubrics is large and the others of fair size, only such remedies as run through all the component rubrics of this symptom should be taken. Certain symptoms have so large a group of remedies that they are almost useless, except as eliminating symptoms. Such a one is cold-bloodedness of the patient, which appears under GENERALITIES, HEAT, lack of vital, and would serve to eliminate any markedly hot-blooded remedies which had otherwise come through the generals high in a given case.

The student will recall that the common symptoms, or the unqualified big, main rubrics, such as SADNESS, VOMITING, etc., are of little or no use in repertorizing, and that among both GENERALS and PARTI-CULARS, a strange, rare and peculiar symptom ranks high. A strange, rare and peculiar general would be 'During cold stage craves cold', or 'During hot stage craves heat', as in Camphor; a strange, rare and peculiar particular would be 'Thirst for ice water only during chill' (Eupatorium Perf.).

We have said that the beginner should locate in the *Repertory* his eight or more main GENERALS, and chart the remedies appearing under each of these, putting 3 for the bold face (heavy black type), 2 for italics and 1 for roman (plain type). This being done for all the symptoms chosen, the remedies appearing in more than half the rubrics are listed with their fractions, the numerator of the fraction being the numerical totality of the remedy grades, and the denominator being the number of symptoms in which the remedy appears.

Now the PARTICULARS come into play, beginning with the most peculiar ones, and care should be taken not to use rubrics that are too small. In fact, it is safer to use a more general, medium-sized rubric than the more exact particular rubric. The occurrence of these particulars in the few remedies which have stood highest in the GENERALS, and in these only, being taken, you can now see which few remedies are fairly similar to the GENERALS of your case, and which few of those most resemble the PARTICULARS of the case. Add the particular to the general fraction and reduce your list to the three to five remedies which stand highest in their grand total. If one remedy totals 16/7 and another 15/8, the former is to be preferred. As you have taken your symptoms in the strict order of their importance according to the Kentian schema, your first two or three symptoms should appear in the remedies that come high, and where they do not the remedy should be looked on with suspicion. It is to be remembered that certain remedies, like Sulphur, Calc. Carb., Nux Vomica, Pulsatilla, almost always come out high numerically, because they have been so thoroughly proved. Unless the beginner discounts this and bases his final judgement on materia medica, and especially the mentals and type of the patient, he will prescribe these well-proved polychrests too often. Conversely, it must not be forgotten that some remedies, like Tuberculinum, have but a fragmentary part of their proving in the *Repertory*. Only a little more than five hundred remedies are mentioned in the *Repertory*, and very few of the nosodes and double salts are adequately stressed. When the remedies have been reduced numerically to three to five, these must then be read in the materia medica, especially their MENTALS, and the original case as taken reviewed and compared to each of the remedies. The miasmatic relationships of the patient, and also of the remedies that come out high, must be considered. For future reference in treating the case, in acute as well as chronic prescribing, a list should be made on the patient's chart of the constitutional remedies which come high, of the nosodes which most nearly apply, and of the acute remedies ranking highest. These, or complements of them, will often be found to fit any illness of that patient in the future, unless an epidemic remedy be called for.

Ideally, each symptom should be stated on the repertorizing record in the words of the patient in the symptom column, restated in the exactly corresponding rubric in the rubric column, noting the page where this is found. (Repertorizing sheets are available at a nominal cost from the National Center for Homeopathy, 1500 Massachusetts Ave, N.W., Washington, DC 20005, USA.)

THE BOENNINGHAUSEN REPERTORY: ITS CONSTRUCTION

Boenninghausen's *Therapeutic Pocket Book*, one of the earliest repertories, is based largely on Hahnemann's *Materia Medica Pura*, and the idea of it was approved by Hahnemann himself. The book falls into seven distinct parts. Although each of these is complete in itself, 'yet each one gives but one portion of a symptom, which can be completed only in one or several other parts'. For example, the seat of pain is found in the second section, the kind of pain in the third, the aggravation or amelioration according to time or circumstances in the sixth, and the necessary concomitants in the various sections. The seven sections are: 1) The Mind and Disposition; 2) Parts of the Body and Organs; 3) Sensations and Complaints in alphabetical order, in general and then specially, of the glands, of the bones, and of the skin and exterior parts; 4) Sleep and Dreams; 5) Fevers with Chill, Circulation and Sweat (the 2nd, 4th and 5th sections have concomitants); 6) Aggravations and

Ameliorations from time and circumstances; 7) Relationship of Remedies. In section (7) under each drug the previous section headings, (1) through (6) are given, and under each of these the remedies applying in that section which are related to the particular remedy in question. At the end of each remedy there is a list of other related remedies plus the antidotes.

THE BOENNINGHAUSEN REPERTORY: ITS USE

This repertory is based on GENERALS much more even than the Kent. The rubrics in the different sections dealing with the different aspects of one symptom are used to eliminate all remedies except those that run through them all. This is a swifter, easier method than the Kent, but too general, and a great many symptoms cannot be found in it at all. Also, there are very few rubrics under MIND – only seven pages out of 482. Boger's *General Analysis* is based on this repertory, and his unique method of working cases by it is also deserving of study.

THE BOERICKE REPERTORY

The Kent repertory in its present form is unwieldy for the physician to carry with him to the bedside. Neither the Boenninghausen nor Kent repertories have any materia medica. Two books which combine materia medica and repertory are handy in the pocket or medical bag. One of these is Boger's *Synoptic Key*, of which his *General Analysis* is an abridged form, and the other is Boericke's *Materia Medica with Repertory*. The Boericke repertory resembles the Kent rather than the Boenninghausen, although Boericke has reclassified some of the anatomical sections. For instance, vertigo appears under HEAD; sinuses are grouped together under NOSE; lips are under MOUTH instead of FACE; tongue has a section to itself, as have gums; oesophagus is under THROAT instead of STOMACH; foods that disagree are in STOMACH with the cravings and aversions; rectum and stool are under ABDOMEN; all the URINARY SYSTEM is together under that heading; breasts are rightly classed under the FEMALE SEXUAL SYSTEM; there is an admirable section on PREGNANCY, LABOUR and LACTATION; after GENITALIA comes the section on the CIRCULATORY SYSTEM, including pulse; then comes the LOCOMOTOR SYSTEM, including extremities, gait, neck, inflammatory rheumatism and arthritis, back and axillae; then comes RESPIRATORY SYSTEM, including lungs, cough, expectoration, larynx, voice and respiration; following this is the SKIN. The FEVER section includes chill and sweat, the exanthemata and various fevers such as influenza, typhoid, malaria. The NERVOUS SYSTEM follows and includes epilepsy, paralysis, sleep, dreams, weakness, convulsions, goitre, sea-sickness, neuralgia, sciatica, spine, meningitis, etc. The GENERALITIES section is much reduced and contains mainly diseases, tissues, poisonings, suppressions (under CHECKED discharges), glandular affections including mumps, goitre, a very interesting section on COMPLAINTS from winds, damp places, sudden, gradual, injuries, prophylactics, and tumours. This section has been relieved of much misplaced matter and has added to it a great deal of interesting and valuable material. The last section is MODALITIES, first aggravations and then ameliorations; time under these appears in alphabetical order under morning, night, periodicity, etc., instead of altogether at the beginning of the section, as in Kent.

Under all extensive headings, such as HEADACHE, appear definite captions in the following order: Cause, Type, Location, Character of Pain, Concomitants, Modalities, i.e., Aggravations and Ameliorations.

This book is a clinical rather than a symptomatological index and has many technical terms as main headings. A tremendous number of remedies are given in the materia medica section, and well given, with plentiful mentals. Owing to its small size, a great many symptoms have had to be omitted from the repertory. Its pretensions are not great but its usefulness within its sphere is tremendous.

This provides a bird's eye view of three of the most useable general repertories. It is strongly advised that every student should master the Kent method, as it will reward familiarity more than any other. To the advanced student it should be added that many strange and peculiar symptoms cannot be found in these three repertories, and must be searched for in Gentry's *Concordance*, Knerr's *Repertory*, Lippe, Jahr, or some of the special repertories.

These different methods of repertorizing will appeal to different types of minds and will also be suitable for different types of cases; the Boger method suiting those with much pathology and few other symptoms; the Kent method suiting those with marked mentals and an intricate anamnesis; the Boenninghausen method suiting conditions with acute pains and clear-cut modalities – cases without subtleties.

I would however reiterate: *Study the Kent method first, last, and all the time.*

Potency Selection

After thoroughly digesting the preceding sections of this Brief Course, and doing wide collateral reading and studying, one should be able to select the most similar remedy. The most similar remedy, however, does not become the simillimum until the potency is adjusted to the plane of the individual during his or her illness at the time of prescribing. Our philosophy teaches us that pathology, and even bacteria, are the ultimates of disease, and that the true cause is far deeper and less material than these. In order to truly wipe out the cause of a so-called disease, one must administer the remedy on or near the plane of the cause. It follows that for mental distresses and disease of manifestly psychic origin the high potencies (10M and upward) would be employed, other things being equal; and that for grossly material conditions, such as marked organic and pathological changes, the lower or medium potencies would be selected. In general, functional diseases – where the symptoms are subjective or physiological, and where the vital force is labile – respond well to high potencies; and the organic conditions respond well to lower ones. It makes some difference whether the conditions are acute or chronic. For instance, diphtheria has marked pathology, as does pneumonia, yet the pathology is recent and swift in pace and the high potencies are suitable.

In general, acute diseases respond well to high potencies, especially of acute remedies. High potencies of deep-acting chronic remedies, when these are indicated in an acute condition, may be dangerous. Certain acute crises based on chronic trouble, such as cardiac asthma, would have to be treated with medium or low potencies, because the high potency could stir up more than the vital force could cope with in the face of the advanced chronic pathology.

In chronic prescribing it is a safe rule to begin with the 200th centesimal, unless this is dangerous because of the nature of the remedy, the degree of the pathology or the depth of the miasm. One great object in starting at the 200th in chronic cases is that you then have an ascending series of potencies to use as the treatment progresses. The Kentian ideal is to exhaust the action of one potency (see the section on 'Repetition', below) and then to step up to the next, exhausting that, and so on to the highest known potency of that remedy if no change of remedy is indicated. Hahnemann defines the highest suitable potency as that one which will produce a very slight aggravation of the symptoms in any given case. In my experience you can usually use the highest known potency of the true simillimum and still get action, although at times action will cease with, say, the CM potency. When the top of the series has been exhausted and yet the same remedy is still called for, you begin again at the 200th and repeat the ascending series.

Series of homoeopathic potencies have been made by many famous people, either by hand, as in the case of the Jenichen potencies, or by various machines. As a general rule it is best to stick to the potencies made by one person as you go up the series in any one case, as for instance Kent's 200c, 1M, 10M, 50M, CM. On the other hand, if a jolt is needed, although the same remedy is called for, a change from, say, the Skinner to the Fincke potencies may whip up the case. For those who understand rhythms and cycles it may be well, after a patient has been through an ascending series of a remedy from one source, to change to one of the irregular potencies of the same remedy from another source. For instance, we have seen Skinner's Lycopodium 2M beneficial instead of Kent's 1M, or Fincke's 43M in place of a 50M. This change seems to start a new rhythm or cycle – it is as though the vital force became bored with the first system and responded with a renewed spurt to the alteration of potency. (This is advanced doctrine.)

In acute and desperately ill cases, where the fight for life is active, the high potencies are indicated. Where the desperate illness is the terminal stage of a chronic disease, the very high potencies will induce euthanasia. In chronically incurable cases, unless the vitality is very good and the pathology not yet too extreme, low or medium potencies are suitable. Here the deep-acting simillimum must usually be avoided and a palliative remedy given. If such a palliative is not too searching a remedy, for example Sanguinaria, Rumex or Pulsatilla, it may be given even to incurable patients in a fairly high potency.

One snag is the problem of potency selection in acute disease incident to chronic treatment. Patients long under correct chronic prescribing show fewer and fewer acute diseases; in other words, their susceptibility is eradicated. However, explosions of latent psora do occur sometimes, particularly when the general vigour is increased by the proper chronic remedy, as a sort of vent or effort on the part of the vital force toward house-cleaning. The first problem for the prescriber in this connection is to determine whether the acute symptoms arising during chronic treatment are an aggravation following the remedy; and if so, whether they are an aggravation due to the reactive curative power of the body, or else a remedy aggravation due to oversensitivity or to a wrong potency. If either of these should be the case and the aggravation is not too severe, no remedy should be given – merely placebo. If the aggravation threatens life or is unbearably painful, and may therefore have to be antidoted, or for some social reason is particularly intolerable for the moment, an acute remedy may be given in the medium-low potencies, preferably the 30th or 200th; this will probably not interfere with the action of the chronic remedy. In acute exacerbations or explosions of active chronic disease you can often give the acute complement or cognate of your chronic remedy. In this case too the chronic remedy may continue to act undisturbed. In very severe acute diseases during the course of chronic treatment it will sometimes be better to give the acute remedy high. After the acute condition has subsided retake the chronic case, which will then often show a new picture. The new prescription takes into account the original chronic symptoms but lays more stress on the recent developments.

In many conditions with marked tissue change, such as adhesions or chronic cardiac decompensation, very low potencies, even tinctures, may be useful. Potencies as low as the 12th or even the 6th are occasionally invaluable in single dosage in such grave conditions as tuberculosis, where even a 30th or a 200th of such a remedy as Phosphorus or Silica might set the economy on the downgrade.

From this brief outline of the possibilities of potency it will be seen that in general we uphold the use of the high potencies. The question of potency is the most moot point in all homoeopathy, and even today many strict homoeopaths are low potency prescribers. These follow Hughes and are more pathological in their prescribing. The strict Kentians, almost without exception, are preponderantly high potency.

The degree of susceptibility of your patient also influences potency selection. Certain persons are oversensitive, often owing to improper homoeopathic treatment, and will prove any remedy you give them. They therefore require medium-low potencies. Other patients are very sluggish, often as a result of much allopathic drugging. These will often take a very high potency to get any action at all, or they may need a low potency repeated every few hours until a favourable reaction sets in. A third type of patient is the feeble one, where the vital force can easily be overwhelmed. Repetition is the greatest danger here. Robust but acutely ill patients will stand repetition of high potencies until a favourable reaction commences, although the ideal is the single dose. Children take high potencies particularly well, and in general the very aged required medium potencies, except in the case of euthanasia. Some individuals have idiosyncrasies in respect of homoeopathic potencies of certain substances. Some degree of idiosyncrasy to a remedy must be present or the patient will not be sensitive enough to be cured, but where this is extreme the rule of medium potencies should be preferred.

Where patients have been poisoned by a crude substance it is not in general advisable to give that substance in very high potency, but better to give an antidotal substance high. For instance, patients formerly dosed with calomel were not relieved by high potencies of Mercurius but may have been by Hepar Sulph. On the other hand exceptions to this occur, as in the case of a chronic susceptibility to poison ivy poisoning, where Rhus Tox. CM may eradicate the tendency. If not, a deeper antipsoric in accordance with the totality of the symptoms is indicated. Certain remedies are noted for their power to restore order after chronic poisoning with crude drugs, such as Natrum Mur. after the misuse of quinine or silver nitrate. When accurately chosen, the very low potencies, such as 3x and 6x, can be very dangerous. This may be mainly due to the repetition that is customary in low potency prescribing.

Great care must be taken in potency selection of certain very deep-acting remedies in serious chronic cases. For instance, Kali Carb. in gout; Sulphur, Silica, Tuberculinum or Phosphorus in tuberculosis; Psorinum in asthma; and Arsenicum Alb. and Lachesis in many conditions. These remedies should be carried in the 30th potency even by those who give almost entirely the higher degree.

Repetition

The single remedy is the third member of the essential homoeopathic trilogy. The reason for this is obvious: only one remedy can be the most similar at any given time to the condition of any given patient. If the prescriber is unable to decide between two remedies, he has not identified the totality of the symptoms, or else the remedies he has chosen are merely superficially akin to fragments or aspects of the case. Furthermore, the simillimum is a personality with a rhythm – one might almost say a permeating aura of its own – and in the fleeting instant of its administration it takes complete possession of the patient, thereby buoying up the vital force so that it can carry on the restorative process. To have two or more remedies would be to introduce two separate rhythms, partial and disharmonious factors. Moreover, if more than one remedy is used, the prescriber cannot know which element was curative and one source of future guidance is thereby obscured. Lastly, since only one remedy can possibly be proved at a time, so only can one remedy cure at a given moment. Some homoeopaths do give mixed prescriptions when in doubt, but this is merely prescribing symptomatically, one remedy for one symptom or organ, and another for another. Each of these, if homoeopathically chosen, may wipe out the fragmentary illness at which it was aimed. But that which is profound, total and primal, of which all these several symptoms are but manifestations, will remain untouched and simply crop out through other channels as subsequent symptoms. Other half-hearted homoeopaths, and even some with a wide knowledge of the materia medica but a relatively feeble grasp of the philosophy, alternate remedies. This practice cannot be too strongly condemned, as it seesaws the patient into temporary improvements without real progress. Many French homoeopaths give a main deep-acting remedy and one or more so-called drainage remedies with it – the chronic remedy in high potency and the drainage remedies in low potency, the idea being that the drainage remedy opens up an outlet for the exodus of the disease. These drainage remedies aim at the production of a discharge or the stimulation of the secretory organs. This is a recent variant and does not appear in Hahnemann, the old masters or Kent.

The subject of the intercurrent remedy may well be mentioned here.

Many pure Kentians hold that there is no such thing, and that when, after a series of potencies of the same remedy a new one is called for to stir up or develop the case, this is not an intercurrent remedy but rather the simillimum at that moment.

There is some division of practice as to whether the single remedy should be given in one or more doses. High potentists favour the single dose, although two, three or more doses of a high potency may be given at short intervals – every four, eight or twelve hours – especially in very acute cases with fever, as the increased metabolism appears to 'eat up' the remedy fast. In slow diseases such as typhoid, high potencies may also be repeated close together, but in every instance *it is an absolute rule that when favourable reaction sets in, the administration of the remedy must cease.* So long as improvement is visible in the patient himself the remedy should not be repeated. Not only is there no need of 'more of a good thing', but repeating a remedy which is still acting successfully defeats itself and actually hinders cure. Very occasionally, however, we have found that when a certain potency is aiding to some extent, a higher potency of the same remedy will lift the case to speedier cure. In this connection it is of interest to mention the theory of double dosage promulgated by Gordon of Edinburgh. Gordon gives his remedy in two doses, eight hours apart, the first dose of a lower and the second of a higher potency of the same remedy – for example, Phosphorus 200c at bedtime and Phosphorus 1M on rising. Some of the masters use a lower potency after a higher one and claim good results. This seems in accord with the order of the progress of disease, from within and above, outward and downward. This latter method has been even less used than the former, and we have no statistics as to whether the cases would have done as well or better on the lower potency originally.

Another method of multiple dosage, which almost amounts to divided single doses, is that of plussing. Plussing means dissolving your dose in a third of a glass of water, taking two teaspoonfuls, throwing away most of the rest, adding water up to the original quantity, stirring, succussing and again taking two teaspoonfuls as the second dose, and so on. This process raises the potency very slightly between each of the doses, giving a somewhat wider range of plane, and is particularly indicated in stubborn and refractory cases. If very low potencies are used in ordinary acute illness, repeated doses are necessary in most cases until improvement sets in. For instance, a decompensated cardiac case calling for Crataegus might need two drops of tincture in water night and morning for a week. Where there is more pathology than vitality, this might open the case better than a single high potency dose of Crataegus, although the latter might follow

313

later. According to low potency prescribers Bryonia 3x should be given as pellets or in water, at intervals of one to four hours according to the pace of the case, in acute cases calling for Bryonia. We would wholeheartedly advocate a single dose of Bryonia high under the same conditions. So much for the administration of the first dose or doses prior to the setting in of a favourable reaction.

Next comes the problem of when to prescribe again. *The rule here is: never repeat or change the remedy while the patient himself is improving.* When improvement has apparently ceased in acute diseases you may need to repeat the same remedy in the same or a higher potency; or, if your remedy was not a true simillimum, you may need another remedy to round out the cure. You must be sure that the cessation of improvement is not due to an emotional, mechanical or hygienic cause, or merely to the aggravation or outcropping of single symptoms. In chronic work you should wait some time, from three or four days to two or three weeks or more, because the vital force has cycles even on the upward grade, and true curative action must not be interrupted until it is certain that the reactive force is exhausted. Kent admirably stresses this in his injunction to 'watch and wait'.

As to the interval between repetition of prescriptions, this may vary from a few minutes to a year or more, and is entirely dependent on the general amelioration of the patient. When you have had true improvement and if, particularly in chronic cases, you have observed the working of Hering's law of cure, sit tight. More cases are bungled by too frequent repetition than by anything else. In this connection it is of course necessary to know which are the long-acting remedies, although we have known of the good effect of Bryonia 30c, one dose, continuing for two years in a chronic condition. Every student should own the little pamphlet by R. Gibson Miller on *The Relationship of Remedies*. This gives approximate durations of action, but the only true guide to the duration of action of a remedy in a given potency on any patient is the cessation of that patient's general sense of wellbeing. In general, if you are a good prescriber, one dose, single or divided as above, should cope with brief diseases, to be followed at the termination of the disease with a chronic remedy to set the economy in order. If a change of remedy is indicated in acute disease, there will often be a reversion to the primary remedy towards the close of the disease.

The subject of the second prescription and of aggravations is taken up in the next chapter. It remains only to mention the place of placebo in prescribing. A famous doctor said that 'Sac. Lac. is the second best remedy'. Patients who understand homoeopathy deeply may often be content with a single dose at long intervals without placebo, but it is good policy to give even these persons a single powder of placebo at every visit. Most patients require medicine often, not only so that they feel something is being done but also that they may have powders for emergencies, and it is both honourable and indeed necessary to give plentiful placebo. It is wise to train patients to take placebo powders or pellets which are similar in appearance to the actual remedies, and not to give them tempting brown, pink or green blank tablets.

Complicated as these elementary rules may sound, they are but the beginning of homoeopathic wisdom. Every student should own and read at least once a year Kent's *Lectures on Homoeopathic Philosophy*. He should also be conversant with the writings of Stuart Close, Gibson Miller and John Weir, as well as with the *Lectures on Therapeutics* by Dunham and by Joslin and, of course, with that keystone of our art, Hahnemann's *Organon*.

Aggravation

Having learned how to select the remedy and the potency, and in how many doses to give it, the next step is to know how to watch your case. The homoeopath must be able to determine whether the remedy is acting at all, and if so, whether favourably, and what prognosis may be expected. He must know how to determine the length of action of his remedy in each individual case; in short, having started the journey to cure, he must be sure he is in the right train and that he knows when and where to change.

Two things above all help in these decisions and both are determined by careful observation based on seeing the patient, for what the patient will tell you is often misleading. The first signpost to guide you is the aggravation. A discussion of this is best given in Chapters 34 and 35 in Kent's *Lectures on Homoeopathic Philosophy*, from which I have taken much of what follows.

The types of aggravation which may be observed are:

1) A prolonged aggravation with subsequent decline. This means either that the patient is incurable or that he has been overwhelmed by the turmoil ensuing on too high a potency. This usually occurs in cases of marked pathology, where the patient's vitality is nevertheless able to emit symptoms. In our discussion of the second prescription we take up what to do in such exigencies, but the doctor must be sure, before resorting to a second prescription, that he truly has an aggravation of the first and not the second type.

2) This second type is a long aggravation followed by slow improvement. It indicates a serious case on the border of incurability, but caught just in time.

3) The third type of aggravation is quick, brief and vigorous, followed by speedy relief of the patient. This type is much to be desired. It is a sign that the improvement will be of long duration and that any structural changes are in non-vital organs. Abscesses and suppurating glands appear at times in these cases as part of the aggravation. This is a good sign and should not be interfered with.

4) The fourth type is where there is practically no observable aggravation and yet the patient recovers steadily. This is the ideal. It shows

that there is no great organic disease and that the potency chosen exactly fitted the case, especially if during recovery the symptoms follow Hering's laws, discussed later.

5) The fifth type is where brief amelioration comes first and aggravation afterwards. This can mean that your remedy was only palliative and did not touch the true constitutional state of the patient, or that the patient was incurable, or yet again that some deeper miasmatic remedy is needed – like a mordant to enable the indicated remedy (or dye, to follow our simile through) to take hold. For example, a Silica case of ours would be markedly ameliorated for a week or ten days and then slip back, nor did a change of potency hold longer. However, Tuberculinum took hold and kept it, and after that other remedies were effective.

6) Another type of aggravation is where the symptoms that develop turn out to be a proving of the remedy. This may be an idiosyncrasy to the particular remedy on the part of your patient, or else the patient may be an oversensitive person who proves everything that is given to him. These patients need the medium-low potencies and are often incurable.

7) Another apparent form of aggravation is where new symptoms appear after the administration of a remedy. This suggests that the prescription was incorrect. We will deal with this under the second prescription.

8) There is a type of aggravation in which the individual symptoms stand out clearer while the patient himself feels better. This is often followed by old symptoms reappearing in the reverse order of their coming (Hering's laws of cure). This is highly favourable. The direction of the reappearing symptoms must be noted. If they go wrongly, i.e., from without inward, it is dangerous; if from within outward, it is favourable.

Another variant is a too short relief of symptoms without any special aggravation. This is very similar to the fifth type of aggravation and causes the prescriber to cast about for a miasmatic remedy.

Sometimes there is a full amelioration of symptoms without any special relief of the patient himself. This shows that the case is open only to palliation and that the vital force cannot make the grade to cure.

An unnecessarily severe aggravation will be caused by too high or too low a potency. A well-chosen potency will give, as above, either no aggravation or else a quick short one. Too prolonged an aggravation may be caused by giving too low a potency, or by repeating. In the aggravations after high potencies, such as CM in curable cases, the patient feels distinctly better even during the aggravation, as it is the characteristic symptoms and not the disease of the patient which are aggravated.

A very feeble vitality may not be able to throw out an aggravation. Such a case must be given a single dose of a really high potency and watched for the minutest signs. On the other hand, a strong vitality may have marked tissue changes which will produce a violent aggravation, so that the physician must bear in mind the two factors – the vitality of the whole and the pathological changes – and balance these carefully in his choice of potency.

If there is no aggravation in cases of vigorous vitality it is probable that your remedy was only partially similar. The ideal cases of recovery without perceptible aggravation are usually not those with especially marked vitality. In acute diseases, an amelioration without a slight initial aggravation often means that your remedy is not deep enough and that another dose of it will probably be needed.

The Second Prescription

Kent defines the second prescription as 'the one after the one that has acted'. This means that a bungling prescriber may have given four or five remedies and that the sixth, if it really takes hold, should therefore be classed as the first prescription. Granted that your remedy was well chosen and has acted, according to the above observations on aggravation, *let it alone*. 'Watch and wait.' Before making any second prescription *re-study the case*. According to Kent, there are three possibilities for the second prescription: either *repetition, antidoting* or *complementing*.

The prime indication for the second prescription to be a *repetition* is the return of the original symptoms of the patient. They have been better, with or without aggravation, and they tell you (and you observe) that the original symptoms have reappeared, whether identical, less severe or more severe than at first. This calls for repetition in the same potency after you are sure that the symptoms have returned to stay. It should be added that if the patient returns telling you that their general sense of wellbeing has come to a standstill, but that their original symptoms have not yet returned, you should wait. Improvement often goes in cycles and the good work will begin again of itself. Even if they tell you that they themselves feel worse, wait and watch for the return of the original symptoms before repeating. Moreover, even if the symptoms change, but the patient feels and seems still improved, do not change your remedy. It would be chasing will-of-the-wisps to do so and you would ruin your case. While wellbeing increases, wait; when it comes to a standstill, wait. If the general state is worse and the symptoms have changed, then consider a new second prescription, as follows.

The prime indication for a change of remedy in the second prescription is where new symptoms crop up after your first prescription, without amelioration in the general wellbeing of the patient, and then remain. This means that the first prescription was unfavourable and that you must antidote it. The selection of this antidotal second prescription is based on the original symptoms plus the new symptoms, with more emphasis on the new ones. The second prescription, then, should wipe out the new symptoms and modify the old.

The prime indication for a change to a complementary remedy is where your first prescription, especially in acute disease or if it was not a deep-acting remedy, does not seem to have fathomed the case. Here a complementary remedy will take deeper hold. Belladonna may have been the simillimum in an acute throat, for instance, but after the acute attack passed a chaser was needed to prevent recurrence and eradicate predisposition. If the symptoms agree, your second prescription would be the chronic complement of Belladonna, which is Calc. Carb.

There is another indication – which goes deep into the philosophy – for a change of remedy in your second prescription, which is likely to be a remedy from a different miasmatic group. This will entail a change in the plan of treatment consequent upon the cropping-up of a different miasm, after the first prescription has cleared away the miasm which was originally at the top of the case.

The subject of the second prescription has been for me the most difficult in homoeopathy. Every beginner should read and re-read his Kent's *Philosophy*, re-study his cases, and above all 'watch and wait'.

Remedy Relationships

The subject of the relationship of remedies is one of the most fascinating in homoeopathy. Long before Hahnemann, Paracelsus wrote much on the Doctrine of Signatures and the old herbalists determined the uses of their remedies partly from those suggested signs. A vast amount of work on the relationship of remedies to each other, rather than to symptoms, has been done by such homoeopaths as Boenninghausen, Hering, Clarke, Gibson Miller, the Allens, Kent, Guernsey and Lippe. Most of this work has been along one main line, that of complementary remedies; in other words, those remedies which carry on or complete most successfully the action of other given remedies. The following are among the best sources in the literature. No homoeopathic practitioner should be without Gibson Miller's little pamphlet, *The Relationship of Remedies*. When your case has repertorized out to three or four remedies and it seems evident that no simillimum will unravel the whole condition, and if at the moment it is impossible to decide which of two to give first, Miller's tables will often indicate the one that follows the other to better advantage. The fourth volume of Clarke's *Dictionary*, the *Clinical Repertory*, contains the same type of tables and material on a greater number of remedies, although I feel that Gibson Miller has pruned wisely. (See also Olds' 'Complementary Remedies' in the *Homoeopathic Recorder* for April 1928, page 205.) There are very suggestive groupings of remedies by Teste in his *Materia Medica*, although unfortunately he does not explain how he arrived at them.

There are several classes of complementary relationships, and a word of explanation about the practical application of each is in order. A plain complementary remedy, such as those listed immediately below, is related (i) by symptomatology, (ii) sometimes, as in the case of Arsenicum Alb. – Phosphorus, by occurrence in nature, and (iii) sometimes by constituents, for example Badiaga – Iodum. In explaining this type of complementary remedy it may be said that ideally 'one remedy, one dose' should cure; but most cases are so mixed, so confused by miasms or by drugging, that one must tack against the wind, using more than one remedy. Some of the main complementary relationships of this type are as follows:

Antimonium Tart. – Ipecac.	Iodum – Lycopodium
Apis – Natrum Mur.	Lachesis – Lycopodium, Nitric Ac.
Argentum Nit. – Natrum Mur.	Medorrhinum – Sulphur
Arsenicum Alb. – Phosphorus	Mezereum – Mercurius
Baryta Carb. – Dulcamara	Natrum Sulph. – Thuja
Berberis Vulg. – Lycopodium	Opium – Plumbum
Bryonia – Rhus Tox.	Petroleum – Sepia
Calc. Carb. – Rhus Tox.	Phosphorus – Carbo Veg.,
Chamomilla – Magnesium Carb.	Arsenicum Alb.
China – Ferrum	Pulsatilla – Kali Sulph.
Conium – Baryta Mur.	Sabina – Thuja
Cuprum – Calc. Carb.	Stannum – Pulsatilla

A more specialized class of complementary remedies is the *acute* complements of chronic remedies or the *chronic* complement of acute remedies, according to whether your patient is first seen as an acute or chronic case. For instance, an acute Belladonna throat may need the chronic complement Calc. Carb. to prevent recurrence and finish off the case; or a chronic Natrum Mur. case may develop an acute cold which will call for its acute complement, Bryonia. One of the confusing points is that a chronic remedy may have more than one acute complement. For example, Natrum Mur. has Bryonia, Ignatia and Apis; Lycopodium has Rhus Tox, Chelidonium and Pulsatilla, and sometimes Iodum. Some of the best known examples, putting the acutes first, are:

Aconite – Sulphur	Colocynth – Staphysagria
Arsenicum Alb. – Thuja	Hepar. Sulph – Silica
Bacillinum – Calc. Phos.	Nux Vomica – Sepia
Belladonna – Calc. Carb.	Pulsatilla – Silica
Bryonia – Aluminium, Natrum Mur.	

The third type of complementary remedies is the one on which the least work has been done, most of the data being found sprinkled around in Kent's *Materia Medica*. These are remedies *in series*; for instance, Calc. Carb. – Lycopodium – Sulphur. (Note that all three of these are chronic remedies. They must be used in this order and not in the opposite one.) Other examples are: Ignatia – Natrum Mur. – Sepia; Pulsatilla–Silica – Fluoric Ac.; Arsenicum Alb. – Thuja – Tarentula; Allium Cepa – Phosphorus – Sulphur; Aconite – Spongia – Hepar Sulph.

Of course, only a few examples from among those listed in the suggested study books have been given here. The reader will notice that for the most part the nosodes have been omitted, as have the tissue salts; also, certain notable remedies, like Kali Carb., for which many complements have been suggested but where none seems wholly satisfactory.

In the above sources certain remedies are listed as *incompatible*. This does not only mean that the remedies cannot be given together – for no two remedies are ever given together by the true Hahnemannian homoeopath – but it means that they must not follow each other without either an intervening remedy or else considerable time. Some of these are as follows:

Aconite – Acetic Ac.	Ferrum *after* Digitalis
Ammonium Carb. – Lachesis	Ignatia – Coffea, Nux Vomica,
Apis – Rhus Tox.	Tabacum
Aur. Mur. Natr. – Coffea	Lachesis – Dulcamara, Psorinum
Belladonna – Dulcamara	Ledum – China
Calc. Carb. *after* Kali Bich. or	Lycopodium *after* Sulphur
Nitric Ac., and *before*	Mercurius – Silica
Baryta Carb. or Sulphur	Phosphorus – Causticum
Causticum – Phosphorus	Psorinum – Sepia
Chamomilla – Nux Vom., Zinc	Rhus Tox. – Apis
Cocculus – Coffea	Sepia – Lachesis

The subject of *remedy analogues* in the animal, vegetable and mineral kingdoms has been very little studied and offers a fruitful field. (Some prescribers hold that there should theoretically be a remedy in each of the three kingdoms for every ill.) Examples of these are: Ignatia is the vegetable analogue of Natrum Mur., and Phytolacca of Mercury.

The relationships of remedies according to their chemical constituents is a highly interesting and also undeveloped subject. It illuminates relationships – for instance, Pulsatilla contains Kali Sulph., Belladonna has much Magnesia Phos., Allium Cepa and Lycopodium contain Sulphur. Quantitative chemical analyses should be done on all our vegetable remedies. Among the animal remedies, Badiaga and Spongia contain Iodine.

The botanical relationships of the vegetable remedies are also very suggestive. These are to be found in Clarke's *Clinical Repertory*. The student would do well to familiarize himself with the better-known remedies in this group, a few of which are given here:

BERBERIDACEAE:
  Berberis
  Caulophyllum
  Podophyllum

LOGANIACEAE:
  Brucea
  Curare
  Gelsemium
  Hoang Nan
  Ignatia
  Nux Vomica
  Spigelia
  Upas

MELANTHACEAE:
  Colchicum
  Helonias
  Sabadilla
  Veratrum Alb.
  Yucca

RANUNCULACEAE:
  Aconite
  Actea Racemosa (Cimicifuga)
  Actea Spicata
  Adonis
  Aquilegia Vulg.
  Caltha Pal.
  Clematis

  Helleborus
  Hepatica
  Hydrastis
  Peonia
  Pulsatilla
  Ranunculus Bulbosus
  Ranunculus Sceleratus
  Staphysagria

RUBIACEAE:
  Cahinca
  China
  Coffea
  Galium
  Ipecacuanha
  Mitchella
  Rubia Tinctorum

SOLANACEAE:
  Belladonna
  Capsicum
  Duboisin
  Dulcamara
  Hyoscyamus
  Lycopersicum (tomato)
  Mandragora
  Pichi
  Solanums (potato, etc.)
  Stramonium
  Tabacum

Some of the therapeutic snags in connection with the relationship of remedies are taken up in the following chapter on the dangers of homoeopathic prescribing.

The Dangers of Homoeopathic Prescribing

The greatest danger for any homoeopath is that he or she shall not be truly Hahnemannian. Mongrelism defeats not only the doctor and the patient but also the cause of homoeopathy. The specific pitfalls most frequently met are as follows:

1) The physician does not bear in mind his homoeopathic philosophy.
2) He fails to take a complete enough case from which to deduce the true remedy. He omits the mentals, or the profoundly important generals, or fails to elicit the modalities of the particular symptoms.
3) He lacks patience. Having given the remedy, he forgets that he must *wait* and *watch*. He repeats the remedy, in unwise zeal, before the definite slump comes after the improvement which has followed his remedy – more of a good thing does not mean a better thing in homoeopathic prescribing.
4) He fails to look for the action of Hering's three Laws of Cure: that the remedy works *from within outward, from above downward*, and *in the reverse order of the occurrence of the symptoms*. (This never happens except under the action of the curative remedy.)
5) He omits to make use of the 'second-best remedy' – Sac. Lac. Thereby he sometimes loses the patient's confidence, especially in those who are accustomed to taking much medicine.
6) He fails to make sure that the patient has actually taken the remedy. (Whenever possible, always administer the dose yourself.) Or he fails to find out what other remedies the patient may be taking, or what dietetic interferences there are. The physician must be cognizant of the substances which interfere with the action of our different remedies, such as coffee with Nux Vomica or acids with Aconite.
7) He does not search out the psychological and sociological deterrents to cure, and teach the patient how to evade and overcome these.
8) He sometimes does not recognize soon enough when the remedy is *not* working, and is then often too busy to revise the case and try again to find the most similar remedy.
9) He permits himself to give minor remedies for trivial or temporary

ailments incident to chronic treatment, when Sac. Lac. or sensible adjuvants such as hydrotherapy would suffice.

10) He changes the remedy because of the outcropping of other symptoms without discriminating between: (i) aggravation symptoms; (ii) symptoms due to idiosyncrasy; (iii) symptoms returning under the chronic remedy (symptoms which the patient may not recall ever having had before); (iv) actual new symptoms which occur because the remedy was only partially similar; and finally (v) symptoms of some discharge – such as coryza, leucorrhoea or perspiration – which represent a curative vent and are due to the action of the remedy.

11) He gives the wrong potency of the right remedy. (If you are sure of the remedy, it is well to try another potency, or, first, three doses of the original potency at two or four hour intervals.) Always instruct the patient to stop taking the remedy as soon as appreciable amelioration sets in, and to switch to the 'second' remedy, i.e., Sac. Lac.

12) He gives too high a potency in an incurable case, or in one with marked pathological changes, and so induces an aggravation with which the vital force cannot cope. (If he has done this and the patient is going downhill, he must antidote.)

13) He gives a profound constitutional remedy to a case which is too sick to stand it and which should merely have a related palliative remedy. For instance, in incipient tuberculosis it is dangerous to give Sulphur, Silica or Phosphorus, at least in high potency. A single dose of the 30th is as high as he should venture. If the case is far gone in tuberculosis these remedies must not be given, but rather a palliative for the most distressing symptoms, such as Rumex, Sanguinaria, Pulsatilla or Senega.

14) He must remember that certain remedies are dangerous to mishandle. For instance: Kali Carb., especially in cases of advanced arthritis; Silica, where an abscess, if suppuration were brought on, would break out in a dangerous location such as in the lungs; some of the nosodes, like Psorinum in deeply psoric cases, say of asthma, may induce a terrific aggravation; Lachesis, whose improper repetition may engraft a permanent unfavourable mental state on the patient. Arsenicum Album is another dangerous remedy. When apparently indicated in the last stages of an acute disease, say pneumonia, it may hasten demise (although it will make the death tranquil), but it will not rally the patient as one might expect. In the terminal stages of chronic disease, where cure is impossible, it will

sometimes bring the patient back long enough to sign a will or see the family, and will ultimately induce a peaceful death.

15) He will often be surprised to find that certain symptoms or groups of symptoms are relieved by his remedy, and yet the patient feels worse or develops more deep-seated trouble. In this case, the prescribing has been superficial and suppressive. Suppression is perhaps the greatest danger of ordinary medicine from the point of view of homoeopathic philosophy, and the deep homoeopath must be constantly on his guard not to produce suppression with his remedies. If he has given an acute remedy for an apparently superficial trouble, which is relieved but where the patient also feels badly, he should do the chronic case at once, and the deep-acting remedy will put the matter right.

16) He may give remedies in the wrong order, or inimical remedies in succession, thereby aggravating the patient and mixing up the case.

Throughout his practice the physician must sell the idea of homoeopathy with brief but helpful explanations to the patient in order to ensure his or her co-operation. He must have the character to sit tight when he knows what he is doing, and not spoil the case by unnecessary and harmful prescribing. Above all, he must consider each patient as an opportunity for service not only to the individual and the community, but also to homoeopathy and the human race.

Pathological Prescribing

Few things are more stimulating than to have our own pet prejudices successfully attacked. One fundamental principle drilled into every good Kentian homoeopathic student is that one must not prescribe pathologically. For the allopath to adopt this point of view is one of the most difficult obstacles to acquiring homoeopathy. By dint of much repetition it finally becomes ingrained. We realize that it is the patient and his individual reaction to the so-called disease for whom we must prescribe. We realize that pathology is an ultimate, an exteriorization, a protective out-throwing, an excrescence, or discharge on the part of the organism.

Our tendency is, then, to throw pathology overboard and to disregard all such symptoms and organic facts that we class under this head. If we do not take great care we find we are not succeeding as we should, that we are giving remedies on functional symptoms only, and that these remedies do not have the power to produce, and so cure, the given pathology. We may stop a haemorrhage from a fibroid uterus with a remedy which does not in its nature have the ability to produce fibroids. This will be suppression. We may relieve pain and fever in a case of pleuritic exudate with a lightweight remedy, but we will not cause resorption of the exudate by such treatment. So, little by little, our own experience, as well as that of many master prescribers, will bring it home to us that *pathology is to be considered in prescribing* – not as a sole basis, but as an important factor in the totality of the symptoms. We come to see that the pathology also reveals the patient. A tendency to polypi is a valuable symptom. We must know our pathology in all our cases, even in those which have abundant non-pathological symptoms – for diagnostic purposes, to satisfy the patient, to govern our prognosis, and especially to determine our choice of potency and remedy.

A safe rule is to give the lower potencies where there is marked organic change, even though a high potency in a vital person, if it is the true simillimum, will often cause great amelioration of the patient and drive the disease faster into or through the pathology. This may alarm or inconvenience the patient, but the true homoeopath will understand the process and explain it to him and his family. It will influence the choice of our remedy in that it will make us give one big enough to cope with the situation; it will teach us when the case in incurable; and warn us away from giving too high a potency in cases where this will cause a severe aggravation from which the economy cannot rally. In incurable and precarious cases of chronic disease, or even in such acute ones as early tuberculosis, it will show us when we must eschew the true simillimum and give a palliative remedy, or a less deep-acting remedy, as a preparative for the true simillimum. In those cases (and there are not so many) where the alert homoeopath cannot find subjective symptoms or modalities, he must resort to prescribing on pathology.

Pathology is often also a general, for Kent himself tells us that a condition appearing in three or more particulars ranks as a general. Such symptoms as excessive discharges, which Dr Boger classes in his *General Analysis* under moistness, may also lead us to the true inner nature of the patient.

There is another type of pathology which Dr G. B. Stearns classes as objective symptoms – in other words, pathology visible to the eye. This may not only mean unalterable organic tissue change, but also includes such rewarding details as redness of the orifices, fissures, herpes, eruptions, skin discolorations, warts, moles, peculiarities of hair, nails, etc. In children especially, these objective symptoms are often our best guide. Even the strictest Hahnemannian amongst us should give the pathological symptom its due!

The Problem of Suppression

A patient said to me, 'Where can I find literature showing the dangers of suppression? My daughter wants to put ointment on her baby's scalp eczema and won't believe me when I tell her it is perilous to do so.' This made me search the literature, which I found very meagre, and hence this attempt to clarify an important problem.

By definition, the term 'suppression' means that a disease manifestation is caused to disappear before the disease itself is cured. Suppression is one of the most important subjects from the homoeopathic point of view, but one of the least familiar to the ordinary medical mind. In conventional medicine we are continually meeting with examples of suppression; indeed, from our point of view, all that part of conventional medicine which is not subconscious homoeopathy is suppressive. There are various types of suppression.

1) Those which are accidental or natural and not due to medication of any kind, such as suppression of strong emotion due to the unnatural exigencies of our collective living. These are more or less conscious suppressions, although the seriousness of their results is not usually known and the individual takes great pride in thrusting down these emotions.

   A second kind of accidental suppression comes from great mental shocks such as mortification or grief.

   A third type of natural suppression is in the physical realm, such as where the menses are checked by injudicious bathing, or the lochia stopped after labour by catching cold, or milk suppressed, or perspiration suddenly inhibited by chilling.

   Then there is also the suppression of one disease by another, which is so frequently spoken of in the *Organon*. This may take the form of one acute disease held in abeyance by another until the 'cure' of the second; or it may be an acute disease suspending a chronic until the acute course is run. The reverse of this, where a chronic disease gives a partial or full measure of protection against acute disease, could really be classed as suppression, although it is more usually thought of as immunity.

2) A second type of suppression, most frequent in conventional medicine, is suppression by local applications. This enters into many fields. For instance: coryzas and sinus troubles are suppressed by local applications of antihistamines and other substances; leucorrhoeal and gonorrhoeal discharges by various medicated douches; eruptions, from such acute ones as scabies and impetigo, through to the chronic ones, such as eczema and psoriasis, by various preparations, including corticosteroids. The rashes due to the exanthems, which may also be classed under natural suppressions in some instances, may be driven in by the unwise use of cold packs. Other secretions, such as foot-sweat are often suppressed by foot powder; conjunctival pus by antibiotic ointments; ulcers by various local dressings, and warts by trichloracetic acid or electrical means. We have further the local suppression of many conditions by different types of irradiation and other such means.

Haemorrhages are suppressed by local astringents such as tannic acid, or by local coagulants such as thromboplastin, or by X-ray. They may also be suppressed by general medication such as calcium lactate and gelatin. This brings up the question as to whether a homoeopathic remedy such as Ceanothus Americanus should be classed as suppressive or curative.

3) Now we come to the conditions suppressed by current internal medication. For instance, malaria, which, if not of the quinine type, is simply suppressed by the massive routine dosage of quinine derivatives. This often results in recurrent neuralgia. In acute rheumatic fever the patient may be overpowered with salicylates, leading to suppression of joint symptoms and the inroads of the disease on the heart; epilepsy and choreas are often driven to cover by saturation with sedatives; and heart disease may be masked by digitalis.

4) Disease is all too frequently suppressed by surgery: the removal of growths, benign or malign, polypi, tonsils, appendices, varicosities, haemorrhoids, fistulae and bone hypertrophies such as turbinates. The trouble here is that modern medicine seeks to remove pathology rather than to cure the underlying causes, not realizing that the ultimates of disease are benign attempts at exteriorization, at protective localization.

5) Most insidious of all are the suppressions by vaccine injections, which are now so prevalent that a child may take seven or eight different kinds in a year. I know a family of seven children of a well-known allopathic physician who were given in one year cold vaccines, diphtheria, scarlet fever, whooping-cough, typhoid, paratyphoid and

5) Most insidious of all are the suppressions by vaccine injections, which are now so prevalent that a child may take seven or eight different kinds in a year. I know a family of seven children of a well-known allopathic physician who were given in one year cold vaccines, diphtheria, scarlet fever, whooping-cough, typhoid, paratyphoid and smallpox, and two of the seven were also given hay fever pollen inoculations.

6) There is the whole question of the suppression of syphilis by antibiotic treatment, which many doctors, even orthodox ones, feel tends to develop later grave nervous tertiaries as well as saddling the patients with drug results.

7) There is another aspect of suppression, which is the suppression of individual symptoms, and this may be done quite as effectively by the use of homoeopathic remedies as by conventional drugs. Never forget that to palliate a curable case is suppression. It will involve you in a continual change of remedies, a sort of 'puss wants a corner' with the symptoms. It will mask the true fundamental picture of the disease and complicate it to the point where it will be incurable. The degree to which this is done by the general run of homoeopathic practitioners is not realized, and is appalling.

I need not go into the bad results of these different kinds of suppression. They include asthma, convulsions, paralysis, insanity, tuberculosis and deep diseases of the vital organs. Dr Stearns gave a paper on *Prodromal Symptoms and Their Importance in Prescribing*. This chapter of mine should be entitled *Prodromal or Prior Suppressions, Their Importance in Prescribing*. In every case we must 'cherchez' not 'la femme' but 'la suppression'. Shall we prescribe for the symptoms before the suppression took place? Shall we use the form of suppression as a symptom in our totality? Shall we prescribe mainly for the present post-suppressive syndrome?

We must remember that suppression in any of its forms drives diseases in, masks symptoms, makes protein changes in the form of the disease, and blocks the natural exit of the disease. Always leave the golden bridge of your pathological ultimates, as by that route only can the disease return to cure. Disease is the Minotaur in the labyrinth. Theseus, the symptom, must find his way back and out of the labyrinth. Do not cut his cord!

The Management of the Homoeopathic Patient

Our duty as homoeopaths to our patients is great. The first in importance is *to pick the right remedy* and to remove obstacles to cure. To stop harmful practices, and give placebo if needed to keep them from taking other things. To give them enough understanding of homoeopathic philosophy to co-operate in their cure. To institute proper diet, hygiene, protection and state of mind.

The second is to win the patient's confidence by what you are – by your profound humanity, by your ability to see them as they could be *whole*. By your painstaking thoroughness in questioning and in examination. By your attitude toward science, using tests when these are harmless and diagnostically helpful.

Many of the most truly homoeopathic doctors object to this on the grounds that they do not need laboratory tests or a diagnosis for cure. They often do not need it for the removal of symptoms; in functional cases, not even for cure. But modern patients are very medicine-conscious and will class you as unscientific if you disregard all this. Moreover, your actual prescribing will be improved if you know the pathological tendencies and conditions.

The second act of our homoeopathic drama is, to me, far more difficult: the determination of the time when another remedy is needed. Many homoeopathically well-trained patients can be allowed to ride on a remedy which is helping until they themselves tell you they need another boost. But many will feel neglected and must be seen daily, even when you know you will not change the remedy. If you have a competent nurse on the case, she can often tell whether you are really needed and help to convince the family if you are not.

One of the recurring questions in case management is whether you should tell a patient if he has a serious or fatal disease. A wise man once said, 'When it is time for them to know, they will know and tell *you*. After that you can discuss it with them.' But for one's own protection, if one is sure of the diagnosis, a near relative must be told. Human resilience is incredible.

Many suggestible patients are convinced that they have (or will have) diseases which they definitely do not have. No amount of reassurance avails with some, although a simple statement that 'You just don't have the symptoms of that', with a little smile, will do wonders. (Never tell such a patient what the symptoms *are*, though!)

To go back to another reason why homoeopaths need diagnosis. I lost a delightful family as patients because I kept my diagnosis to myself. A cocky boy of eleven returned from boarding school where they had mumps, and his mother phoned to say that he had it and asked me to come and see him. I said, 'But you aren't swollen or sore in the mumps gland – the parotid.' 'Oh I have it, though', said he.

He was a very Phosphorus type of child. He had cervical adenitis. I had worried about the possibility of tuberculosis with him and built him up with remedies. I had actually given him Tub. Bov. 1M but had not told the mother, who was very apprehensive, lest I scare her, knowing I could cope with the conditions. She thought he did not get well quickly enough for mumps, called another doctor who diagnosed tubercular glands, and I lost the family. Since then I write a letter containing the diagnosis to myself, and keep it on file unopened in such cases!

The most difficult cases to manage are the new patients who do not yet understand what they must *not* do: that they must not suppress an eruption or discharge that the homoeopath has been trying to bring out again. Always warn your patients with suppressions in their histories, if a rash or discharge recurs, to do *nothing* and let you know.

Aggravations are not so hard to handle if you warn your patients. Tell them that these may occur and that it will be a good sign if they do.

Another problem is the veteran patient with access to homoeopathic remedies. Give cases of remedies by all means to out-of-towners or inaccessibles with children, but *numbered*, not named, and have them phone you which to give. Be sure there are various bottles of placebo under different names. But even then they will vex you. In one kit that I give out, No. 18 is Sepia. My patient found it so effective for her state of mind that she got to taking it on her own. Maybe we should call in the cases for periodic revision and change the numbers.

One of the worst problems is when the patient has a disease considered to be fatal, for which the prescribed treatment at least prolongs life, and where the disease is *rare* and there are no data of treatment by pure homoeopathy in a large series of cases. For instance, I have a case of chronic myeloid leukaemia in a man of 42. Low-dose X-ray therapy of the spleen is *de rigueur*. He and his friends would not consider omitting it. Nor do I consider myself justified in advising against it, as I would the omission of quinine in malaria, sulfa drugs in pneumonia, etc. I *believe* homoeopathy can help *this* case, for the man comes out clearly to a remedy (Phosphorus) and the case has had suppressions enough to give any fatal trouble (psoriasis, sinus, piles, etc.). But am I justified in trying to battle for Phosphorus alone? He has improved on it, although his blood count rises periodically. He is stronger and works more than he should. His postnasal drip has returned, and also an eruption. He then got a sore throat away from New York and a doctor friend gave him a heavy dose of a sulfa drug. He returned looking ghastly. Here is one case surely in which the diagnosis is like a millstone around the neck!

No discussion, however brief, of homoeopathic case management should go without comment on what you may let the patient do while the remedy is working: calendula ointment, echinacea succus, oil of lavender, pinus pumilio salves, hydrotherapy, mullein oil, plantago oil, arnica cerate, postural drainings in ear troubles, normal salt solution as a cathartic and in beginning migraines.

As to the real essence of remedy management, you can read Kent on *The Second Prescription* and the types of aggravations. Philosophy can be learned from books, but I have yet to see a book or take a course on the thousand and one things that make a doctor a great success with his or her patients. In the end, as in all things, the effective management of the patient is dependent on how one manages oneself, for we do not teach or learn by what is said, but from what we feel and sense and know and are.

Timing in Prescribing

Every good mechanic knows the importance of timing in the engine of an automobile. If the cylinders do not synchronize there is loss of power. In diplomacy, timing is of the most vital importance. To philosophers as well as to athletes, rhythm, which is really timing, is paramount. A beginner in homoeopathic prescribing may take his case magnificently but have no sense for chronology, for the sequence of cause and event. Always put dates opposite the illnesses, operations or catastrophes in the patient's history. After a while you get a sixth sense of how one thing follows another; you will see the life of the patient, and even of his forebears and progeny, as an organic whole. Try to connect the ills to which he is heir with seasons, periodicity, time, meteorological phases. Learn to sense how each individual person swings in or out of the master rhythms of the universe.

This same perception of timing applies to the physical examination. It is not sufficient that a man's heart shows no gross organic disturbances on an electrocardiograph. Using more senses than we give ourselves credit for, one must enter into the rhythm of his pulse, his breathing. We must understand the metabolic rhythms of eating, digestion and elimination, and use such means as will help us determine where in his physiology the lag or the spurt is. We must observe with instruments, with our eyes, ears, noses and fingers the delicate aberration of human functionings. We must realize how a tiny change in phase or current or magnetic field may have an apparently disproportionate counterpart in health and harmony.

When we have somehow pervaded the patient with a sense of the necessity of order and rhythm, we are then ready to come to the giving of our healing agent, the similar remedy. An old professor of mine used to say that curing is like peeling an onion – you must begin at the top layer; and it is a sound principle of homoeopathy that, in an untreated case which requires an acute prescription, the most recent symptoms are the guide to the remedy that you should start with. When you have taken a chronic case from birth on, you should be able to see what remedy this human being needed as an infant, as a child, at puberty, in young adulthood, in maturity and in old age. At some time in the complete cure

336

of a personality you may work back to the basic remedy or element lacking many years before, but if you give this substance prematurely you will put your timing off. Only the nosodes can be given with profit, either first or intercurrently, as timing regulators. To borrow a botanical analogy, the nosodes are like the genus and the remedy like the species.

The most perilous moment in any homoeopathic cure is that of the second prescription. If you cut in zeal, or panic before your first dose has run its course to the full, you will mix up your case. On the other hand, if you wait too long, you will lose valuable time and may alienate your patient. The expert homoeopath should be able to 'smell' when a repetition, change of potency or another remedy is indicated, and should have the character not to be stampeded or misled by the disease, the patient, the family, the consultant, the nurse or the family retainers!

Remember your cardinal principles: Never repeat a remedy when the patient himself is improving. Never change a remedy when the symptoms are following Hering's law of cure in the reverse order of the symptoms. Never change your remedy when a discharge or eruption follows the administration.

But there is more to timing than just repetition or change. One can almost include potency selection under timing. The patient's vitality is rhythm, and his pathology or suppressions are obstacles. A homoeo-pathic cure is something of a steeplechase; clock your remedies and your potencies, and may the best timing win.

337

The Relation of Diet to Homoeopathic Remedies

Homoeopathy is so rich in remedial agents that its practitioners often tend to rely on their remedies alone, disregarding hygiene and other adjuvants to cure. Especially do they fail to work out diets in detail for their patients. It is essential that they bother to do this for a number of reasons. In the first place, for the *psychological effect* upon the patient. Patients want to feel that every scientific care is being given them, and that the doctor takes flattering pains with them; and secondly, they need something to *do*, a call to *active* co-operation on their part. And further, without any remedy of any kind, diet can do wonders for many types of cases.

Let us consider for instance the value, without any remedy, of strict diets in such diseases as: diabetes, nephritis, high blood pressure, renal colic and the uric acid diathesis, arthritis, gallstones and jaundice, gastric and duodenal ulcer, mucous colitis, visceroptosis, constipation, obesity, and last but by no means least, tuberculosis and cancer. Every homoeopathic physician must be grounded in the classical dietary treatments. He must know how to influence acidity, strong urine, asthma and eczema by dietary means.

It is good training for us, and a method of experimental control of our remedies, to start chronic patients who have some one of the above mentioned diagnoses, on diet and regimen plus Sac. Lac. without any remedy, and see how far you can improve their condition. Thus do we learn what scientific commonsense will and will not do. Meanwhile you are getting closer to the patient's true simillimum, and can give it in prepared ground, with startling and enlightening effect.

Diet can often replace the use of remedies – a valuable help for the homoeopath. Take a patient who has been 'living on' soda bicarbonate for years. Teach them that soda, chemically alkaline, produces acid physiologically in the stomach, and train them to substitute lemon juice and the citrus fruits in general, and watch. You will be amazed that so simple a means will work so well. Meanwhile the soda intoxication symptoms will pass off, and your case values will begin to be clarified.

From the start the physician must also remove articles of diet and habits of eating which hold the patient back from cure, and which cover

338

the spoor on the trail to a 'totality', and thus to healthful progress. He learns in this quest the patient's idiosyncrasies to food. As every homoeopath knows, these are of great help and import. In this connection there is a wise rule: chronic cases should *not* eat to excess that substance which they especially crave, whereas acute patients *may* – and *should* – eat largely of what they crave, if the craving comes on with the illness. The most extraordinary lapses from classical procedure show admirable results when this rule is followed. But be sure that it is a true craving, an unusual circumstance, individualizing the patient's reaction to the (so-called) acute disease. The craving for and aversions to food in chronics will, of course, give you sound generals for your hierarchy of symptoms. If the remedy is given in chronic cases it will, little by little, enable the patient to assimilate the food he craved, at the same time modifying the craving. For example, I have an Argentum Nitricum patient who craved sugar and was ill from it, and who, under that remedy no longer craves it but can eat it with impunity. Similarly, I have a Calcarea child, who, after Calc. Carb. ceased craving chalk and indigestibles and can assimilate lime from the food.

Several interesting points arise in connection with being made ill by specific articles of food. Try at first to see whether it is a combination of foods which disagree, or just one given element of diet. A wise teacher once told me that almost anyone could eat almost anything if they ate it by itself. Next, in the case of certain acids, try giving cream cheese or cottage cheese with them. For instance, those with whom strawberries disagree can often take strawberries if cream cheese is eaten at the same time; and similarly with tomatoes. This also applies to shellfish in some patients. Beware the combinations of acids and sugars, or starches with meat, in people with delicate digestions. Buttermilk will often so alter the colon's flora and fauna that putrefaction is regulated and much can be digested which hitherto did not agree. The famous German homoeopath, Dr Schegel the elder, told me that if everyone would drink buttermilk the race would profit enormously, and if they would add honey (formic acid) and radishes (which are anti-uric acid), even more trouble would be saved. Remember that onions help to keep blood pressure down (Italians with their garlic and onions rarely have hypertension).

In idiosyncrasies of preference, rather than actual aggravations, ingenuity will save much trouble. Your child or patient who will not take milk may enjoy it if carbonated water is added, or if milk and cream are mixed half-and-half with ginger ale or sarsaparilla. The difference between hot and cold milk may also change the dislike.

Those who need iron, who also claim that cabbage gives them gas, can often take raw cabbage with sour cream dressing. Spinach puréed with egg chopped on it will tempt the anti-green child. Cider and raw apples are marvellous for thinning the arthritic patient. Brown sugar, molasses, maple syrup and honey will not harm him in the way that other sweets will. These hints may seem trivial but they work.

In addition to buttermilk and lemon juice, there is another sphere where diet aids materially in cleansing the system. White of egg with lemon or orange juice makes a detoxifying liver wash for the bilious. The egg albumen forms albuminates with the toxins which accumulate in the liver. Tea made from red clover blossoms and drunk, two quarts daily, can help the cancer patient and appears to cleanse the system (an old German adjuvant).

Then there is the important relationship between certain foods and the best action of our remedies. For example, Aconite and acids do not agree, coffee antidotes the action of Nux Vomica. These relationships are legion and can be found in Clarke's *Dictionary of Materia Medica* and in many other of our classics, under the separate remedies.

Other theoretical problems of interest come up under this subject. For instance, we use articles of food as remedies. What reaction, if any, may these have on patients sensitive to them, even in the crude, comestible form? And vice versa, can we aid the suitable remedy by giving its unpotentized counterpart as a food simultaneously? Should we not prove the whole range of vegetables, fruits and other foods, so that when we find a patient with an idiosyncrasy to a food we can compare his case with the proving of the offending substance, and see whether it may not fit and aid? These foods should be proved on those with a sensitivity to them.

A Classical Homoeopathic Bibliography

Dr Hubbard recommended the following list of fundamental books that every homoeopath should have, and study:

Boenninghausen's *Philosophy of Homoeopathy*
Boericke's *Materia Medica*
Boger's *Synoptic Key*
Clarke's *A Dictionary of Practical Materia Medica*
Guernsey's *Keynotes to the Materia Medica*
Hahnemann's *Nature of Chronic Diseases*
Hering's *Guiding Symptoms*
Kent's *Materia Medica*
Kent's *Philosophy of Homoeopathy*
Kent's *Repertory*
Pulford's *Key to the Homoeopathic Materia Medica*
Roberts' *Practice and Principles of Homoeopathy*
Roberts' *Sensations As If*
Tyler's *Homoeopathic Drug Pictures*
Ward's *Sensations As If*
Wheeler's *Principles and Practice of Homoeopathy*
Woodbury's *Materia Medica for Nurses*

Index of Remedies

343